Sports
Physiology

wcb
Wm. C. Brown Publishers
Dubuque, Iowa

Sports Physiology

**Second
Edition**

Edward L. Fox
**Professor of Physical Education
Director, Laboratory of Work Physiology,
School of Health, Physical Education and
 Recreation
The Ohio State University
Columbus, Ohio**

Illustrated by Nancy Allison Close

RC 1235 F67 1984

Dedicated with Love to My Three Beautiful Girls
My Wife, Ann
Our Children, Eva Virginia and Catherine Cary

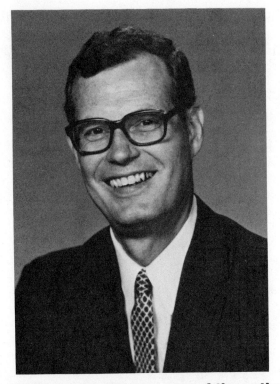

**Rededicated to the memory of the author
EDWARD L. FOX
May 30, 1938–April 1, 1983**

A devoted and respected scholar, author,
teacher, and researcher of exercise physiology
A trusted friend and inspiration to his
colleagues and students

Preface

One of the major revisions of this second edition of *Sports Physiology* is a thorough updating of all materials. For example, menstrual disorders have now been recognized in some female athletes, and the materials relating to this problem have been correspondingly updated. Also, several new studies have been conducted on blood doping and its effects on endurance performance. These have also been incorporated into this edition.

A second major revision is inclusion of new materials, thereby expanding the applied concepts. Concepts relating to energy production, lactic acid accumulation and muscular fatigue, basic anatomy and physiology of the heart, the effects of alcohol ingestion on sports performance, and body composition and weight control have all been expanded in relation to their direct applications to sports and sports activities. While no entirely new chapters have been added, additional chapters have been generated through "splitting" of existing chapters.

The last major revision is the reorganization of the chapter materials. It is never possible to organize a textbook to everyone's satisfaction. However, I hope that this edition is better organized than the last edition.

For purposes of clarification, it seems appropriate to comment on the major differences between this text and my other text, *The Physiological Basis of Physical Education and Athletics*. Both texts, of course, relate to exercise physiology as applied to sports and physical education. However, *The Physiological Basis of Physical Education and Athletics* emphasizes more basic physiology. In *Sports Physiology*, on the other hand, the emphasis has been placed on the *applications* of physiology rather than on physiology itself. Accordingly, only those physiological principles deemed most necessary for direct applications to sports and performance are included. Often the applications do not require extensive explanations of the scientific principles, but only a practical presentation along with an explanation of what is safe and effective. These two textbooks, then, provide students a choice depending upon their science backgrounds. For example, with more science background, *The Physiological Basis of Physical Education and Athletics* might be the better choice. For those students with a lesser background in science and with a keener interest in coaching, *Sports Physiology* should "fill the bill."

Finally, the coaching of a sport or the teaching of a motor skill is both an art and a science. As such, coaches and physical educators must have competency in both teaching and scientific application. It is to this latter point that this book is dedicated; I sincerely hope that the applied physiological material presented here will significantly contribute to teaching, coaching, and athletic success.

Acknowledgments

I would like to thank my editor, John Butler of Saunders College Publishing, for his encouragement and guidance relating to the second edition of this book. I would also like to acknowledge Lou Close for her excellent art work, not only for this book but for my other books as well. I also thank my colleagues and students, past and present, for their many helpful suggestions for revision. In this regard, I especially thank Dr. Melvin H. Williams, of Old Dominion University, and Dr. James R. Morrow, Jr., of the University of Houston for their most helpful critical reviews of the manuscript. Finally, I once again thank my family, including Eva B. Roberts, for their help, patience, and most of all their love.

Edward L. Fox
Upper Arlington, Ohio

To the Student

Although each student has his or her own "best" way of studying, the following study guidelines are recommended for full comprehension of the materials contained within this textbook:

- Read the chapter outline to get an idea of what topics are contained within the chapter.
- Read the summary of major concepts at the end of the chapter.
- Skim through the chapter and read the emphasized materials which are in boldface type and contained within boxes.
- Read the chapter in full from the beginning, including re-reading the summary.
- Read the questions and answers relevant to the chapter materials that are found in Chapter 13.

Contents

ix

1

Energy— The Name of the Game

Introduction

Perhaps the most valuable concept relating science to physical education and athletics is human energy production. The importance of this concept becomes obvious when one stops to think about how versatile the human body is with respect to the kinds of movements and sports activities it is capable of performing. The activity spectrum, for example, spans the range of human movements from those requiring large bursts of energy over short periods of time, such as in the case of the sprinter, the running back, and the base stealer, to name but a few, to those activities requiring a steady but sustained energy production as in the case of the marathoner, the distance swimmer, and the cross-country skier. Even within the same activity, the energy requirements may change from one moment to the next. Take sports such as basketball, soccer, baseball, and tennis: one moment the athlete is maintaining a steady pace of energy expenditure, whereas a moment later he or she is sprinting all-out.

The purpose of this chapter is to show how the understanding of energy concepts can be applied to sports and physical education.

Applications of Energy Concepts

Five important applications of energy concepts to sports and physical education will be outlined here.

1

The Construction of Physical Training Programs (Fig. 1-1)

In order for a training program to have the most beneficial effects, it must be constructed to develop the specific physiological capabilities required to perform a given sports skill or activity. One of these capabilities involves supplying energy to the working muscles. For example, the way in which energy is supplied during sprinting differs from the way it is supplied during the running of a marathon. As a consequence, training programs designed to improve a given type of performance must be constructed so as to increase the type of energy supply specific to that performance.

On the other hand, different sports can require the same type of energy supply. For example, the way in which energy is supplied to a 400-meter swimmer is very similar to the way it is supplied to a mile-runner. In this case, the two training programs would be similar except that swimmers would swim during their training sessions and runners would run. More detailed background for understanding the energy concept as related to physical training programs is presented in Chapters 2, 3, 7, 8, and 9.

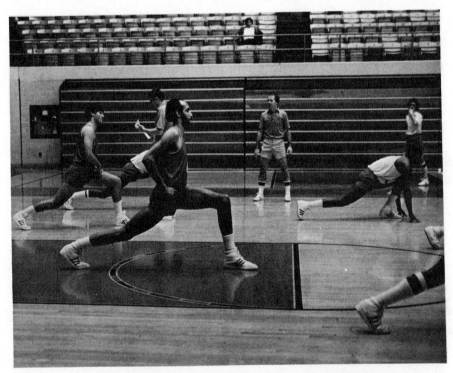

Figure 1-1 The understanding of how energy is produced in the body is extremely important to the coach when constructing physical training programs for his or her teams. (Photograph courtesy of Chance Brockway, Buckeye Lake, OH.)

Training must also take into account physiological capabilities involving specific kinds of muscle fibers found in most human muscles. Basically, there are two types of fibers or motor units—one suited for high power output activities (called fast-twitch, or FT) and the other for low power output activities (called slow-twitch, or ST). For our purposes, we may think of most human muscles as containing a mixture of "sprint" and "endurance" fibers. This kind of specificity is in part related to the difference in energy potential between the two fiber types. This aspect of the application of energy concepts to the construction of physical training programs will be detailed in Chapters 6 and 9.

The Prevention, Delay, and Recovery from Fatigue (Fig. 1–2)

Understanding how energy is produced within the body will provide us with some insight into what fatigue is and how it can be delayed or in some instances even avoided during performance. As an example, almost everyone has seen a runner lead the pack for the first part of a race but end up nearly last

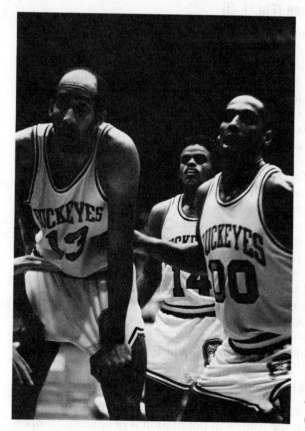

Figure 1-2 Understanding how energy is produced and how the body recovers from fatigue is important in preventing and/or delaying fatigue. (Photograph by Tom Malloy, Courtesy of the Department of Photography, The Ohio State University, Columbus, OH.)

at the finish. In this case, running too fast at the beginning of the race causes fatigue to set in, preventing the runner from "kicking" at the finish. This kind of "early" fatigue is related to the way in which energy is produced and can be avoided or at least delayed through proper pacing. For example, from a physiological standpoint, the runner should maintain a steady but sufficient pace throughout the majority of the race, then finish with an all-out effort. This delays the onset of fatigue until the end of the race.

The prevention of and recovery from fatigue are also related to the understanding of how energy is supplied to the muscles. In some instances, fatigue can be completely prevented merely by allowing a small amount of recovery between heavy bouts of work. For example, working at a very heavy load that causes fatigue in a few minutes, when performed continuously, can be performed intermittently for several hours without fatigue by alternating 10-sec work bouts with 20-sec recovery periods. This kind of information is valuable in planning for the most intensive training and competitive schedules and also in understanding why the interval training technique is such an effective training method. These applications of the energy concept will be further studied in Chapters 5 and 6.

Nutrition and Performance (Fig. 1–3)

Recently, new information regarding nutrition and performance in humans has become available. For example, it has been found that endurance performance can be improved following several days of diets rich in carbohydrates. Likewise, the ingestion of glucose in low concentrations during extremely long performances (e.g., 3 or more hours) has been found to correlate with improved endurance performance and the delay of fatigue. Even the ingestion of a fatty meal several hours prior to exercise has been experimentally shown to increase endurance performance and delay fatigue. Applying these findings to sports involves an understanding of which foods are preferentially used for energy by the muscles and how the dietary regulation of these foods affects their availability as energy fuels.

Even with the latest research, serious questions regarding nutrition and performance remain. Several may have come to your mind. What, for instance, is the protein requirement of athletes engaged in heavy physical training? What about surplus iron, salt, vitamins, and so on? Do they affect energy production? Are they essential for good athletic performance? What should the pregame meal consist of? It is hoped that an understanding of the complexities of nutrition will help you appreciate why such questions can sometimes have differing answers and why not all the answers are yet known.

Background information for the study of energy as related to nutrition and performance is contained in Chapters 4 and 10.

The Control of Body Weight (Fig. 1–4)

Closely associated with nutrition are the problems of obesity and body weight control. Obesity in the American population is of epidemic propor-

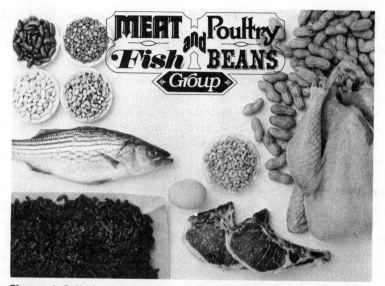

Figure 1-3 Understanding how energy is produced in the body and which foods are preferentially used for energy by the muscles is essential in understanding how good nutritional habits lead to improved performance. (From Food. *Home and Garden Bulletin, 228.* Prepared by the Science and Education Administration, U.S. Department of Agriculture, 1979.)

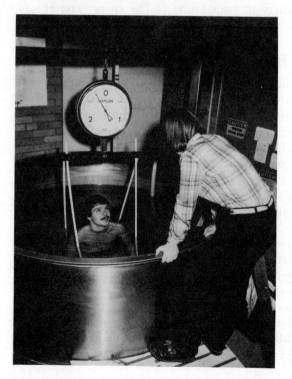

Figure 1-4 The understanding of the energy balance concept is basic to the understanding of the control of body weight. (Photograph by Tom Malloy. Courtesy of the Department of Photography, The Ohio State University, Columbus, OH.)

tions. Its major cause is lack of physical activity. It has been said that if you intend to maintain an average body weight and, at the same time, lead a sedentary way of life, you will have to literally starve yourself for the majority of your life. How true this is.

One of the most important concepts regarding the control of body weight is energy balance. Quite simply, if more energy in the form of food is taken in than is expended in the form of activity or exercise, the body weight will increase. The converse is also true. In most sports, maintenance of a desirable body weight is essential for continued good performance.

However, the principles of body weight control apply to the nonathlete as well as to the athlete, but for different reasons. The nonathlete must always be concerned with the problem of obesity, whereas the athlete is more concerned with gaining muscle mass or fat-free weight. In either case, the "do's and don'ts" of body weight control must be learned and thoroughly understood by the coach and physical educator.

Controlling energy balance and body weight necessarily involves principles of nutrition and body composition. For example, understanding the energy value of foods, the difference between weight loss due to dehydration and that due to loss of body fat, and the hazards of too rapidly achieving the desired weight in wrestling, will enable you to adopt scientifically sound practices regarding desirable body weight and nutritional habits. In particular, recognizing the difference between weight reduction due to water loss and that due to fat loss will allow you to recommend exercise programs that will not jeopardize the health and safety of your athletes. The energy concept as applied to body weight control is presented in Chapter 11.

The Maintenance of Body Temperature (Fig. 1–5)

A stable body temperature requires that the amount of heat (energy) produced by the body equals the amount of heat given off to the environment. During exercise, heat production increases in direct proportion to the amount of work performed. To prevent an excessive rise in an athlete's body temperature during exercise, the coach has to recognize that the effectiveness of the heat loss mechanisms, particularly the evaporation of sweat, must not be inhibited by excessive clothing or athletic equipment. Football coaches who insist that their players wear full uniforms during practice sessions on hot, humid days are greatly increasing the chances of heat stroke, which if severe enough can be fatal.

Serious heat disorders in athletics are not confined to football. Any sport or physical activity is potentially hazardous insofar as heat illness is concerned. This includes wrestling because the wrestler frequently loses large quantities of water in order to "make weight," and track and field events, particularly those held outdoors. For example, heat stroke in novice long-distance runners is now quite common. Certainly no coach would ever knowingly jeopardize the life of any athlete. The maintenance of body temperature will be discussed in greater detail in Chapter 12.

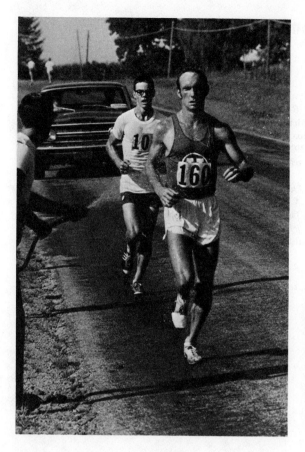

Figure 1-5 The understanding of how the body prevents an excessive rise in body temperature during exercise is not possible without an understanding of how energy is produced by the body and how it is lost to the environment.

Summary

- One of the most important concepts relating science to sports and physical education is human energy production.
- The energy concept applies to sport in understanding how to construct physical training programs.
- The energy concept applies to sport in understanding how to prevent, delay, and recover from fatigue.
- The energy concept applies to sport in understanding the relationship between nutrition and exercise performance.
- The energy concept applies to sport in understanding how body weight is controlled.
- The energy concept applies to sport in understanding how a nearly constant body temperature is maintained.

Selected References and Readings*

Bergstrom, J., et al.: Diet, muscle glycogen and physical performance. *Acta Physiol. Scand., 71*: 140–150, 1967.

Costill, D. L., et al.: Effects of elevated plasma FFA and insulin on muscle glycogen usage during exercise. *J. Appl. Physiol.: Respirat. Environ. Exercise Physiol., 43*:695–699, 1977.

Fox, E. L.: Physical training: Methods and effects. *Orthop. Clin. N. Am., 8*:533–548, 1977.

Fox, E. L., et al.: Effects of football equipment on thermal balance and energy cost during exercise. *Res. Quart., 37*:332–339, 1966.

Hickson, R., et al.: Effect of increasing plasma free fatty acids on endurance. *Fed. Proc., 36*:450, 1977.

Fox, E. L., and D. K. Mathews: *The Physiological Basis of Physical Education and Athletics.* 3rd ed. Philadelphia, Saunders College Publishing, 1981.

Mathews, D., E. L. Fox, and D. Tanzi: Physiological responses during exercise and recovery in a football uniform. *J. Appl. Physiol., 26*:611–615, 1969.

Shaffer, T. E., and E. L. Fox: Guidelines to physical conditioning for sports. *Pediatric Basics, 18*: 10–14, 1977.

*For full titles of journals, see Appendix A.

2
The Energy Systems

Introduction

As was mentioned earlier, various sports activities involve specific demands for energy. For example, sprinting, jumping, and throwing are high-power output activities, requiring a relatively large production of energy over a short period of time. Marathon running, distance swimming, and cross-country skiing, on the other hand, are mostly low-power output activities, requiring energy production over a prolonged period of time. Other sports activities, as we shall soon see, demand a blend of both high- and low-power output. These various energy demands can be met because there are three distinctly different ways in which energy can be supplied to the skeletal muscles.

The major purpose of this chapter is to develop the concept of human energy production.

9

Definitions

Three components of human energy production require formal definitions: energy itself (and some of its forms), work, and power.

Energy

Energy is described as the capacity or ability to perform work. While the definition is simple, the concept of energy is not necessarily easy to grasp.

We are interested mainly in only two of the six forms of energy—**mechanical** and **chemical**. In baseball, a swinging bat performs mechanical work by virtue of its motion. The same is true of the golf club, the tennis racket, or other such sports tools. In like manner, mechanical work can be performed by acceleration of the center of gravity of the body in a frontal direction, such as in running. Energy associated with motion is known as **kinetic energy**. Mechanical work performed by virtue of position, such as a bent bow in archery or lifting the body against gravity, is a result of **potential energy.**

Chemical energy also represents a source of potential energy. For example, in the body, foodstuffs are degraded through chemical reactions, releasing chemical energy, which in turn is used to synthesize other chemical compounds. Some of the latter compounds are called "energy-rich" compounds; when broken down, these compounds release chemical energy that is used by the skeletal muscles in performing mechanical work. Notice that we are back to mechanical work or energy. In other words, some of the chemical or potential energy represented by the foods we eat is converted to mechanical or kinetic energy by the skeletal muscles.

The most common unit of measure of energy is the **calorie**. A calorie is the amount of heat energy required to raise the temperature of 1 g of water 1° Celsius (formerly centigrade). A **kilocalorie (kcal)** is equal to 1000 calories and is the unit most often used in describing the energy content of foods and the energy requirements of various physical activities.

Work

Since energy is the capacity to perform work, the definition of work becomes important in understanding the total energy concept. Quantitatively, **mechanical work (W)** is the product of a force (F) acting through a distance (d). In mathematical form:

W $= F \times d$
Work = force times distance

As an example, if you weigh 70 kg (force) and you ascend a flight of stairs 2 m in height (distance), you will have performed 70 kg $\times$ 2 m = 140 kg-m of mechanical work. Energy and work have the same units of measure; in our example, 140 kg-m is equivalent to 0.33 kcal or 1012 foot-pounds.

Although the terms work and energy may be used interchangeably, it should be pointed out that it is possible to expend energy but perform no mechanical work. For example, holding a weight at arm's length requires energy, but no mechanical work is performed while the weight remains stationary.

Power

Power (P) is work per unit time (t), or:

$$P = W/t = (F \times d)/t$$

From our earlier example, if you ascended the flight of stairs in 1 sec (t), then you would have generated (70 kg $\times$ 2 m)/1 sec = 140 kg-m/sec of power.

The importance of power in athletics can be readily appreciated. In most sports activities, the greatest energy produced in the shortest period of time is a prime factor in a successful performance. This is true, for instance, of jumping, running (particularly sprinting), and throwing. One of the most frequently used screening tests for potential success in football at any position is the time of the 40-yd dash (from a standing start). The reason for this, of course, is that the 40-yd dash is a test of power—and the ability to generate power is obviously necessary for football performance.

A summary of the definitions and common units of measure for energy, work, and power is given in Table 2-1.

The Energy Systems

The next step in studying the energy systems is to briefly discuss the immediate energy source—ATP, explaining the important principle of coupled reactions, clarifying what exactly is meant by aerobic and anaerobic metabolism, and finally, reviewing the energy systems themselves.

The Immediate Energy Source—ATP

Adenosine triphosphate, or, more simply, **ATP**, is the immediately usable form of chemical energy for muscular activity. This is one of the most important of the so-called "energy-rich" compounds mentioned earlier. It is

Table 2-1: Definitions and Common Units of Measure for Energy, Work, and Power

Term	Definition	Common Units
Energy	Capacity to perform work	Calorie, kcal
Work	Product of a force acting through a distance	kg-m, ft-lb, kcal
Power	Time rate of performing work	kg-m/sec, ft-lb/sec, kcal/sec, watts

stored in most cells, particularly muscle cells. Other forms of chemical energy, such as that available from the foods we eat, must be transferred into the ATP form before they can be utilized by the muscle cells.

The chemical structure of ATP is complicated but for our purposes can be simplified as shown in Figure 2-1A. As you can see, ATP consists of a large complex of molecules called **adenosine** and three simpler components called **phosphate groups**. The last two phosphate groups represent "high energy

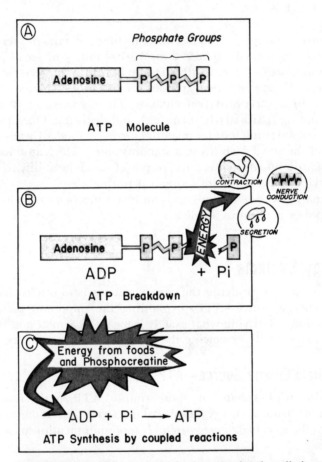

Figure 2-1 A, ATP consists of a large molecule called adenosine and three simpler components called phosphate groups. B, The energy released from the breakdown of ATP is used to perform biological work. The building blocks for ATP synthesis are the by-products of its breakdown, adenosine diphosphate (ADP) and inorganic phosphate (Pi). C, The energy for ATP resynthesis comes from the breakdown of foods and phosphocreatine. This energy is coupled with the energy needs of the reaction that resynthesizes ATP.

bonds." In other words, they store a high level of potential chemical energy. When the terminal phosphate bond is chemically broken, as shown in Figure 2-1B, energy is released, enabling the cell to perform work. The kind of work performed by the cell depends on the cell type. For example, mechanical work (contraction) is performed by muscle cells (smooth, skeletal, and heart muscle), nerve conduction by nerve cells, secretion by secretory cells (e.g., endocrine cells), and so on. All "biological" work performed by any cell requires the immediate energy derived from the breakdown of ATP. (The amount of energy released in the body per mole of ATP broken down is estimated at 7 to 12 kcal. A **mole** is a given amount of a chemical compound by weight; the weight is dependent upon the number and kind of atoms making up the compound.)

The Principle of Coupled Reactions

Since energy is released when ATP is broken down, it is not too surprising that energy is required to rebuild or resynthesize ATP. The building blocks for ATP synthesis are the by-products of its breakdown, adenosine diphosphate (ADP) and inorganic phosphate (Pi) (see Fig. 2-1B). The energy for ATP resynthesis comes from three different series of chemical reactions that take place within the body. Two of the three depend upon the food we eat, whereas the other depends upon a chemical compound called phosphocreatine (see Fig. 2-1C). (As we will soon see, phosphocreatine is similar to ATP and is stored in muscle cells.) The energy released from any one of these series of reactions is coupled with the energy needs of the reaction that resynthesizes ATP. In other words, the separate reactions are functionally linked together in such a way that the energy released by the one is always used by the other. Biochemists refer to these functional links as **coupled reactions**, and it has been shown that such coupling is the fundamental principle involved in the metabolic production of ATP.

In chemical terms, the equations for coupled reactions might look like this:

$$AB \longrightarrow A + B + \textbf{ENERGY}$$
$$\textbf{ENERGY} + C + D \longrightarrow CD$$

Compound AB breaks down into its components A and B and energy is released. This energy is then used to form compound CD from its components C and D.

Aerobic and Anaerobic Metabolism

The term **metabolism** refers to the various series of chemical reactions that take place within the body, including those just mentioned. **Aerobic** refers to the presence of oxygen, whereas **anaerobic** means without oxygen. Therefore, **aerobic metabolism** refers to a series of chemical reactions that requires the presence of oxygen. **Anaerobic metabolism** means just the opposite—a series of chemical reactions that does not require the presence of oxygen. Two of the three series of reactions involved in ATP resynthesis, the ATP-PC series and the lactic acid series, are anaerobic, whereas the other, the oxygen series, is aerobic.

ATP-PC: The Phosphagen System

PC is an abbreviation for **phosphocreatine**, another one of those "energy-rich" phosphate compounds closely related to ATP. PC, like ATP, is stored in muscle cells, and when it is broken down (i.e., when its phosphate group is removed), a large amount of energy is released (see Fig. 2-2). The released energy, of course, is coupled to the energy requirement necessary for the re-synthesis of ATP. In other words, as rapidly as ATP is broken down during

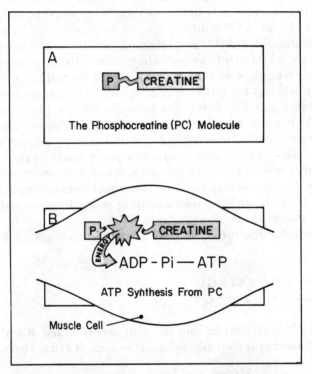

Figure 2-2 The ATP-PC system, also called the phosphagen system. A, Phosphocreatine, which is stored in muscle cells, contains a high-energy bond. B, When ATP is broken down during muscular contraction, it is rapidly reformed by the energy liberated during the breakdown of PC. Activities requiring only a few seconds to complete, such as sprinting, jumping, and kicking, are dependent upon the stored phosphagens for their primary energy source.

muscular contraction, it is continuously reformed from ADP and Pi by the energy liberated during the breakdown of the stored PC. For every mole of PC broken down, 1 mole of ATP is resynthesized.

Again in chemical terms, the coupled reactions look like this:

$$PC \longrightarrow Pi + C + \textbf{ENERGY}$$
$$\textbf{ENERGY} + Pi + ADP \longrightarrow ATP$$

PC breaks down to its component parts, inorganic phosphate (Pi) and creatine (C), releasing energy for the resynthesis of ATP.

The total muscular stores of both ATP and PC (collectively referred to as phosphagens) are very small—only about 0.3 mole in females and 0.6 mole in males. Thus, the amount of energy obtainable through this system is limited. In fact, if you were to run 100 m as fast as you could, the phosphagen stores in the working muscles would probably be empty by the end of the sprint. However, the usefulness of the ATP-PC system lies in the rapid availability of energy rather than in the quantity. This is extremely important with respect to the kinds of physical activities that we are capable of performing. For example, activities such as sprinting, jumping, swinging, kicking, and other similar skills requiring only a few seconds to complete are all dependent upon the stored phosphagens for their primary energy source.

The Lactic Acid System

This system is technically known as **anaerobic glycolysis**. Glycolysis refers to the breakdown of carbohydrate (sugar); anaerobic, as mentioned earlier, means without oxygen. In this system, the breakdown of sugar (a carbohydrate and one of the foodstuffs) supplies the necessary energy from which ATP is manufactured (see Fig. 2-3). When carbohydrate is only partially broken down, one of the end products is **lactic acid** (hence the name lactic acid system).

When lactic acid accumulates in the muscles and blood and reaches very high levels, temporary muscular fatigue results. This is a very definite limitation, and is the main cause of the "early" fatigue mentioned on page 4. Another limitation of the lactic acid system that relates to its anaerobic quality is that only a few moles of ATP can be resynthesized from the breakdown of sugar as compared to the yield possible when oxygen is present. For example, only 3 moles of ATP can be manufactured from the anaerobic breakdown of 180 g (about 6 oz) of **glycogen** (glycogen is the storage form of glucose in the muscle). As we will soon see, the aerobic breakdown of 180 g of glycogen results in enough energy to resynthesize 39 moles of ATP!

The coupled reactions for the lactic acid system can be summarized as follows:

$$(C_6H_{12}O_6)_n \longrightarrow 2C_3H_6O_3 + \textbf{ENERGY}$$
(glycogen)   (lactic acid)
$$\textbf{ENERGY} + 3Pi + 3ADP \longrightarrow 3ATP$$

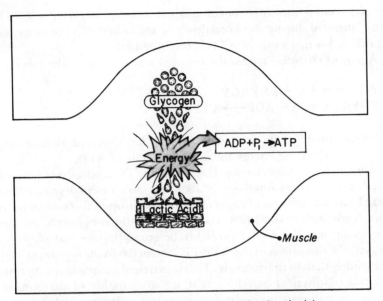

Figure 2-3 The lactic acid system (anaerobic glycolysis). Carbohydrate (glycogen) is broken down anaerobically (without oxygen) to lactic acid. The latter causes muscular fatigue. The energy released during this breakdown is used to resynthesize ATP. Exercises performed at maximum rates for between 1 and 3 min depend heavily upon the lactic acid system for ATP energy.

The lactic acid system, like the ATP-PC system, is extremely important to us, primarily because it too provides for a rapid supply of ATP energy. For example, exercises that are performed at maximum rates for between 1 and 3 min, such as sprinting 400 or 800 m, depend heavily upon the lactic acid system for ATP energy. Also, in some performances, such as running 1500 m or a mile, the lactic acid system is used predominantly for the "kick" at the end of the race.

The Oxygen, or Aerobic, System

In the presence of oxygen, the complete breakdown of 180 g of glycogen to carbon dioxide (CO_2) and water (H_2O) yields enough energy to manufacture 39 moles of ATP. This series of reactions, like the anaerobic series, takes place within the muscle cell, but is confined to specialized subcellular compartments called **mitochondria**. Mitochondria (singular: **mitochondrion**) are slipper-shaped cell bodies often referred to as the "powerhouses" of the cell because they are the seat of the aerobic manufacture of ATP energy. As you might guess, muscle cells are rich with mitochondria (see Fig. 2-4).

A summary of the aerobic resynthesis of ATP is shown in Figure 2-5. Besides the fact that abundant ATP can be manufactured during aerobic metabolism, notice that no fatiguing by-products are formed. The carbon dioxide

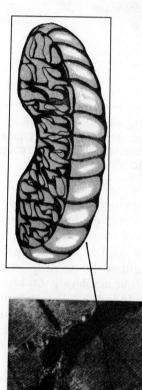

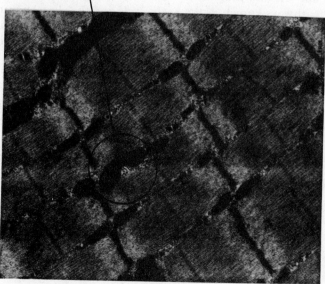

Figure 2-4 Mitochondria. **Left,** An electron micrograph of a longitudinal section of rat skeletal muscle, showing several mitochondria. (Courtesy of Dr. James Cirrito, The Ohio State University, Columbus, OH.) **Right,** A schematic illustration of a mitochondrion. The top has been removed to show its extensive membrane system, which contains the enzyme systems for aerobic metabolism. Notice that the membrane system is also visible in the mitochondria shown in the electron micrograph.

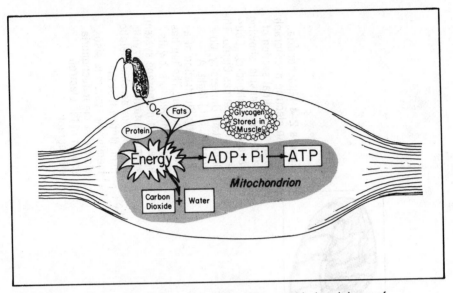

Figure 2-5 The oxygen, or aerobic, system. The aerobic breakdown of carbohydrates, fats, and even proteins provides energy for ATP resynthesis. Since abundant ATP can be manufactured without yielding fatiguing by-products, the aerobic system is most suited for endurance activities.

that is produced diffuses freely from the muscle cell into the blood and is carried to the lung, where it is exhaled. The water that is formed is useful within the cell itself, since the largest constituent of the cell is, in fact, water.

Another feature of the aerobic system that should be noticed is that concerned with the type of foodstuff required for breakdown. Not only glycogen but fats and proteins as well can be aerobically broken down via chemical pathways known as the Krebs cycle and the electron transport system, to carbon dioxide and water, with energy released for ATP synthesis. For example, the breakdown of 256 g (9 oz) of fat will yield 130 moles of ATP. During exercise, both glycogen and fats, but not protein, are important sources of ATP-yielding energy. (For more on the fuels for exercise, see Chap. 4.)

There are hundreds of chemical reactions involved in the aerobic system. While we will not review each one of them, we will discuss the three major series of reactions, namely: (1) aerobic glycolysis; (2) the Krebs cycle; and (3) the electron transport system.

Aerobic Glycolysis

As mentioned earlier, glycolysis refers to the chemical breakdown of glycogen or glucose whereas aerobic means in the presence of oxygen. Therefore, **aerobic glycolysis** means the breakdown of glycogen or glucose in the presence of oxygen. This may come as a surprise, since it was just said that glycolysis is an anaerobic pathway. Actually, there is only one difference between the anaerobic glycolysis discussed earlier and the aerobic glycolysis that occurs when there is a sufficient supply of oxygen: lactic acid does not accumulate in the presence of oxygen. In other words, the presence of oxygen inhibits the accumulation of lactic acid but not the resynthesis of ATP. Oxygen does this by diverting the majority of the lactic acid precursor, pyruvic acid, into the aerobic system after the ATP is resynthesized. Thus, during aerobic glycolysis, 180 g of glycogen are broken down into 2 moles of pyruvic acid, releasing enough energy for resynthesizing 3 moles of ATP. These coupled reactions can be summarized as follows:

$$(C_6H_{12}O_6)_n \longrightarrow 2C_3H_4O_3 \ + ENERGY$$
(glycogen)   (pyruvic acid)
$$ENERGY + 3ADP + 3Pi \longrightarrow 3ATP$$

The Krebs Cycle

Next, the pyruvic acid formed during aerobic glycolysis continues to be broken down in a series of reactions called the **Krebs cycle** after its discoverer, Sir Hans Krebs.* For this important discovery, he won the Nobel Prize in 1953. This cycle is also known as the tricarboxylic acid (TCA) cycle and as the citric acid cycle after some of the chemical compounds found in the cycle. There are two main chemical changes that occur during the Krebs cycle—the production of CO_2 and oxidation (i.e., the removal of electrons). As mentioned earlier, the CO_2 produced diffuses into the blood and is carried to the lungs, where it is eliminated from the body.

Chemically, **oxidation** is defined as the removal of **electrons** from a chemical compound. In this case, the electrons are removed in the form of hydrogen atoms (H) from the carbon atoms of what was formerly pyruvic acid and before that, glycogen. The hydrogen atom, you may recall, contains a positively charged particle called a proton (referred to here as a hydrogen ion) and a negatively charged particle called an electron. In other words:

$$H \longrightarrow H^+ \ + \ e^-$$
(hydrogen   (hydrogen   (electron)
  atom)   ion)

Thus when hydrogen atoms are removed from a compound, that compound is said to have been oxidized.

The production of CO_2 and the removal of electrons in the Krebs cycle are related as follows: pyruvic acid (in its modified form) contains carbon (C), hydrogen (H), and oxygen (O); when H is removed, only C and O (i.e., the chemical components of carbon dioxide) remain. Thus in the Krebs cycle, pyruvic acid is oxidized resulting in the production of CO_2. The Krebs cycle is shown schematically in Figure 2-6.

---

*Pyruvic acid does not enter the Krebs cycle as pyruvic acid. It is first modified to a compound called acetyl-Co-A.

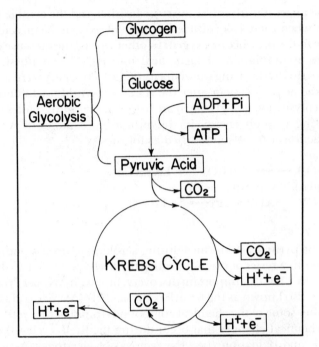

Figure 2-6 The Krebs cycle. Pyruvic acid, the end product of aerobic glycolysis, enters the Krebs cycle after a slight chemical alteration. Once in the cycle, two further chemical events take place: (1) the release of CO_2, which eventually is eliminated from the body by the lungs; and (2) oxidation—that is, the removal of hydrogen ions (H^+) and electrons (e^-), which ultimately enter the electron transport system for further chemical alterations.

The Electron Transport System (ETS)

Continuing in the breakdown of glycogen, the end product, H_2O, is formed from the hydrogen ions and electrons that are removed in the Krebs cycle and the oxygen we breathe. The specific series of reactions in which H_2O is formed is called the **electron transport system** or the **respiratory chain**. Essentially what happens in the electron transport system is that the hydrogen ions and electrons are "transported" to oxygen by "electron carriers" in a series of enzymatic reactions, the end product of which is water. In other words:

$$4H^+ + 4e^- + O_2 \longrightarrow 2H_2O$$

that is, 4 hydrogen ions ($4H^+$) plus 4 electrons ($4e^-$) plus 1 mole of oxygen (O_2) yield 2 moles of water ($2H_2O$). As the electrons are carried down the respiratory chain, energy is released, and ATP is resynthesized in coupled reactions.

For each pair of electrons (2e⁻) carried down the chain, enough energy is released to resynthesize an average of 3 moles of ATP. Overall, 12 pairs of electrons are removed from the breakdown of 180 g of glycogen, and thus 36 moles of ATP are generated. Therefore, during aerobic metabolism, most of the total of 39 moles of ATP are resynthesized in the electron transport system at the same time water is formed.

Summary Equations for Aerobic Metabolism

A summary of the coupled reactions involved in the aerobic breakdown of 180 g of glycogen is as follows:

$$(C_6H_{12}O_6)_n + 6O_2 \longrightarrow 6CO_2 + 6H_2O + \textbf{ENERGY}$$
(glycogen)
$$\textbf{ENERGY} + 39ADP + 39Pi \longrightarrow 39ATP$$

Notice that a total of 39 moles of ATP are resynthesized, 3 from aerobic glycolysis and 36 through the electron transport system.

A summary of the coupled reactions involved in the aerobic breakdown of a typical fat, palmitic acid, is as follows:

$$C_{16}H_{32}O_2 + 23O_2 \longrightarrow 16CO_2 + 16H_2O + \textbf{ENERGY}$$
(palmitic acid)
$$\textbf{ENERGY} + 130ADP + 130Pi \longrightarrow 130ATP$$

A summary of the aerobic system is shown in Figure 2-7.

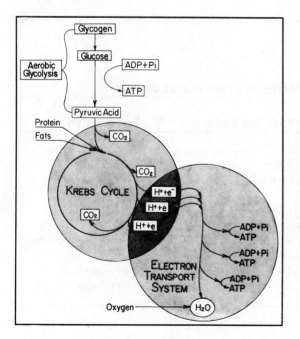

Figure 2-7 Summary of the aerobic (oxygen) system. Glycogen is oxidized in three major series of chemical reactions: aerobic glycolysis, in which pyruvic acid is formed and some ATP resynthesized; the Krebs cycle, in which CO_2 is produced and H^+ and e^- are removed; and the electron transport system, in which H_2O is formed from H^+, e^-, and oxygen, and more ATP is resynthesized.

The amount of oxygen we need to consume from the environment in order to synthesize 1 mole of ATP is approximately 3.5 L if glycogen is the food fuel and about 4.0 L with fat (a liter—1000 ml—is equal to 1.0567 qt). At rest, most of us consume between 0.2 and 0.3 L, or 200 to 300 ml, of oxygen per minute. In other words, a mole of ATP is aerobically manufactured every 12 to 20 min under normal resting conditions. During maximal exercise, a mole of ATP can be aerobically supplied to the working muscles every minute by most of us. For the highly trained endurance athlete, more than 1.5 moles of ATP can be aerobically synthesized and supplied to the muscles every minute during maximal effort.

In summary, then, the aerobic system is capable of utilizing both fats and glycogen for resynthesizing large amounts of ATP without simultaneously generating fatiguing by-products. With respect to sports, it is easy to see that the aerobic system is particularly suited for manufacturing ATP during prolonged, endurance-type activities. For example, during marathon running (42.2 km or 26.2 miles), approximately 150 moles of ATP are required over the 2½ hr the race takes. Such a large, sustained output of ATP energy is possible only because early fatigue can be avoided and large amounts of food (glycogen and fats) and oxygen are readily available.

Some general characteristics of the three energy systems are given in Table 2-2.

Table 2-2: General Characteristics of the Energy Systems

ATP-PC (Phosphagen) System	Lactic Acid System	Oxygen System
Anaerobic	Anaerobic	Aerobic
Very rapid	Rapid	Slow
Chemical fuel: PC	Food fuel: glycogen	Food fuels: glycogen, fats, and protein
Very limited ATP production	Limited ATP production	Unlimited ATP production
Muscular stores limited	By-product, lactic acid, causes muscular fatigue	No fatiguing by-products
Used with sprint or any high-power, short-duration activity	Used with activities of 1 to 3 min duration	Used with endurance or long-duration activities

Relationship between Oxygen Consumption and Energy (Heat) Production

Up to this point in this chapter, we have mentioned oxygen consumption in terms of its functional link to the aerobic release of energy from foodstuffs for ATP synthesis. In Chapter 1, we mentioned energy expenditure and heat production as they relate to the performance of various sports. It is now appropriate to link these diverse elements—to see just what the relationships among oxygen consumption, energy (heat) production, and energy expenditure are.

Oxygen Consumption

The oxygen required for the breakdown of carbohydrates and fats comes from the air we breathe. The breakdown (oxidation) of any particular carbohydrate (e.g., glycogen) or fat will require a specific amount of oxygen. For example, 192 g of oxygen are needed in order to oxidize 180 g of glycogen. In terms of volume, this works out to 134.4 L of oxygen per 180 g of glycogen. With a typical fat such as palmitic acid, 515.2 L of oxygen are required for oxidation of 256 g of the fat.

The quantities of oxygen that go into the breakdown of a foodstuff are of course linked to an overall quantity—the amount of oxygen we consume. At rest we consume oxygen at a rate of approximately 0.2 to 0.3 L per min; during maximal exercise the rate increases to 3 to 6 L per min, depending upon, among other things, sex, age, and level of fitness. The abbreviation for the volume of oxygen consumed per minute is $\dot{V}O_2$; V is the symbol for volume, O_2 refers to oxygen, and the dot over the V ($\dot{V}$) means per unit time, usually per minute. The abbreviations max $\dot{V}O_2$ and $\dot{V}O_2$ max are used interchangeably to refer to the maximal volume of oxygen consumed per minute during exercise (such as the 3 to 6 L per min just mentioned). The $\dot{V}O_2$max is the single most valid measure of the functional power capabilities of the aerobic energy system.

Energy (Heat) Production

When a given amount of oxygen breaks down a given amount of glycogen or fat, a specific amount of energy is released. For example, when 134.4 L of oxygen oxidize 180 g of glycogen, 686 kcal of heat (energy) are released. About half of this is captured as ATP energy; the remaining energy is in the form of heat and is either stored in the body or eventually lost to the environment. Some of the energy released when ATP is broken down is used by the cells in performing biological work. The remaining energy here also appears as heat, being either stored or dissipated.

The amount of energy released when a given amount of oxygen is consumed for the breakdown of a given amount of glycogen or fat can be measured either as the amount of heat produced or as the amount of oxygen consumed. Since in man the latter is easier, it is the method used most often. When 1 L of oxygen is consumed with glycogen as the food fuel, 5 kcal of heat are released. With fats as the fuel, only 4.7 kcal of heat are released per liter of oxygen consumed. **There is a direct relationship between oxygen consumption and energy and heat production in the body.**

Energy Expenditure

Energy expenditure refers to the amount of energy required to perform a given activity. It is usually measured or estimated from the amount of oxygen consumed during performance of the activity. For example, in running, the energy expenditure is 0.2 ml of oxygen per kilogram of body weight and per meter run. Thus, if you weigh 70 kg and run 1500 m, your energy expenditure will be approximately $0.2 \times 70 \times 1500 = 21$ L of oxygen. If it is assumed that glycogen was the major food fuel involved, then 21 L of oxygen would represent $21 \times 5 = 105$ kcal of energy expended during the run. The energy expenditure of various activities, as will be discussed later (p. 300), is generally expressed in kcal. The energy expenditure during rest is between 60 and 85 kcal per hour for a person who weighs 70 kg.

Summary

- Energy is the capacity to perform work. Kinetic energy is associated with motion, such as swinging a bat or club. Potential energy is energy by virtue of position, such as in a bent bow. Chemical energy is potential energy, such as represented by the foods we eat.

- The unit of measure of energy is the calorie, the amount of heat required to raise the temperature of 1 g of water 1° Celsius (centigrade). The kilocalorie (kcal) is equal to 1000 calories.

- Work (W) is the product of a force (F) acting through a distance (d): $W = F \times d$. Power (P) is work per unit time (t): $P = W/t = (F \times d)/t$.

- Adenosine triphosphate (ATP) is the immediately usable form of chemical energy for muscular activity; it is stored in all muscle cells.

- The energy needed to synthesize ATP comes from energy released during the breakdown of foods and other chemicals in the body. The coupling of energy release and energy usage—a system called coupled reactions—is the fundamental principle involved in the metabolic production of ATP.

- Aerobic metabolism refers to a series of chemical reactions in the presence of oxygen. Anaerobic metabolism refers to a series of reactions without oxygen.

- The ATP-PC system is an anaerobic energy system that resynthesizes ATP from energy released when phosphocreatine (PC) is broken down. It is a very rapid but limited source of ATP that is used predominantly during the performance of high-power, short-duration activities.

- The lactic acid system is also anaerobic, resynthesizing ATP from energy released during the breakdown of glycogen (sugar) to lactic acid. Accumulation of the latter causes muscular fatigue. This system is used predominantly during activities that require between 1 and 3 min to perform.

- The oxygen system utilizes both glycogen and fats as fuels for ATP resynthesis. By chemical reactions that take place in the mitochondria of the cells, the system yields large amounts of ATP but no fatiguing by-products. The aerobic system is used predominantly during endurance tasks or low-power output activities.

- Glycogen is oxidized in three major series of chemical reactions, aerobic glycolysis in which pyruvic acid is formed and some ATP resynthesized; the Krebs cycle in which carbon dioxide (CO_2) is produced, and hydrogen ions (H^+) and electrons (e^-) are removed; and the electron transport system in which water (H_2O) is formed from H^+, e^-, and oxygen, and more ATP is resynthesized. Fats and proteins, when used as fuels for ATP resynthesis, also go through the Krebs cycle and the electron transport system.

- A specific amount of oxygen is required in order for a given amount of energy or heat to be released from the breakdown of a given amount of glycogen or fats. About half of the energy released is captured as ATP energy, with the remainder given off as heat. The amount of energy required to perform a given activity is estimated from the oxygen consumed during performance, and is usually expressed as heat (kilocalories).

Selected References and Readings

Fox, E. L. Energy sources during rest and exercise. *In* Stull, G. A. (ed.): *Encyclopedia of Physical Education, Fitness, and Sports*. Salt Lake City, Brighton Publishing Company, 1980, pp. 251–258.

Fox, E. L., and D. K. Mathews: *The Physiological Basis of Physical Education and Athletics*. 3rd ed. Philadelphia, Saunders College Publishing, 1981, pp. 11–32.

3
Sports Activities and the Energy Continuum

Introduction

In the previous chapter, energy was considered in terms of some of its most fundamental properties—how it relates to work, what is meant by potential energy, and so on. At this point, we must examine an aspect of energy that may at first seem to have fewer applications: the continuum concept. As we will see, the idea of an energy continuum is in fact entirely applicable to sports activity, and is well backed by broad observation and specific research.

The Energy Continuum Concept

In the last chapter, we learned that ATP is the immediate form of muscular energy. As shown for review in Figure 3-1, ATP is supplied in three

26

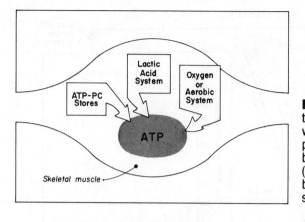

Figure 3-1 ATP is supplied to the muscle in three ways: by the stored phosphagens (ATP and PC); by the lactic acid system (anaerobic glycolysis); and by the oxygen (aerobic) system.

ways: (1) by the stored phosphagens, ATP and PC; (2) by the lactic acid system (anaerobic glycolysis); and (3) by the oxygen, or aerobic, system. We also learned that the ability of each system to supply the major portion of the ATP required in any given activity is related to the specific kind of activity performed. For example, in short-term, high-intensity types of activities, such as the 100-m dash, most of the ATP is supplied by the readily available phosphagen system. In contrast, longer-term, lower-intensity types of activities, such as the 42.2-km marathon, are supported almost entirely by the oxygen, or aerobic, system.

In the middle range of activities are those tasks that rely heavily on the lactic acid system for ATP production—for example, the 400- and 800-m dashes. Also in the middle are those activities that require a blend of both anaerobic and aerobic metabolism—for example, the 1500-m and mile runs. In these latter activities, the anaerobic systems supply the major portion of ATP during the sprint at both the start and finish of the race, with the aerobic system predominating during the middle or steady-state period of the run.

Just from these examples it can be seen that what is at work in physical activities is an energy continuum, a continuum relating the way in which ATP is made available and the type of physical activity performed.

The Energy Continuum and Running and Swimming Activities

Perhaps the best way to further illustrate the energy continuum idea is to look closely at the energetics of track and swimming events. In Figure 3-2, two aspects of the energetics of swimming and running are presented. The first of these, shown in Figure 3-2A, is concerned with energy **capacity**, or the total amount of ATP required during the performance of the various events. The

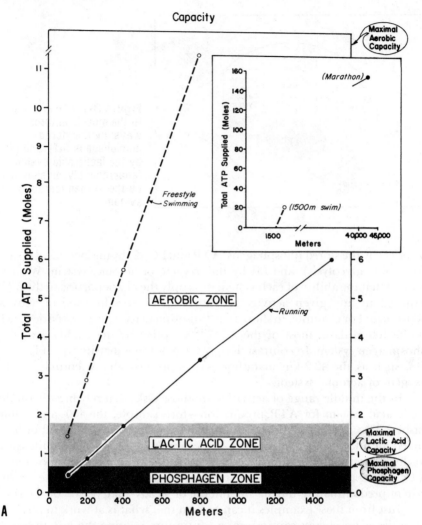

Figure 3-2 Energetics of track and swimming events in relation to the three energy systems. A, The energy capacity or total amount of ATP required during performance of the various events. B, The power or rate at which ATP is supplied during performance. See text for further explanation of capacity and power.

approximate total number of moles of ATP required during an event is shown on the vertical axis and was calculated from energy cost data. Since the amount of ATP required for any given swimming or running event is mainly dependent upon the distance traveled, ATP requirements have been plotted against the distance, in meters, of the event (horizontal axis).

The shaded areas represent the capacities of the various energy systems for supplying ATP. They were estimated from data obtained from a number of

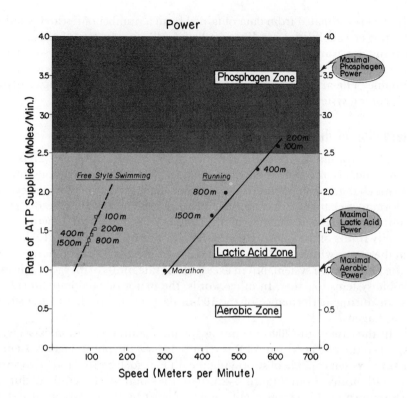

B

different studies performed on human subjects. In the figure, the capacities are "stacked" one on top of the other. From this "stacking," you can see that if (for instance) both the phosphagen and lactic acid systems were used to their capacities during the performance of an event, a total of about 1.8 moles of ATP would be supplied (see Fig. 3-2A). The large arrows on the right side of the figure indicate the absolute capacities of the energy systems. In other words, the values indicated by the arrows represent the maximum amount of ATP capable of being supplied by any one of the three energy systems alone. For example, the most ATP that can be supplied by the lactic acid system alone (maximal lactic acid capacity) is about 1.2 moles.

Figure 3-2B involves **power**, or the rate at which ATP is supplied during performance. Here, the speed of running and swimming is shown on the horizontal axis and is plotted against the rate at which ATP is supplied (vertical axis) during freestyle swimming events of 100, 200, 400, 800, and 1500 m and during running events of 100, 200, 400, 800, 1500, and 42,200 (marathon) m. The speeds were calculated from world records, whereas the rate of ATP demanded during performance was calculated from the energy cost estimates mentioned above.

The shaded areas shown in Figure 3-2B represent the power capabilities of each energy system for supplying ATP. As with the capacities, the power values were estimated from data obtained from a number of research studies. The power capabilities are likewise "stacked" one on top of the other—meaning, for example, that with the aerobic and lactic acid systems supplying ATP at their maximal rates, about 2.5 moles of ATP per min would be available. The arrows to the right indicate the absolute power capability of each energy system alone.

Interaction of the Energy Systems

The most important point to notice from Figures 3–2A and 3–2B is how the dependence on a given energy system as well as the interactions among systems changes as the distance swum or run changes and the power (speed) of performance changes. For example, in Figure 3–2A, notice that the total ATP required during performance of the 100-m running sprint is within the capacity limits of the phosphagen system. In Figure 3–2B, it can also be seen that the rate at which ATP is required during this event is below the rate limit of the phosphagen system, but in excess of the rate limits of the lactic acid and aerobic systems together. In other words, the major or predominant energy system during performance of the 100-m dash is clearly that of the stored phosphagens.

In the case of the 200-m running sprint, a similar situation exists with respect to the rate at which ATP is required—i.e., the phosphagen system is the only system capable of supplying the ATP at such a rapid rate. However, you will notice from Figure 3–2A that the total ATP required during performance of this sprint event cannot be met by the phosphagen system alone; the lactic acid system is also required. Thus, during performance of the 200-m sprint, both anaerobic systems are important contributors of ATP energy.

As the speed of performance decreases, and the duration or distance increases, the major energy system shifts toward the lactic acid and aerobic mechanisms. Thus while there is an interaction of the phosphagen, lactic acid, and aerobic systems during the 400-m running sprint and the 100-m swim, there is a distinct predominance of the lactic acid and aerobic systems in the supply of ATP energy during performance of the 800-m and 1500-m runs and in most of the swimming events. During marathon running and the 1500-m swimming event, it is the aerobic system that predominates, as can be seen in Figure 3–2A.

The Energy Continuum and Other Sports

Where do other sports fit on the energy continuum? As a starting point in answering this question, let's look at Figure 3–3. The track and swimming events just referred to have been included in this continuum along with many other types of sports activities. Again notice that both aerobic and anaerobic

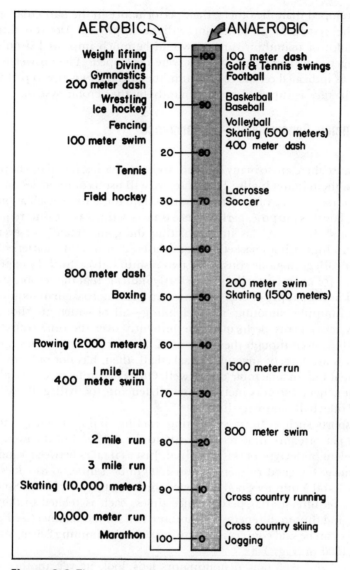

AEROBIC		ANAEROBIC
Weight lifting	0 — 100	100 meter dash
Diving		Golf & Tennis swings
Gymnastics		Football
200 meter dash		
Wrestling	10 — 90	Basketball
Ice hockey		Baseball
Fencing		Volleyball
100 meter swim		Skating (500 meters)
	20 — 80	400 meter dash
Tennis		
Field hockey	30 — 70	Lacrosse
		Soccer
	40 — 60	
800 meter dash	50 — 50	200 meter swim
Boxing		Skating (1500 meters)
Rowing (2000 meters)	60 — 40	
1 mile run		1500 meter run
400 meter swim		
	70 — 30	
2 mile run	80 — 20	800 meter swim
3 mile run		
Skating (10,000 meters)	90 — 10	
		Cross country running
10,000 meter run		Cross country skiing
Marathon	100 — 0	Jogging

Figure 3-3 The energy continuum and various sports activities. Although both aerobic and anaerobic energy systems contribute some ATP during the performance of various sports, one system usually contributes more, as indicated by the aerobic and anaerobic percentages.

systems contribute at least some ATP during performance of all the activities shown. Also notice that one system usually contributes more (as indicated by the aerobic and anaerobic percentages) during given activities than do the other systems. This is quite important in athletics, for if one energy system is more developed than the others, then performance in the particular sport in which the system is predominant will be improved. Do you think the performance of marathon runners would be much improved if only their phosphagen and lactic acid systems were developed? The answer is "no," because, as indicated on the continuum, the necessary energy to perform the 2½- to 3-hr race is supplied predominantly by the aerobic system.

The Common Denominator—Performance Time

Because there are so many different sports activities, it will not be possible to discuss them individually. Therefore, we will use a common denominator, the performance time of an activity, rather than the activity itself as our basis of study. For this purpose, performance time is defined as the time required in executing skills as well as in completing the game, match, or event. For example, a high school basketball game lasts 32 min (four quarters of 8 min each). In college, a game consists of two 20-min halves. Such long performance times for completing the game clearly indicate that the aerobic system is involved in the supply of energy. However, playing basketball requires such skills as jumping, shooting, and defending—all of which are short, high-intensity movements performed intermittently over the time course of the game. Thus, even though the game itself lasts for many minutes, the skills themselves are largely anaerobic. Basketball, then, has not only an aerobic component but an anaerobic one as well. Other examples of sports falling in this same general category include baseball, fencing, football, golf, ice hockey, tennis, volleyball, and wrestling.

In sports such as track, swimming, cycling, skiing, rowing, and speed skating, performance time refers mostly to the duration of the event, being independent of the type of skill involved. Just as it takes between 4 and 5 min, for instance, for good runners to run 1500 m or a mile, so too does it take between 4 and 5 min for good freestyle swimmers to swim 400 m. Since both activities require similar performance times, each is related to the energy systems, and thus to the energy continuum, in a similar manner (see Fig. 3-2). The same can be said concerning running 800 m, swimming 200 m, and speed skating 1500 m (Fig. 3-3).

Using the common denominator, let's look at yet another way to illustrate the energy continuum. Figure 3-4 shows the percent energy in the form of ATP contributed by the three energy systems as related to performance time or power output. Remember, the shorter the performance time of an activity, the greater the power output of the activity and the more rapid the energy requirement. (The converse should also be recalled.) Figure 3-4 shows, once again, the interaction among the three energy systems. Notice, for example, that the ATP-PC and oxygen systems are mirror images of each other; as the percentage of ATP supplied by the one system increases, it decreases in the other. Both systems are responsible for supplying nearly all of

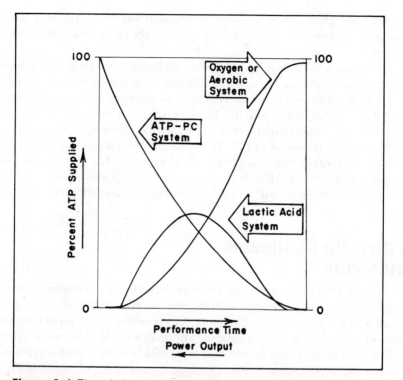

Figure 3-4 The relationship between the percent ATP contributed by the three energy systems as related to performance time or power output. The shorter the performance time, the greater the power output and the more rapid the energy (ATP) requirement. (Based on data from Fox and co-workers, 1969.)

the ATP for activities at the extremes of the continuum; if these systems are improved through training, then improvement in performance will follow.

Of special interest in Figure 3-4 is the curve of the relationship between energy contributed by the lactic acid system and performance time. During very high intensity activities with short performance times, the lactic acid system contributes very little, if any, energy. The same holds true for the lower intensity activities with longer performance times. Only for activities between these extremes does the lactic acid system contribute a large portion of the total ATP requirement. The overall pattern is thus quite different from that of the phosphagen and aerobic systems.

The reason for the difference is twofold. First, it requires time to "activate" the lactic acid system. This means that when the performance times of activities are less than or equal to this "activation" time, scant amounts of energy can be supplied by the lactic acid system. Second, you will recall that the lactic acid system limits, to a certain extent, the time of performance because muscular fatigue results from the accumulation of lactic acid.

Therefore, in order to delay fatigue brought on by lactic acid during prolonged activities, the energy contribution via the lactic acid system must be kept low.

As indicated by the height of the lactic acid curve, the energy contribution of this system is lower, even when in full use, than that of the other systems. This indicates that the lactic acid system alone does not usually predominate as an ATP supplier in any activity. Thus, even in activities in which the lactic acid system is important, there is at least one other system acting as a significant contributor of ATP. Training of two energy systems is thus required for greatest improvement in performance. For this reason, such activities are often very difficult to perform well, and require a most difficult training program. More will be said about this in a later chapter (see p. 206).

Setting Up Continuum Guidelines

Although the continuum concept is essential to a good understanding of the interactions of the energy systems, the continuum itself is not easily applied to the various sports. Therefore, let's construct some guidelines from which we can more readily determine the major energy system or systems involved during the performance of most sports activities. Such information is vital to the development of proper training programs. As shown in Figure 3–5 and Table 3–1, the continuum of performance times can be divided into four distinct areas.

Area One

The first area includes all activities requiring performance times of less than 30 sec. In these activities, the predominant energy system is the phosphagen (or ATP-PC) system. Examples of some of the sports activities falling under Area One of the continuum are the shot-put, 100-m sprint (running), base stealing, the golf and tennis swings, and the running plays of backs in football.

Area Two

This area includes those sports activities requiring between 30 sec and 1½ min to perform. The predominant energy systems in this case will be both the ATP-PC and the lactic acid systems. Examples of sports activities in this area are the 100-m freestyle swim, 200- and 400-m runs, and 500-m speed skating.

Area Three

The third area takes into account those sports activities requiring between 1½ and 3 min to perform. Here, as in Area Two, there are two major energy systems involved—in this case the lactic acid system (or anaerobic

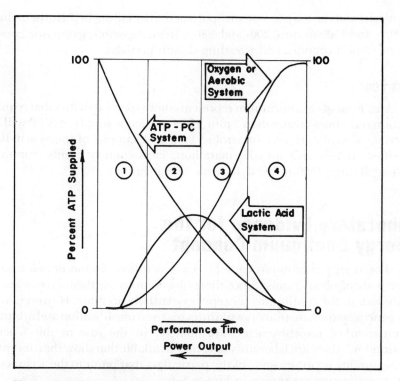

Figure 3-5 Division of the relationships shown in Figure 3-4 into four areas of activity. Specific sports covered by these energy continuum guidelines are cited in Table 3-1.

Table 3-1: Four Areas of the Energy Continuum

Area	Performance Time	Major Energy System(s) Involved	Examples of Type of Activity
1	Less than 30 sec	ATP-PC	Shot-put, 100-m sprint, base stealing, golf and tennis swings, running plays of football backs
2	30 sec to 1½ min	ATP-PC and lactic acid	200- to 400-m sprints, speed skating, 100-m swim
3	1½ min to 3 min	Lactic acid and O₂	800-m dash, gymnastics events, boxing (3-min rounds), wrestling (2-min periods)
4	Greater than 3 min	O₂	Soccer and lacrosse (except goalies), cross-country skiing, marathon run, jogging, distance swimming

glycolysis) and the oxygen system. Sports activities falling in this area include the 800- and 1500-m runs, 200- and 400-m freestyle swims, gymnastic events, boxing (3-min rounds), and wrestling (2-min periods).

Area Four

Area Four of the continuum represents those sports activities that require performance times greater than 3 min. Here the major supply of ATP will be contributed by the oxygen, or aerobic, system. Examples of sports activities classified in this area are the marathon, cross-country events (running, cycling, skiing), 1500-m freestyle swim, and jogging.

Laboratory Evidence for the Energy Continuum Concept

The energy continuum concept is a generalized notion drawn from a large body of observations. Since these observations are themselves scientifically sound, the continuum concept is essentially accurate. However, as in any generalization, there are possibilities for oversimplification and arbitrary elimination of inconsistencies. Fortunately, in the case of the "energy continuum," there are laboratory data now available that show the concept to be measurably accurate; some of the particulars that point to the accuracy of the generalization are shown in Figure 3–6.

Maximal oxygen consumption ($\dot{V}O_2max$) values for 19 different groups of athletes are shown in Figure 3–6A. You will recall that $\dot{V}O_2max$ is the single most reliable indicator of the power of the aerobic energy system. The athletes, both male and female, were members of the Swedish national teams. (The data for females are not as complete because at the time of testing, 1967 to 1968, few female teams were organized for national and international competition.) Note how the $\dot{V}O_2$ max values are high in those groups of athletes whose sport requires aerobic endurance, and low in those athletes who participate in anaerobic events. Also notice that in the middle are those sports that demand both aerobic and anaerobic metabolism.

In Figure 3–6B, a different measure is used: the lactic acid accumulation in the blood after exhaustive exercise involving arm and leg work, performed by 11 groups of athletes. In this case, the athletes, mostly males, were members of the Finnish national teams during the 1972 and 1974 world and European championships and Olympic games. Those athletes involved in aerobic events (e.g., long-distance running and cross-country skiing) were found to have low values for lactic acid accumulation, whereas those involved in activities relying heavily on both anaerobic and aerobic power (e.g., alpine skiing, running 800 m, and canoeing) had much higher values. Low values can also be seen for athletes engaged in sprint-like events such as ice hockey and speed skating.

A stair-climbing test, which lasts for only a few tenths of a second, was used on the Finnish national team members for evaluation of the phosphagen system. The results are shown in Figure 3-6C. Athletes participating in the short-term, high-intensity events had high anaerobic (phosphagen) power values, whereas those in endurance events had relatively lower values.

The contours of the lines given in Figure 3-6 should be compared to those given in Figures 3-4 and 3-5. Although the match is not "smooth," they are in good agreement.

Summary

- The energy continuum idea is based on the fact that the ability of each energy system to supply ATP is related to the specific kind of activity performed.

- On one end of the continuum are the short-term, high-intensity sports activities, such as the 100-m dash, in which the major portion of ATP is supplied by the phosphagen system.

- On the opposite end of the continuum are the longer-term, lower-intensity sports activities—such as marathon running—which are supported almost entirely by the aerobic system.

- In the middle of the continuum are those sports activities that rely heavily on the lactic acid system for ATP energy. The 400- and 800-m dashes are examples of such activities.

- Also in the middle of the continuum are those activities that require a blend of both anaerobic and aerobic metabolism—e.g., the 1500-m and mile runs.

- In evaluating sports activities on the basis of their relative position on the energy continuum, two aspects of energetics should be considered: capacity, or the total amount of ATP required during performance, and power, or the rate at which ATP is required during performance. For track and swimming events, a rather sophisticated evaluation can be made from known energy cost data and world performance records.

- Relative positions of other sports on the energy continuum can be estimated from performance times. The performance time of an activity is defined as the time required in executing skills as well as in completing the game, match, or event.

- The energy continuum of performance times can be divided into four distinctive areas:

  Area One includes activities requiring less than 30 sec to perform. The major energy system is the stored phosphagens (ATP and PC).
  Area Two includes activities requiring between 30 and 90 sec to perform. The major energy systems are the ATP-PC and lactic acid systems.
  Area Three includes activities requiring between 1½ and 3 min to perform. The major energy systems are the lactic acid and aerobic systems.
  Area Four includes activities requiring performance times greater than 3 min. The major energy system is the aerobic, or oxygen, system.

- Laboratory data are now available that confirm the energy continuum concept.

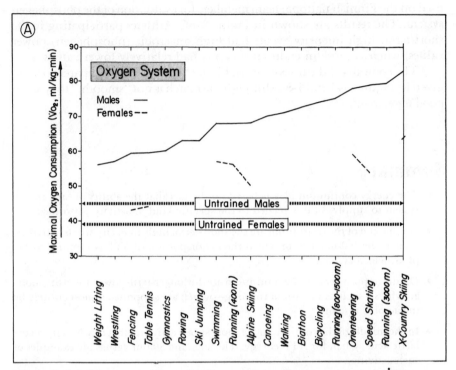

Figure 3-6 Laboratory evidence for the energy continuum concept. A, $\dot{V}O_2$max values for 19 different groups of athletes are shown. Note how the values are high in those who participate in endurance events and low in those who participate in anaerobic events. B, Maximal blood lactic acid levels following exhaustive exercise are shown for 11 different groups of athletes. Note that those involved in aerobic events have low values and those involved in anaerobic events have high values. C, Values for a stair-climbing test (involving the phosphagen system) are shown; the same trend shown in B is evident. (Data in A from Saltin and Astrand, 1967; data in B and C from Komi and co-workers, 1977.)

Selected References and Readings

Dill, D. B.: Oxygen used in horizontal and grade walking and running on the treadmill. *J. Appl. Physiol., 20*:19–22, 1965.

di Prampero, P. E., D. R. Pendergast, and D. W. Rennie: Energetics of swimming in man. *J. Appl. Physiol., 37(1)*:1–5, 1974.

Fox, E. L.: Physical Training: Methods and effects. *Orthop. Clin. N. Am., 8(3)*:533–548, 1977.

Fox, E. L., and D. K. Mathews: *Interval Training: Conditioning for Sports and General Fitness.* Philadelphia, W. B. Saunders Company, 1974.

Fox, E. L., and D. K. Mathews: *The Physiological Basis of Physical Education and Athletics.* 3rd ed. Philadelphia, Saunders College Publishing, 1981.

Fox, E. L., S. Robinson, and D. L. Wiegman: Metabolic energy sources during continuous and interval running. *J. Appl. Physiol., 27*:174–178, 1969.

Hultman, E.: Studies on muscle metabolism of glycogen and active phosphate in man with special reference to exercise and diet. *Scand. J. Clin. Lab. Invest.* (Suppl. 94), *19*:1–63, 1967.

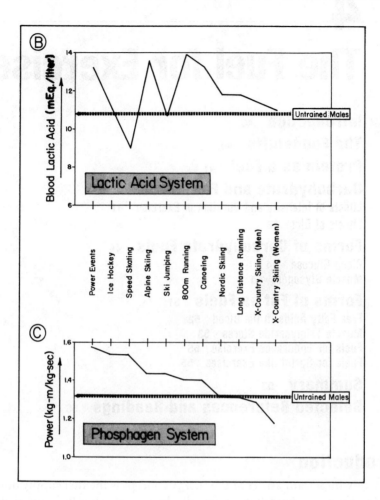

Karlsson, J.: Lactate and phosphagen concentrations in working muscle of man. *Acta Physiol. Scand.* (Suppl. 358):1-72, 1971.

Komi, P., H. Rusko, J. Vos, and V. Bihko: Anaerobic performance capacity in athletes. *Acta Physiol. Scand.*, *100*:107-114, 1977.

Margaria, R., et al.: Energy cost of running. *J. Appl. Physiol.*, *18*:367-370, 1963.

Pendergast, D. R., et al.: Quantitative analysis of the front crawl in men and women. *J. Appl. Physiol.: Respirat. Environ. Exercise Physiol.*, *43(3)*:475-479, 1977.

Saltin, B., and P. O. Astrand: Maximal oxygen uptake in athletes. *J. Appl. Physiol.*, *23*:353-358, 1967.

*For full titles of journals, see Appendix A.

4

The Fuel for Exercise

Introduction

A very important aspect of the energy concept is the fuel supply during exercise. Knowing something about the fuel (food) supply to the skeletal muscles during exercise is essential in helping you understand the nutritional needs of your athletes. The information presented in this chapter, then, will cover what foods serve as fuels, and how these fuels are selectively used in athletic performance.

The Foodstuffs

What is generally meant by "fuel supply" is the type of foodstuff used for ATP production during exercise. There are three foodstuffs: (1) protein; (2) carbohydrate (i.e., glucose and its storage form glycogen); and (3) fat. You will recall that the energy released from the breakdown of all three foodstuffs can be used in the oxygen system for generating ATP, and that carbohydrate serves as the sole source of energy for ATP formation by anaerobic glycolysis (the lactic acid system).

Protein as a Fuel

As mentioned in Chapter 2, although protein can be used as an energy fuel for the aerobic system, it is not normally a significant fuel during exercise of any kind. The significant use of protein as a metabolic fuel occurs only when the other foodstuffs are unavailable, such as during prolonged and severe starvation. We will see how important this information is in Chapter 10, when we discuss the efficacy of coaches encouraging their athletes to eat large quantities of protein in hopes of increasing energy capacity.

Carbohydrate and Fat as Fuels

There are two major factors that significantly affect the preference for and interaction of carbohydrate and fat fuels during exercise: (1) the intensity and duration of exercise and (2) the diet.

Effects of Intensity and Duration of Exercise

As shown in Figure 4-1, as the intensity of exercise increases and the duration decreases, the predominant food fuel shifts toward carbohydrate. One of the reasons for this is that ATP production shifts toward anaerobic metabolism (the lactic acid system) during short-term, heavy exercise. As just mentioned, carbohydrate is the only fuel for this system. (It should be pointed out here that during very heavy but very brief exercise, such as sprinting 100 m,

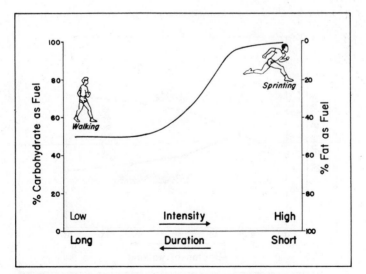

Figure 4-1 As exercise intensity increases and duration decreases, the predominant food fuel shifts toward carbohydrate.

the major "fuel" for ATP resynthesis is phosphocreatine (PC). Only an insignificant amount of carbohydrate can be broken down in the muscle in such a short period of time.)

Again referring to Figure 4-1, as the exercise intensity decreases and duration increases, fat becomes the major source of fuel. Although fat is a major fuel during prolonged efforts, carbohydrate is still important, particularly during the beginning or early portion of the performance. This is shown in Figure 4-2. Notice how the usage of carbohydrate is greater at first, then slowly but steadily yields to fat as the performance continues. One aspect of fuel usage not shown in the figure is the role of carbohydrate in those endurance races that require a "kick" at the finish. During this "kick," carbohydrate is an important fuel because the lactic acid system is involved.

The importance of carbohydrate during prolonged exercise is underscored by the fact that depletion of the intramuscular stores of carbohydrate is almost always coincident with muscular exhaustion. This is true even though there is plenty of fat still available to the muscle as fuel. However, whether the depletion of muscular stores of carbohydrates and muscular fatigue under these circumstances are causally related is not known for sure at this time.

Effects of Diet

The kind of food we eat affects which fuel—carbohydrate or fat—will be more or less available during exercise. Evidence for this relationship can be seen in Figure 4-3, which shows findings from a series of experiments contrasting the effects of a normal diet with those of a high-carbohydrate diet

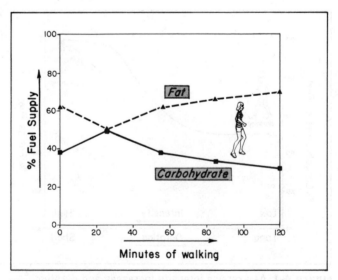

Figure 4-2 During prolonged exercise, the usage of carbohydrate is at first greater than that of fat; fat usage slowly becomes predominant as performance continues, however.

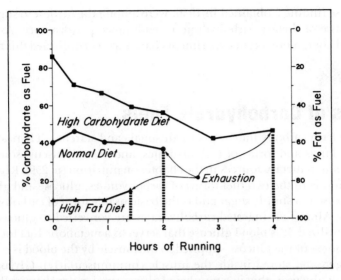

Figure 4-3 The kind of food we eat affects which fuel—carbohydrate or fat—will be more or less available during subsequent exercise. (Based on data from Christensen and Hansen, 1939.)

and a high-fat diet. A normal diet, also called a mixed diet, contains approximately 55% carbohydrate, 30% fat, and 15% protein. As you can see, during endurance exercise (in this case running), the pattern of fuel usage associated with the normal diet (middle line) is one we have already described: at first carbohydrate is used preferentially, but then fat is favored. Subjects who ate the normal diet for a period of several days were able to run for 2 hr before exhaustion set in.

As shown by the lower line in Figure 4-3, after several days on a high-fat, low-carbohydrate diet, the preferred fuel during exercise was fat, even during the first part of the run. This clearly indicates that the availability of a fuel as determined through the diet is an important factor in fuel preference. Notice also that when the subjects on the high-fat diet ran, exhaustion set in in only 85 min, 35 min sooner than on the mixed diet. The upper line shows the fuel preference and exhaustion time for subjects who for several days were on a high-carbohydrate, low-fat diet. Three important features are apparent:

1. Carbohydrate was used in much greater quantities, particularly during the start of exercise.
2. Even with this large availability of carbohydrate, there still was a preference for fat metabolism as the exercise continued.
3. Following the high-carbohydrate diet, the subjects could run for 4 hr before exhaustion set in. This endurance time is twice that associated with the mixed diet and almost three times that associated with the high-fat diet!

These findings, obtained in 1939, were among the earliest to suggest the significance of dietary carbohydrate in endurance performance. As will be discussed later, more recent experiments have further confirmed this relationship.

Forms of Carbohydrate Fuels

The term carbohydrate refers to all sugars and starches. There are many different kinds and forms of carbohydrates, and we will discuss some of the more common dietary sources in the chapter on nutrition (p. 259). Right now, our interest is in the two fuel forms of carbohydrates, glucose and glycogen.

Glucose is a simple sugar and is the basic usable form of carbohydrate in the body. Almost all ingested carbohydrates are converted to glucose before they are utilized. It is **blood glucose** that serves as a metabolic fuel for skeletal muscle. Some of the glucose supplied to the muscle by the blood is converted to glycogen and stored inside the muscle (intramuscularly). Glycogen is a polymer of glucose—that is, a number of glucose molecules chemically linked together. In humans, glycogen represents the storage form of glucose and also serves as a metabolic fuel for skeletal muscle.

Blood Glucose

As shown in Figure 4-4, glucose uptake from the blood by skeletal muscle during rest is rather small. However, during prolonged exercise bouts, glucose uptake from the blood increases substantially, accounting for as much as 30 to 40% of the total fuel used by the oxygen system during the course of the

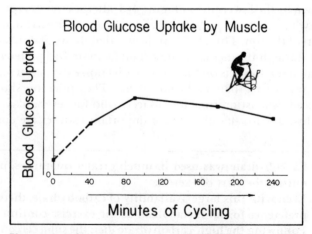

Figure 4-4 Glucose uptake from the blood by skeletal muscle is small during rest but increases during prolonged exercise. (Based on data from Wahren, 1977.)

exercise. Later in our discussion of nutrition we will see that the uptake of glucose by the working muscles can be further enhanced if carbohydrate is ingested either prior to or during exercise.

Maintenance of an adequate blood glucose level is essential at all times because glucose is the major source of fuel for the brain. Levels of glucose in the blood are obviously tied to the carbohydrate portion of the diet, but there is, in addition, some regulation of these levels by the liver. The liver stores relatively large quantities of glycogen; when blood glucose levels are low, liver glycogen is broken down and glucose is released into the blood. When blood glucose levels are high, the liver takes up the glucose from the blood and stores it as glycogen. A major source of blood glucose during prolonged exercise comes from the breakdown of liver glycogen. Of course, exercise can reach a point of straining the mechanisms for maintaining glucose levels; it has been known for some time, for instance, that physical exhaustion, particularly following endurance efforts, can be accompanied by a low blood glucose level (hypoglycemia). Prevention of hypoglycemia during and following exercise will be discussed later on in this book.

The glycogen stored in the muscle cannot directly supply the blood with glucose. Instead, it must first be broken down to lactic acid through anaerobic glycolysis. The lactic acid then diffuses into the blood and is carried to the liver. Here, it can be converted to glucose and can be either stored as liver glycogen or dumped back into the blood.

Muscle Glycogen

The intramuscular stores of glycogen represent another form of carbohydrate that is used as a metabolic fuel. Depletion of these stores appears to play an important role in muscular fatigue. As will be discussed in detail in a later chapter (p. 274), the muscle glycogen stores can be greatly increased through dietary manipulation, an effect which has been shown to enhance endurance performance.

The use of muscle glycogen during exercise is dependent upon a number of factors, including intensity, duration, and mode of exercise. As might be expected, as both the intensity and duration of exercise increase, so does the amount of muscle glycogen utilized. This is shown in Figure 4–5. The data in Figure 4–5A were obtained by having subjects perform several 2-hr bouts of cycling, each at a different intensity. The exercise was measured on a bicycle ergometer, a stationary bicycle in which the work rate and load can be precisely controlled (the term ergometer means work [erg] meter). The data in Figure 4–5B represent cycling at a constant submaximal intensity on the ergometer. In this series of experiments, the subjects were stopped for a few seconds every 20 min, at which times needle biopsies were taken. A biopsy is the removal of a small piece of tissue, in this case a piece of tissue taken from one of the quadricep muscles, the vastus lateralis. The tissue was subsequently analyzed for glycogen content. Notice how the glycogen was virtually all used up at exhaustion. In this cycling activity, as well as that performed at varying

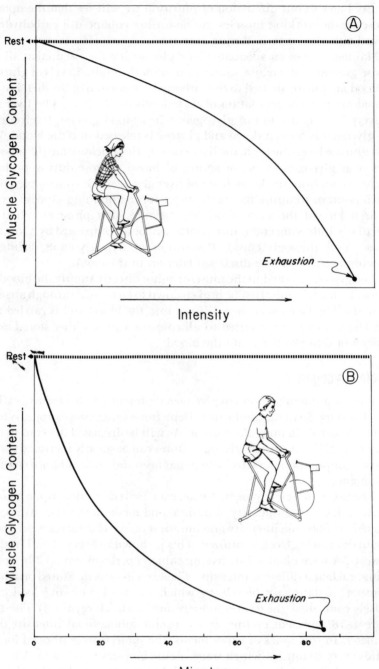

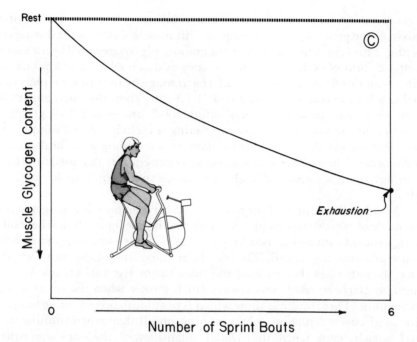

Figure 4-5 As both the intensity (A) and duration (B) of exercise increase, so does the amount of muscle glycogen utilized. In (C), although glycogen is a primary fuel during sprint bouts, plenty of glycogen remains at exhaustion. (Data in C from Gollnick and co-workers, 1973.)

intensities (Fig. 4–5A), the glycogen was used mainly as a fuel for the oxygen system, since this is the predominant energy system for prolonged exercise.

In Figure 4–5C, the amount of glycogen used by the vastus lateralis muscle is plotted against the number of all-out sprints performed on a bicycle ergometer. Each sprint was 1 min in duration, with the work load being the most intensive cycling the subjects were capable of in that time. Ten min of rest followed each 1-min bout of cycling. After six sprints, the subjects were exhausted. The decrease in glycogen shown in the figure resulted mainly from its use as the only fuel for the lactic acid system. You will recall that this is the primary energy system for short-duration (1 min) high-intensity exercise. In this respect, it should be emphasized that exhaustion following this kind of exercise was not accompanied by total depletion of the glycogen stores. In fact, as can be seen from the figure, a considerable amount of glycogen was still available after exhaustion had already set in. Fatigue in this case was most likely directly attributable to the large accumulation of lactic acid in the blood and muscles, resulting from dependence on the lactic acid energy system.

The mode of exercise itself can influence the degree to which glycogen is used in the muscles. For a given muscle, the amount of glycogen used will depend upon the involvement of that muscle during the exercise. If the vastus lateralis muscle, for instance, is more active during cycling than during other activities, the greatest glycogen usage by this muscle should occur during the cycling. This is just the case; in fact, the amount of glycogen used by the vastus during 20 min of cycling is about the same as that used for a 30-km race (19 miles)—and in 60 min of cycling, glycogen usage by the muscle equals that during a 100-km run (62 miles). Figure 4-6A shows how the runs compare to each other—and to cross-country skiing for 7 hr—in terms of glycogen depletion in the vastus. Cross-country skiing is included as an example of a sport that involves heavy activity by many muscles; along with the depletion in the vastus (7 hr uses up an amount of glycogen equal to that used in 12 hr of running), there is considerable glycogen usage in the arm muscles (e.g., the deltoid).

A further illustration of the relationship between muscle glycogen usage and mode of exercise is presented in Figure 4-6B. The figure shows the results of experiments involving two very similar activities—running on a level course and running uphill. The metabolic intensities of the runs were the same in both cases. For each of the three major leg muscles involved in running, glycogen usage was always much greater when the running was done uphill. These findings show why it is possible to become more fatigued (due to glycogen depletion) when running uphill than when running on a level stretch, even when the overall intensities of the runs are equal. Incidentally, this kind of information also lends some scientific support to not recognizing world records in the marathon race because of variations in terrain of the many different courses.

Another factor that is related to mode of exercise and that affects muscle glycogen usage is the type of muscle fiber or motor unit recruited during the exercise. It was mentioned earlier (p. 3) that most human muscles contain two basic types of fibers or motor units, **fast-twitch (FT)** and **slow-twitch (ST)**. The FT fibers are metabolically and physiologically suited for high-intensity, short-duration work. Sprinting, for instance, involves contraction of the FT fibers of the muscles almost exclusively. These fibers contract quickly and have a high capacity for production of ATP by the lactic acid system (anaerobic glycolysis); their aerobic capabilities are rather low. Because of these properties, they are sometimes referred to as fast, glycolytic fibers (FG). Slow-twitch fibers, on the other hand, are characterized by a high aerobic capacity and a low anaerobic capacity; they have a slower contraction time as well. These fibers are thus sometimes referred to as slow, oxidative fibers (SO). From their characteristics it is easy to see that ST fibers are best suited for performing endurance or aerobic exercise.

While more about the metabolic capacities of these fiber types will be mentioned later (p. 100), right now take a look at Figure 4-7A. Here the pattern of muscle glycogen usage for the two fiber types in the vastus lateralis muscle is shown during and following a 30-km (19-mile) running race. In the runners used as subjects, the vastus lateralis contained approximately 60% ST fibers and 40% FT fibers. The average performance time of the runners was just under 2½ hr (147 min). The much greater rate of glycogen depletion in the ST fibers of the vastus muscle clearly indicates that these fibers were more

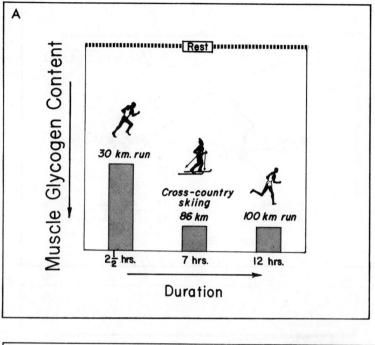

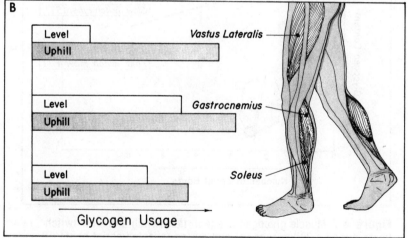

Figure 4-6 The mode of exercise influences the degree to which glycogen is used in the muscles. This is true for different activities (A) as well as for variations of the same activity (B). (Data in A from Essén, 1977; data in B from Costill, 1974.)

active during the endurance run than were the FT fibers. Just the opposite has been demonstrated with bicycle sprints, as shown in Figure 4–7B. In this case, the FT fibers were preferentially recruited in performing the high-intensity, short-duration work, with the ST fibers showing minimal involvement, as indicated by their slight glycogen depletion.

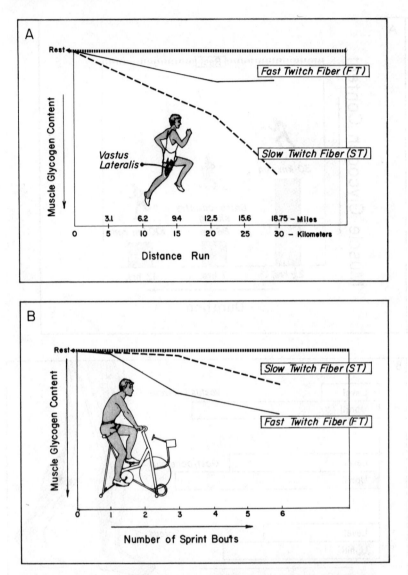

Figure 4-7 Muscle glycogen usage in fast-twitch and slow-twitch fibers during a 30-km race (A) and during repeated sprint bouts (B). Glycogen depletion in the slow-twitch fibers was greatest during the 30-km race; glycogen depletion in the fast-twitch fibers was greatest during the sprint bouts. From this pattern it may be concluded that slow-twitch fibers are preferentially recruited during prolonged work and fast-twitch fibers during sprint work. (Data in A from Costill and co-workers, 1973; data in B from Gollnick and co-workers, 1973.)

The above information is critical with respect to understanding the role of nutrition in athletics. Also, it vividly demonstrates one aspect of the specificity of training—it is not enough for training programs to include activities similar to those involved in the sport being trained for; if the greatest benefit is to be derived, training must involve the activity itself.

A summary of the relationships among blood glucose and liver and muscle glycogen is shown in Figure 4-8. The fate of glucose and glycogen is also shown.

Forms of Fat as Fuels

Like carbohydrate, fat has a basic "usable form" in the body—**free fatty acids**, abbreviated **FFA**. Fats taken in through the diet are digested, producing fatty acids and a substance called glycerol. After the fatty acids are absorbed by the intestinal cells, they are converted to **triglycerides**. Triglycerides contain 1 unit (mole) of glycerol and 3 units (moles) of fatty acids. When triglycerides are broken down, 1 mole of glycerol and 3 moles of free fatty acids are released (see Fig. 4-9).

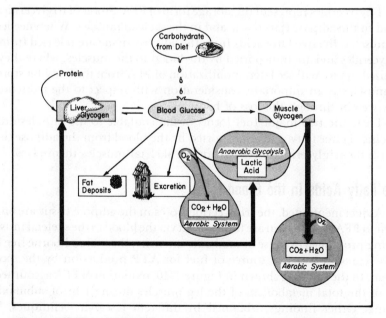

Figure 4-8 The relationships among blood glucose and liver and muscle glycogen. The fate of glucose and glycogen is also shown.

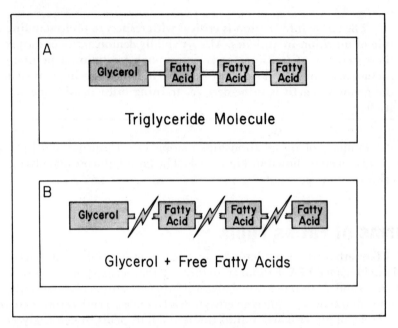

Figure 4-9 A, Triglycerides, the storage form of free fatty acids, contain one mole of glycerol and three moles of fatty acids. B, When broken down, one mole of glycerol and three moles of fatty acids are released.

Triglycerides represent the storage form of FFA. Stores of triglycerides are found in the adipose (fat) tissue and in the skeletal muscles. When needed by the muscles, the free fatty acids from the adipose tissue are released from the triglycerides and are transported by the blood to the muscles, where they are oxidized. As we will see later, mobilization of FFA from the body-fat stores to the muscles is an important consideration with respect to the reduction of body weight through the loss of body fat.

There are two major fuel forms of fat available to the muscles during exercise: (1) free fatty acids transported by the blood from the adipose tissue; and (2) the triglyceride stores within the skeletal muscles themselves.

Free Fatty Acids in the Blood

As just mentioned, the triglyceride stores in the adipose tissue are broken down to FFA, which then are transported via the blood to the skeletal muscles. During prolonged exercise of moderate intensity, these blood-borne free fatty acids represent a major source of fuel for ATP production by the oxygen system. In the findings shown in Figure 4-10, oxidation of FFA accounted for 11% of the total metabolism of the leg muscles during 1 hr of submaximal cycling. Other findings, obtained by different research techniques, have indicated that FFA can account for between 25 and 90% of the total exercise metabolism.

The uptake (use) of FFA by working muscles appears to be related to how much free fatty acid is in the blood. If this is true, then elevation of FFA by dietary intake of fat should enhance FFA utilization. Such an effect has in fact been demonstrated both in rats and in humans. An increased blood FFA level induced through the diet coupled with at least normal muscle glycogen stores has also been shown (in rats) to enhance endurance performance. The increased endurance performance induced in this manner is due to a process referred to as **glycogen sparing**. In this process, the now available free fatty acids are preferentially used as a fuel, thus sparing the muscle glycogen stores. This in turn delays fatigue. Note: Although procedures relating to the dietary intake of fatty meals appear practical, they are not recommended (see further discussion on p. 277).

Muscle Triglyceride Stores

Information concerning the triglyceride stores in muscle is not nearly as complete as that concerning glycogen stores. Nevertheless, recent experiments have indicated that muscle triglycerides are used to a considerable extent during prolonged endurance activities. By looking at Figure 4-10 again, you can see that the triglyceride stores supplied enough fuel to account for 32% of the total metabolism of the leg muscles during an hour of submaximal cycling—an amount that is 75% of the total fat metabolism.

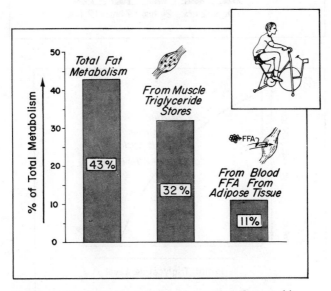

Figure 4-10 Oxidation of blood-borne free fatty acids may account for 11%—and muscle triglyceride stores for 32%—of the total metabolism of the leg muscles during one hour of submaximal cycling. (Based on data from Essén and co-workers, 1977.)

Figure 4-11A shows the depletion of muscle triglycerides following several different activities ranging in duration from 1 to 12 hr. Notice that the depletion of the triglyceride stores, unlike that of the glycogen stores, does not appear to be related to the duration of the activity. What does affect the usage of muscle triglycerides is the level of triglyceride in the muscle before exercise. This is shown in Figure 4-11B. It is easy to see that triglyceride usage following the selected activities (the same as shown in Fig. 4-11A) is dependent upon how much fat is initially stored in the muscles; that is, if the fat stores are higher prior to exercise, then a larger amount of triglycerides will

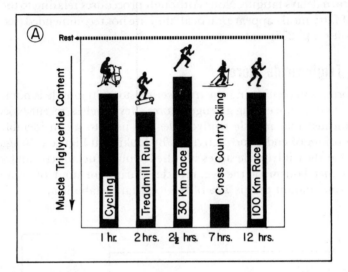

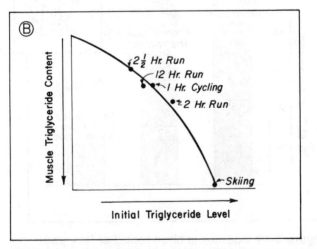

Figure 4-11 Muscle triglyceride depletion does not appear to be related to the duration of the activity (A) but rather to the initial triglyceride levels in the muscles (B). (Data from Essén, 1977.)

be used during the exercise. It has not as yet been scientifically determined if or how the triglyceride stores in the muscles can be significantly altered through the diet so as to beneficially affect endurance performance.

Fuels for Endurance Exercise

Finally, let's put all the fuels together and take a look at how much each contributes to the total metabolism during an endurance performance such as submaximal cycling for 1 hr. The relative contributions under these exercise conditions have been calculated in Figure 4-12. The muscular stores of triglyceride and glycogen supply about 75% of the fuel, whereas the blood-borne fuels—free fatty acids and glucose—account for the remaining 25%.

Fuels for Sprint-like Exercises

The picture for very short, high-intensity efforts is less complicated. The major food fuel in this case is the stored muscle glycogen. Also, as mentioned before, in activities lasting for only a few seconds, the major "fuel" is PC, with neither the blood-borne fuels nor stored food fuels having time to participate.

Summary

- There are three foodstuffs: protein, carbohydrate (sugar), and fat. Each is capable of serving as a fuel for generating ATP energy during exercise.

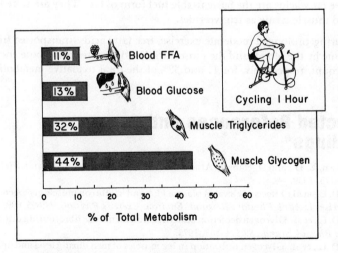

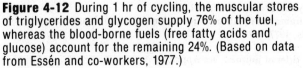

Figure 4-12 During 1 hr of cycling, the muscular stores of triglycerides and glycogen supply 76% of the fuel, whereas the blood-borne fuels (free fatty acids and glucose) account for the remaining 24%. (Based on data from Essén and co-workers, 1977.)

- Protein is not normally used as a fuel during exercise; carbohydrate and fat serve as the two major fuels.

- During prolonged, lower intensity exercise, carbohydrate serves as the major fuel at first, then fat predominates later in the exercise.

- Diet affects the availability of the food fuels. In one study, subjects who ate a high-fat diet for several days experienced early exhaustion when they performed prolonged exercise. After several days on a high-carbohydrate diet, though, endurance time was increased threefold.

- Glucose is the basic usable form of carbohydrate. As a fuel, glucose is transported to the muscle by the blood. The storage form of glucose is glycogen, which is stored in the skeletal muscles and liver.

- Uptake of glucose from the blood by the muscles is increased during exercise and can account for 30 to 40% of the fuel oxidized during prolonged exercise.

- Muscle glycogen usage is dependent upon intensity, duration, and mode of exercise and involvement of different muscle groups.

- Depletion of muscle glycogen during exercise usually results in fatigue even though plenty of fat is still available as a fuel.

- From muscle glycogen depletion patterns, it is evident that slow-twitch fibers or motor units are preferentially recruited during prolonged, low-intensity work, and that fast-twitch fibers are preferred during high-intensity, short-term work.

- The fact that different fiber types have different rates of work is a compelling reason to make training specific—that is, programs must involve the activity being trained for (and hence the fiber types to be used) if maximal benefits are to be derived.

- Free fatty acids are the basic usable fuel form of fats. They are stored in adipose and muscle tissue as triglycerides.

- During prolonged moderate exercise, free fatty acids (transported from adipose tissue by the blood) and the muscle triglyceride stores contribute enough fuel to account, respectively, for 11 and 32% of the total oxidative metabolism.

Selected References and Readings*

Christensen, E. H., and O. Hansen: Arbeitsfähigkeit und Ehrnahrung. *Skand. Arch. Physiol.,* 8: 160–175, 1939.

Costill, D. L., et al.: Effects of elevated plasma FFA and insulin on muscle glycogen usage during exercise. *J. Appl. Physiol.: Respirat. Environ. Exercise Physiol.,* 43:695–699, 1977.

Costill, D. L., et al.: Glycogen depletion pattern in human muscle fibres during distance running. *Acta Physiol. Scand.,* 89:374–383, 1973.

Costill, D. L., et al.: Glycogen utilization in leg muscles of men during level and uphill running. *Acta Physiol. Scand.,* 91:475–481, 1974.

Essén, B.: Intramuscular substrate utilization during prolonged exercise. *Ann. N.Y. Acad. Sci.* 301:30–44, 1977.

---

*For full titles of journals, see Appendix A.

Essén, B., L. Hagenfeldt, and L. Kaijser: Utilization of blood-borne and intramuscular substrates during continuous and intermittent exercise in man. *J. Physiol.*, *265*:489–506, 1977.

Gollnick, P. D.: Free fatty acid turnover and the availability of substrates as a limiting factor in prolonged exercise. *Ann. N.Y. Acad. Sci.*, *301*:64–71, 1977.

Gollnick, P. D., et al.: Glycogen depletion pattern in human skeletal muscle fibers after heavy exercise. *J. Appl. Physiol.*, *34*:615–618, 1973.

Hermansen, L., E. Hultman, and B. Saltin: Muscle glycogen during prolonged severe exercise. *Acta Physiol. Scand.*, *71*:129–139, 1967.

Hickson, R. C., et al.: Effects of increased plasma fatty acids on glycogen utilization and endurance. *J. Appl. Physiol.: Respirat. Environ. Exercise Physiol.*, *43*:829–833, 1977.

Langley, L. L.: *Outline of Physiology.* 2nd ed. New York, McGraw-Hill Book Company, 1965.

Pirnay, F., et al.: Glucose oxidation during prolonged exercise evaluated with naturally labeled (^{13}C) glucose. *J. Appl. Physiol.: Respirat. Environ. Exercise Physiol.*, *43*:258–261, 1977.

Wahren, J.: Glucose turnover during exercise in man. *Ann. N.Y. Acad. Sci.*, *301*:45–55, 1977.

Wahren, J., L. Hagenfeldt, and P. Felig: Glucose and free fatty acid utilization in exercise. *Israel J. Med. Sci.*, *11*:551–559, 1975.

5

The Recovery Process

Introduction

The processes occurring during recovery from exercise are just as important as those occurring during exercise itself. For example, incomplete recovery between exercise bouts or athletic contests will ultimately lead to a decrement in performance.

It is a not uncommon practice nowadays to schedule several athletic contests per week, often with only a day or two of rest between games. Indeed, it is not unusual for athletes to participate in several contests over a weekend or even in one day, particularly during tournament time. The purpose of this chapter will be to highlight how you as a coach can make sure your athletes recover quickly and fully from one performance to another.

Probably the most familiar concept associated with recovery from exercise is the oxygen debt. There are several misconceptions surrounding the oxygen debt concept, so we will start our discussion of the recovery process with a brief review of the oxygen debt. Several other important factors in the recovery process also will be discussed, including: (1) restoration of the muscular stores of phosphagen (ATP and PC); (2) replenishment of myoglobin with oxygen; (3) replenishment of muscle glycogen stores; and (4) the removal of lactic acid from the muscles and blood.

The Concept of the Oxygen Debt

We all know that during recovery from exercise our energy demand is considerably less because we are no longer exercising. However, our oxygen consumption continues at a relatively high level for a period of time, the length of which is dependent on the intensity of the preceding exercise. The amount of oxygen consumed ($\dot{V}_{O_2}$) during recovery—above that which would have ordinarily been consumed at rest in the same time—is called the **oxygen debt**. This is shown schematically in Figure 5-1. The term oxygen debt was first used in 1922 by the eminent British exercise physiologist A. V. Hill. This was the same year that he received a Nobel Prize for Physiology.

The concept of the oxygen debt, as originally developed by Hill, means that the oxygen consumed above the resting level during recovery is primarily used to provide energy for restoring the body to its pre-exercise condition, including replenishing the energy stores that were depleted and removing any lactic acid that was accumulated during exercise. Many erroneously interpret the oxygen debt to mean that the extra oxygen consumed during recovery is being used to replace oxygen that was borrowed from somewhere within the body during exercise. Actually, during maximal exercise, depletion of the oxygen stored in the muscle itself (in combination with myoglobin) and in the venous blood would amount to only about 0.6 L. Oxygen debts, on the other hand, have been found to be nearly 30 times larger than this in athletes during maximal exercise.

As shown in Figure 5-1, the oxygen debt has two components. The slower portion of the debt, called the lactacid oxygen debt component, is primarily

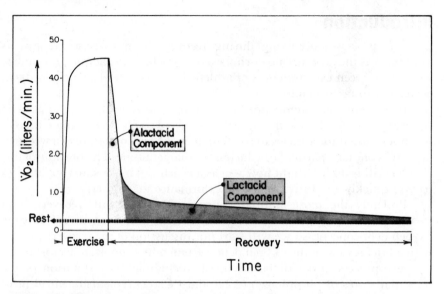

Figure 5-1 The oxygen debt is defined as the amount of oxygen consumed during recovery from exercise above the amount that ordinarily would have been consumed at rest in the same time period.

related to the energetics involved in the removal of the lactic acid from the muscles and blood. The fast portion of the oxygen debt is called the alactacid oxygen debt component. The term "alactacid" means not related to lactic acid. The term came about when it was discovered in 1933 that not all of the oxygen debt was related to the removal of lactic acid from the muscles and blood. To name that part of the debt not related to the removal of lactic acid, the word "alactacid" was coined. Although it was not known at the time of naming the alactacid component, it is now known that the alactacid oxygen debt component provides the necessary oxygen for the energy needed for the restoration of the muscle phosphagens. If this had been known earlier, perhaps the term phosphagen debt component would have been used. Both of these oxygen debt components will be discussed later in this chapter as they relate to the various recovery processes.

Restoration of Muscle Phosphagen Stores

You will recall that the muscular stores of ATP and PC represent immediate energy sources. ATP is the primary energy source—it is used directly by the muscles—whereas the energy donated by PC is used to immediately resynthesize ATP. Although the phosphagen system provides the major energy required for sports activities lasting only a few seconds, it also is involved to various extents in every kind of muscular activity. The restoration of the phosphagen compounds from one performance to another is thus of obvious importance.

Speed of Phosphagen Replenishment

The replenishment of the phosphagen stores is rapid, as shown in Figure 5-2A. The exercise shown in the figure consisted of 10 min of continuous, submaximal cycling. Muscle biopsies were taken before and immediately after exercise, and at minutes 1, 2, 5, and 10 of recovery. The muscle samples were analyzed for ATP and PC concentrations. As can be seen, the major portion of the ATP and PC used during exercise was restored to the muscles within 2 min; it was completely restored in 3 min.

Estimates of the half-time for phosphagen replenishment range between 20 and 30 sec. The half-time is defined as the time required to replenish, during recovery, one half of the phosphagen used during exercise. Using the 30-sec estimate, phosphagen restoration would have the pattern shown in Figure 5-2B. From a practical standpoint, the rapid replenishment of the phosphagen stores means that recovery from athletic performances that depend heavily on the ATP-PC system for energy (such as those represented in Area One of Table 3-1, p. 35) will also be very rapid. Therefore, athletes participating in such performances should have no trouble recovering fully in only 2 or 3 min.

Figure 5-2B and its accompanying table also point out the importance of phosphagen restoration during **intermittent exercise**. Intermittent exercise is closely related to the pattern in which many sports activities are played—i.e., periods of hard work alternated with periods of relief. The latter usually range from complete rest to light or moderate exercise. Even though they may be brief, the relief periods provide time for at least partial restoration of the phosphagen stores. These stores can then be used during subsequent work periods or performances. The availability of the stored phosphagens during each work interval is sometimes important in preventing or delaying fatigue due to lactic acid accumulation.

The pattern of phosphagen depletion and repletion during intermittent exercise is shown in Figure 5-3. The exercise (cycling) intervals were 30 sec long and the relief (rest) intervals 60 sec.

Energetics of Phosphagen Replenishment

The restoration of the ATP and PC stores in the muscles during recovery from exercise requires energy. This energy is derived for the most part from the oxygen system through the breakdown of carbohydrates and fats. It has been suggested that the lactic acid system might also be involved in providing energy for this purpose. Whatever the case, some of the ATP that is synthesized is restored directly to the muscles and some is broken down, with the energy released in the latter process being used to synthesize PC. The PC is then stored

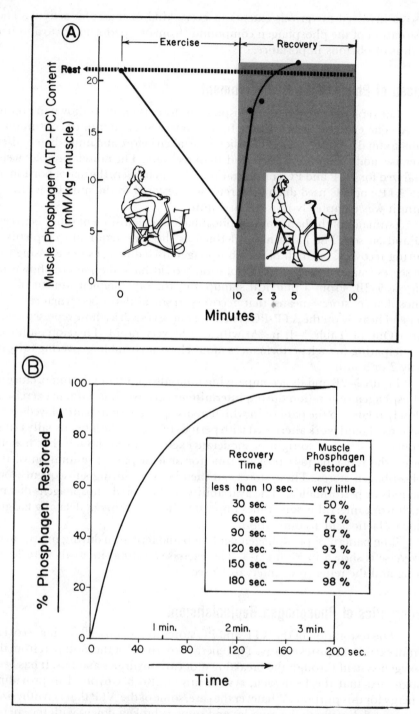

Figure 5-2 Replenishment of the phosphagen stores is rapid. A, Most of the ATP and PC used during exercise is restored to the muscles within 2 to 3 min. (Based on data from Hultman and co-workers, 1967.) B, The half-time for phosphagen replenishment ranges between 20 and 30 sec.

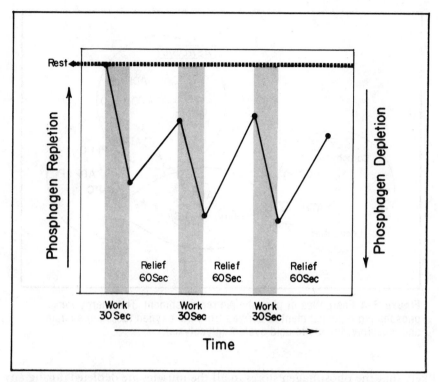

Figure 5-3 The pattern of phosphagen depletion and repletion during intermittent exercise. The work (cycling) intervals were 30-sec long and the relief (rest) intervals were 60-sec long. (Based on data from Saltin and Essén, 1971.)

in the muscle. Phosphocreatine is not synthesized directly by the energy released from the breakdown of foodstuffs; only ATP is synthesized in this manner. To reiterate: during recovery, ATP is directly synthesized—and PC indirectly synthesized—by the oxygen system and, possibly, the lactic acid system. A summary of this process is shown in Figure 5-4.

The Alactacid Oxygen Debt and Phosphagen Replenishment

As mentioned earlier, the involvement of the oxygen system in the restoration of muscle phosphagen is reflected in an increased oxygen consumption, which makes up the alactacid portion of the oxygen debt. The alactacid oxygen debt is completed or "repaid" within 2 to 3 min. One of the things the size of the debt reflects is how much phosphagen has been restored to the muscles. It was mentioned earlier that the total amount of stored phosphagen is about 0.6 mole in untrained males and 0.3 mole in untrained females (see p. 15). If all the stores were completely depleted during exercise, it would take less than 4 L of oxygen for their restoration. Of course, it is not

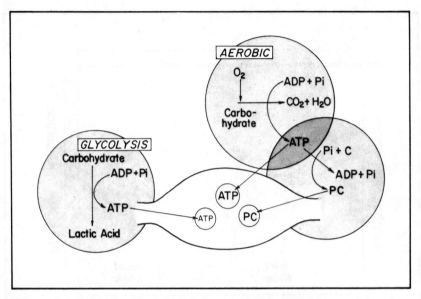

Figure 5-4 Energetics of phosphagen replenishment. The energy for phosphagen replenishment is derived from the oxygen (aerobic) system and, possibly, the lactic acid system (glycolysis).

likely that the phosphagen stores in all the muscles are depleted during any single exercise bout or performance; indeed, the size of the alactacid debt component is usually between 2.0 and 3.5 L of oxygen. This is shown in Figure 5-5. Notice that the largest alactacid debts are found in male and female rowers. These athletes are required to put the greatest work demands on both their arms and legs. The values given in the figure were obtained in simulations of rowing in an eight-oared shell. On a rowing ergometer, females performed exhaustive work equivalent to that involved in a 1000-m race, and male rowers simulated a 2000-m race. Such races, which last about 4 min for females and 6 min for males, require both anaerobic power and aerobic endurance.

Replenishment of Myoglobin with Oxygen

Myoglobin, a protein found in skeletal muscle, binds (stores) oxygen and facilitates the transport of oxygen (diffusion) into the muscle cell. It is similar both structurally and functionally to the hemoglobin found in red blood cells. Often, in fact, it is referred to as muscle hemoglobin. Myoglobin is found in larger quantities in slow-twitch muscle fibers than in fast-twitch muscle fibers—which is one reason for the greater aerobic potential of the slow-twitch fibers. Myoglobin also gives the slow-twitch fibers their red color.

The Size of the O₂-Myoglobin Stores

The amount of oxygen stored by myoglobin is about 11 ml per kg of muscle tissue. Thus, assuming 30 kg of muscle (66 lb) in a 70-kg person (154 lb), the total body stores of oxygen bound to myoglobin would be 330 ml (30 kg of muscle $\times$ 11 ml of O_2 per kg of muscle). Taking into consideration the fact that athletes generally have more muscle mass than the average person, the oxygen-myoglobin (O_2-myoglobin) stores for athletes would probably be around 500 ml, or 0.5 L. While this does not appear to be a significant amount of oxygen, the O_2-myoglobin stores play an important role during exercise in general and during intermittent exercise in particular.

Role of Myoglobin during Exercise

The O_2-myoglobin stores provide a very rapid source of oxygen for the muscles. For example, during the initial phases of exercise, before the oxygen transport system (respiration and circulation) can supply additional oxygen, the oxygen bound to myoglobin is consumed. This supply of oxygen, although small, helps to delay the accumulation of lactic acid in the muscles

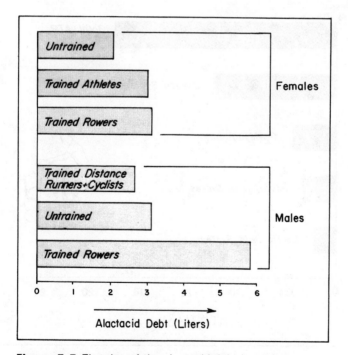

Figure 5-5 The size of the alactacid debt in various athletes and untrained males and females following exhausting exercise. The debt is generally larger in athletes. (Based on data from Hagerman and Fox, 1973; Fox, 1973; and Lesmes, 1976.)

and blood. This is particularly evident during intermittent exercise, in which the oxygen bound to myoglobin can be replenished during the rest periods and then reused during subsequent work periods. An example of this can be seen in Figure 5-6. The values shown in the figure were obtained in experiments in which the ATP requirement during a work interval of intermittent cycling lasting 1 hr was calculated. The hour was divided into cycling intervals lasting 15 sec followed by rest intervals lasting 15 sec. Of the total ATP required in the hour, nearly 20% was supplied by the oxygen bound to myoglobin. This was a larger contribution than that made by either the phosphagen system or the lactic acid system.

A second function of myoglobin, and perhaps the most important, is its facilitation of the diffusion of oxygen from the blood (capillaries) to the mitochondria within the muscle fibers (once in the mitochondria, the oxygen is consumed). The mechanism involved in such a facilitory process has not as yet been determined exactly. However, a "shuttling" from one molecule of myoglobin to another until the oxygen reaches the mitochondria is probably involved.

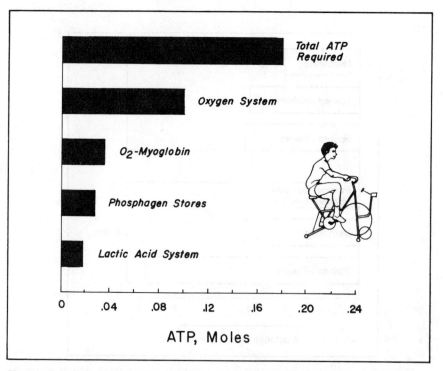

Figure 5-6 During intermittent exercise, the oxygen bound to myoglobin is replenished during rest periods and reused during subsequent work periods. Of the total ATP required during this particular exercise, nearly 20% was supplied by the oxygen bound to myoglobin. (Based on data from Essén and co-workers, 1977.)

Speed and Energetics of Replenishment of the O₂-Myoglobin Stores

Like the phosphagen stores, the oxygen-myoglobin stores are replenished very rapidly during the recovery period. In fact, it is likely that they are restored more quickly than the phosphagens. One of the reasons for this is that the O_2-myoglobin complex does not involve a metabolic source of energy. In other words, the restoration of myoglobin with oxygen does not depend on the metabolic production of ATP per se. The oxygen is chemically bound to myoglobin in much the same way that oxygen is bound to hemoglobin. This chemical binding is primarily dependent upon the availability of oxygen in the blood and tissues.

The relationship between oxygen availability and the binding of oxygen to myoglobin is shown in Figure 5-7. Oxygen availability is represented on the horizontal axis as the **partial pressure** of oxygen. The partial pressure of oxygen, which will be discussed in detail later on, is dependent upon both the concentration of oxygen in the air and the barometric (atmospheric) pressure. In the figure, note that at low oxygen partial pressures (shaded area), the curve is quite steep. This means that when the partial pressure of oxygen in this range changes slightly, the amount of oxygen bound to myoglobin changes a great deal. For example, during exercise, the oxygen partial pressure decreases inside the muscle fiber where myoglobin is stored. As a consequence, oxygen is released from myoglobin and eventually given up to the mitochondria where it is consumed. Just the opposite is true during the recovery period: the partial pressure of oxygen increases, causing a rapid recharging of myoglobin with oxygen.

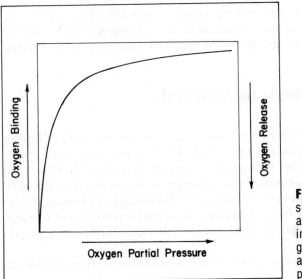

Figure 5-7 The relationship between oxygen availability and the binding of oxygen to myoglobin. The curve is steep at low oxygen partial pressures (shaded area).

Relationship of O₂-Myoglobin Replenishment to the Repayment of the Alactacid Oxygen Debt

We have noted earlier that the alactacid oxygen debt is repaid when oxygen taken in during recovery is used by the aerobic energy system for replenishment of the muscle phosphagen stores. Since the oxygen taken in during recovery is also used for replenishment of myoglobin, O_2-myoglobin replenishment is considered part of the repayment of the alactacid oxygen debt. Though the two recovery processes are related by their use of oxygen (and, as we have mentioned, by their rapidity), it should be remembered that the repayment of the alactacid debt involves a metabolic process (synthesis of ATP) while O_2-myoglobin replenishment does not. As just discussed, replenishment of myoglobin depends mainly on the availability (partial pressure) of oxygen.

Restoration of Muscle Glycogen Stores

In the last chapter, the role of muscle glycogen was discussed as a fuel for exercises differing in type, intensity, and duration. Since glycogen is important both as a fuel for the oxygen and lactic acid systems and as a factor in the delay of muscular fatigue during prolonged exercise, a thorough discussion of the restoration of muscle glycogen stores during recovery from exercise is clearly warranted.

Speed of Muscle Glycogen Replenishment

Much has been learned in the last 10 years concerning how much time is required to fully restore the working muscles with glycogen. Among the factors that affect the rate and amount of muscle glycogen synthesis during recovery from exercise are diet and the intensity and duration of the exercise performed.

Effects of Diet and Intensity and Duration of Exercise

The effect of diet on the rate of muscle glycogen replenishment following prolonged exercise is shown in Figure 5-8. The data presented in the figure were obtained in experiments in which subjects exercised for 2 hr in order to reduce their muscle (vastus lateralis) glycogen stores as much as possible. During the first hour, the exercise consisted of endurance swimming, skiing, running and cycling; in the second hour, the exercise consisted of repeated periods of brief maximal cycling (exercise to exhaustion) on a bicycle ergometer.

During the subsequent recovery period, some subjects received no food,

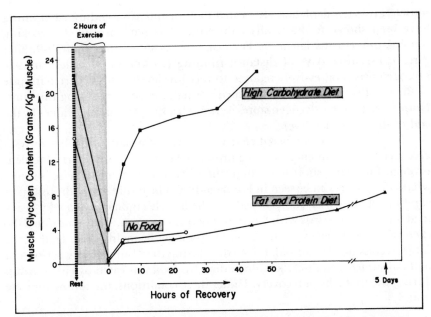

Figure 5-8 The effect of diet on the rate of muscle glycogen replenishment following prolonged exercise. See text for further explanation. (Based on data from Hultman and Bergström, 1967, and Piehl, 1974.)

others ingested a high-fat diet with protein, and still others were given a high-carbohydrate diet. The following information concerning muscle glycogen replenishment after prolonged exercise is observable from the figure:

Following Prolonged Exercise:

1. Complete repletion of muscle glycogen requires a high-carbohydrate diet.
2. Only an insignificant amount of muscle glycogen is replenished, even after five days, if no carbohydrate is taken in through the diet.
3. Even with a high-carbohydrate diet, it requires 46 hr to completely replenish the muscle glycogen.
4. Replenishment of muscle glycogen is most rapid during the first 10 hr of recovery.

The relatively long period of time required for complete muscle glycogen replenishment following prolonged exercise has some important implications for coaches and endurance athletes. One implication involves the training schedule: with an extremely strenuous schedule, the endurance athlete may experience a state of chronic exhaustion that could be related to muscle glycogen depletion. Repeated days of intensive endurance training have been shown to drastically reduce the glycogen stores in the working musculature (vastus lateralis). For example, as shown in Figure 5-9, after three consecutive days of distance running (16 km, or 10 miles), muscle glycogen was progressively reduced to very low levels. This occurred in spite of the fact that the runners consumed normal, mixed diets during this time. Notice also that the glycogen stores were not back to pre-running values by the end of the week (day five).

It should be remembered that the above information applies only to glycogen replenishment following prolonged exercise. The pattern of replenishment following short-term, high-intensity, intermittent exercise is somewhat different, as can be seen in Figure 5–10A. The figure shows the results of experiments in which subjects pedaled the bicycle ergometer at a very heavy load for 1-min intervals with 3-min rest periods between. They continued the exercise until 30 sec of pedaling could no longer be maintained. Half of the subjects consumed a normal, mixed diet during the 24-hr recovery period and half consumed a high-carbohydrate diet. No food was eaten by either group during the first 2 hr of recovery. Under these conditions, the following were found:

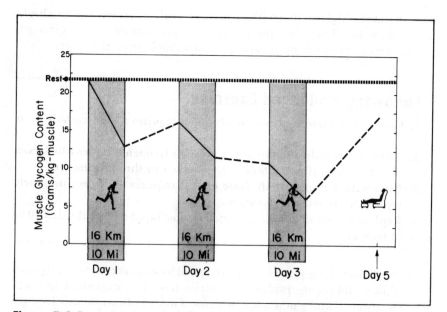

Figure 5-9 Repeated days of intensive endurance training reduce the glycogen stores in the working musculature. (Based on data from Costill and co-workers, 1971.)

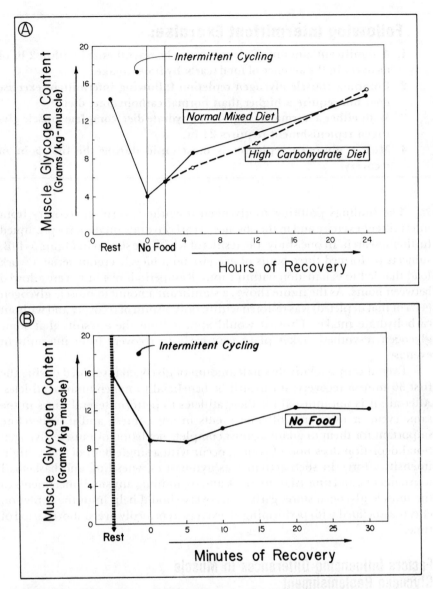

Figure 5-10 The effect of diet on the rate of muscle glycogen replenishment following short-term, high-intensity, intermittent exercise. The time required for complete restoration is shown in A; the extent of restoration immediately after exercise is shown in B. (See text for further explanation.) (Data in A from MacDougall and co-workers, 1977; data in B from Hermansen and Vaage, 1977.)

Following Intermittent Exercise:

1. A significant amount of glycogen can be resynthesized within 2 hr of recovery in the absence of food (carbohydrate) intake.
2. Complete muscle glycogen repletion following intermittent exercise does not require a higher than normal carbohydrate diet.
3. With either a normal or high-carbohydrate diet, complete muscle glycogen replenishment requires 24 hr.
4. Muscle glycogen repletion is most rapid during the first 5 hr of recovery.

The findings pointing to glycogen resynthesis early in recovery from intermittent exercise and in the absence of carbohydrate intake have prompted further research. In one study, the results of which are shown in Figure 5–10B, subjects performed three bouts of exercise on a bicycle ergometer at a work load that led to exhaustion within 1 min. Rest periods of 4 min were allowed between bouts. As the figure shows, a significant amount of muscle glycogen (44% of that depleted) was restored within only 30 min of recovery and without carbohydrate intake. Thus, it would appear from these results that some glycogen resynthesis takes place very early in recovery from intermittent exercise.

Even if only a relatively small amount of glycogen is restored during the first 30 min of recovery, it can still be beneficial to nonendurance athletes. After all, it is not unusual for these athletes to perform several times in the same event or in several different events in one contest, and it is therefore important for them to guard against complete depletion of muscle glycogen (total depletion does not, of course, occur with a single bout of short, high-intensity effort). In such activities as gymnastics, wrestling and basketball tournaments, and time trials for track and swimming, any small increments in the muscle glycogen stores early in recovery should help limit the depletion effects associated with performing an exercise repeatedly over a short period of time.

Factors Influencing Differences in Muscle Glycogen Replenishment

We have established that muscle glycogen replenishment following short-term, high-intensity, intermittent work differs greatly from that following prolonged endurance exercise, but possible reasons for the difference have not been touched on. We will explore this area now. (Keep in mind that not all the factors involved have been satisfactorily identified.) First, the amount of glycogen that is depleted may be a factor in regulating how quickly glycogen is restored. During prolonged exercise, glycogen depletion is always greater. Second, following prolonged exercise, it is common to find low blood glucose levels due to depletion of liver glycogen. However, during high-intensity, intermittent exercise, liver glycogen is seldom if ever depleted. Consequently, blood glucose levels during recovery are at least normal and oftentimes even higher than normal. Therefore, the availability of carbohydrate (glucose), which is necessary for glycogen resynthesis, would be greater following intermittent exercise. This would help explain why there is a significant amount of glycogen replenishment in the absence of dietary intake of carbohydrate following this kind of work but not after prolonged exercise. Finally, there is some evidence that muscle glycogen replenishment is faster in fast-twitch muscle fibers (FT) than in slow-twitch fibers (ST). Since FT fibers are preferentially recruited for high-intensity exercise, and ST fibers are used in prolonged, lower intensity exercise, this may be why glycogen replenishment following the former kind of exercise is faster than following the latter.

Some Applications

The preceding information should be useful to coaches and athletes in promoting adequate recovery of the glycogen stores as quickly as possible between performances. Specifically, the information on glycogen replenishment should be helpful when scheduling athletic contests and when deciding on weekly spacing of difficult training sessions and intrasquad scrimmages. Some applications along these lines are presented:

Concerning Muscle Glycogen Replenishment:

Wise coaches should allow several days and insist on a high-carbohydrate diet for full recovery of the glycogen stores in their endurance athletes. If several days are not possible, then at least 10 hr should be allowed.

For nonendurance athletes, only one day and a normal amount of dietary carbohydrate should be sufficient for full recovery of muscle glycogen after high-intensity, intermittent exercise. If this is not possible, then allow at least 5 hr.

With intermittent exercise, some glycogen resynthesis can be expected within the first 2 hr of recovery (some will occur within just 30 min) even in the absence of food intake. This should help delay progressive glycogen depletion resulting from repeated performance over a short period of time.

Muscle Glycogen Loading (Supercompensation)

Of all the recently available scientific information concerning sports physiology, that relative to muscle glycogen loading, or "supercompensation," has been most widely used by coaches and athletes. Muscle glycogen loading is an exercise-diet procedure that leads to unusually high muscle glycogen storage. In one of the first studies to produce the supercompensation effect, glycogen stores in the vastus lateralis muscle were doubled. The procedure was relatively simple. Two subjects were placed on either side of a bicycle ergometer. Exercise was performed with one leg while the other leg was at complete rest. Thus, both subjects worked simultaneously, one with the left leg, the other with the right (see Fig. 5–11). The vastus lateralis was exercised to exhaustion in order to reduce its glycogen stores to near zero. For three consecutive days following the exercise, both subjects consumed a diet which consisted almost exclusively of carbohydrates. No exercise was performed during this time. As shown in the figure, after the three days of this diet, the glycogen stores in the previously exercised leg muscles were twice those in the resting leg muscles.

Subsequent research has established that further enhancement of local muscle glycogen stores could be promoted if, following exercise-induced glycogen depletion, the subjects consumed a fat and protein diet for three days before consuming the high-carbohydrate diet. More will be said about muscle glycogen loading, including recommended diets and possible side-effects, in Chapter 10 (p. 274).

Energetics of Muscle Glycogen Replenishment

The chemical reactions and enzyme systems involved in glycogen synthesis are quite complex. For our purposes, it will not be necessary to discuss them in detail. There is only one more aspect of muscle glycogen replenish-

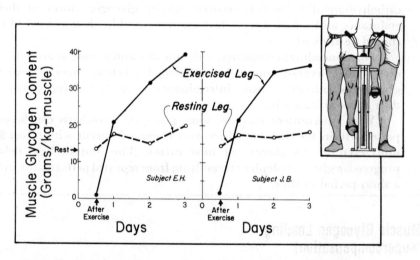

Figure 5-11 Muscle glycogen loading (super compensation). The muscle glycogen stores increase to two to three times their normal levels if the muscles are first depleted of glycogen through exhaustive exercise and are then rested while the individual follows a high-carbohydrate diet for several days. (Based on data from Bergström and Hultman, 1966.)

ment that needs our attention, and that is the energy requirement. Since energy is released when glycogen is broken down, energy is required for glycogen's resynthesis. For the most part, this energy is supplied by the aerobic system.

Relationship to the Lactacid Oxygen Debt Component

Earlier, the two components of the oxygen debt were mentioned. The oxygen consumed during the lactacid component was said to be linked to the removal of lactic acid accumulated in the muscles and blood during exercise. Lactic acid, you will recall, is a by-product of the anaerobic breakdown of glycogen. It is therefore a precursor of glycogen. In other words, given the required energy, lactic acid can be reconverted to glycogen. There is some evidence that glycogen synthesis in the early portion of recovery (within 30 min, as shown in Fig. 5-10B) results at least in part from such reconversion of lactic acid. In this case, the necessary energy is more than likely supplied by the oxygen consumed during the lactacid oxygen debt component.

Perhaps it should be mentioned here that lactic acid is only one of several glycogen precursors. For example, essentially all carbohydrates taken in through the diet are potential glycogen precursors, since most are converted to glucose first before they are used for any purpose. The major source of "fuel" for the rather slow glycogen resynthesis following prolonged exercise is apparently the carbohydrate taken in through the diet (see Fig. 5-8).

Removal of Lactic Acid from Muscle and Blood

As will be pointed out in Chapter 6, accumulation of lactic acid in blood and muscle is implicated in causing temporary muscular fatigue. Thus, its removal from muscle and blood is essential for complete recovery from athletic performances that depend heavily on the lactic acid system for energy (examples of these kinds of performances were given in Chapter 3).

Speed of Lactic Acid Removal

The decrease in levels of lactic acid in blood and muscle during recovery from exercise is shown in Figure 5-12. In the experiments that produced the results shown in the figure, the subjects exercised to exhaustion, whether on a treadmill (Fig. 5-12A) or on a bicycle ergometer (Fig. 5-12B). In the treadmill exercise, both the speed and grade of the treadmill were varied from subject to subject so that fatigue set in at different times (between 2 and 6 min). In the cycling exercise, the subjects performed intermittent work until exhausted on the bicycle ergometer. In both cases, the subjects rested during the recovery

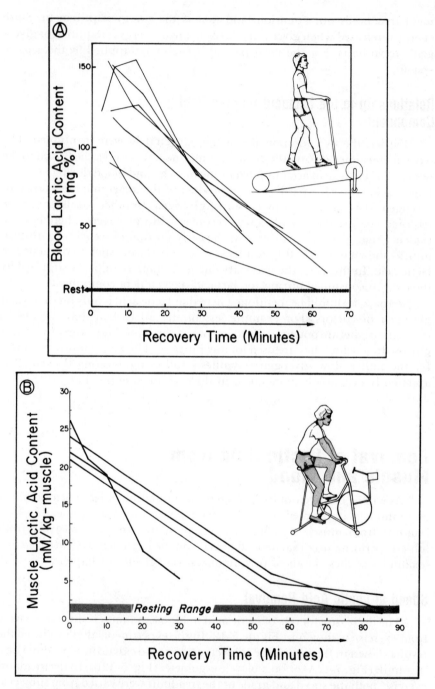

Figure 5-12 A, Decreases in the level of lactic acid in the blood during recovery from an exhausting bout of running on a treadmill. B, Decreases in the level of lactic acid in the muscle during recovery from intermittent work performed to exhaustion on a bicycle ergometer. (Data in A from Fox and co-workers, 1969; data in B from Karlsson and Saltin, 1971, and Hermansen and Vaage, 1977.)

period either by sitting in a chair or by lying down on a cot. As can be seen, it required at least an hour or more for levels of lactic acid in both blood and muscle to approach resting values.

Effects of Exercise-Recovery on the Speed of Lactic Acid Removal

It has been demonstrated that following exhaustive exercise, lactic acid can be removed from the blood more rapidly if one performs light exercise (e.g., walking or jogging) than if one rests during the recovery period. The results of an experiment establishing this fact are shown in Figure 5-13A. In these experiments, the subjects ran a mile on three separate days. As shown in the figure, the blood lactic acid levels were substantially increased following each of the runs. During the recovery periods after each of the runs, the subjects either rested (rest-recovery), or performed continuous jogging at a self-selected pace, or performed intermittent exercise of the kind normally practiced by many athletes. Both exercise-recoveries resulted in substantial increases in the rate of lactic acid removed from the blood and presumably from the muscles. Also note from Figure 5-13A that the lactic acid removal rate was fastest during the continuous jogging recovery.

In a similar experiment, the subjects first performed intermittent exercise until exhausted. The exercise consisted of 1-min runs on the treadmill with 4-min rest periods between runs. In one case, the subjects rested during the 30-min recovery period (rest-recovery); in another, they performed light exercise (jogging). The results were the same as those above—that is, lactic acid was removed from the blood much more rapidly during the exercise-recovery. For example, as shown in Figure 5-13B, the half-time for lactic acid removal during rest-recovery was 25 min, compared to only 11 min during exercise-recovery. Based on these half-times, complete removal of lactic acid from blood would require about 2 hr during rest-recovery, but less than 1 hr during exercise-recovery.

Exercise-Recovery and "Warm-Down"

It is a usual practice of athletes to "warm down"—that is, perform light, intermittent exercise immediately following competition or training sessions. This of course is exercise-recovery, and the above findings that blood lactic acid levels will decrease more quickly under these conditions compared to rest, provide a physiological basis for such a practice. However, since lactic acid is removed most rapidly following continuous exercise-recovery (see Fig. 5-13A), it would be wise to advise athletes to exercise continuously throughout the recovery period rather than intermittently, which is their usual practice. Nevertheless, both coaches and athletes have apparently learned through experience that exercise-recovery will allow them to recover more quickly and thus perform better in subsequent competitions. This method of hastening the removal of blood lactic acid is important in any situation in which a quick recovery between bouts of severe work is essential.

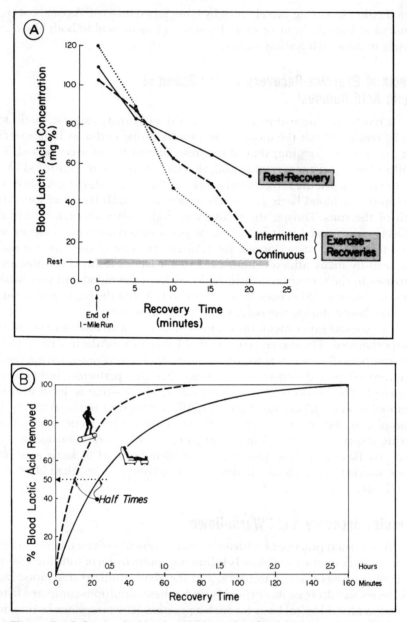

Figure 5-13 Removal of lactic acid from the blood during recovery from exhaustive exercise is more rapid if the recovery period is used for light exercise rather than resting. In A, the actual decrease in blood lactic acid during rest-recovery and exercise-recoveries is shown. In B, the rate of lactic acid removal is shown. The time it takes for one half of the total accumulated lactic acid to be removed during rest-recovery is twice as long as that during exercise-recovery. (Data in A from Bonen and Belcastro, 1976; data in B from Hermansen and co-workers, 1975.)

Lactic Acid Removal and the Lactacid Oxygen Debt Component

The removal of lactic acid from muscle and blood requires energy. Once again, the majority of this energy is made available by the aerobic system.

What happens to the lactic acid? Earlier, we mentioned that lactic acid could be converted to muscle glycogen. However, this represents only one possible fate of lactic acid. As shown in Figure 5-14, other possibilities include conversion to: (1) liver glycogen; (2) blood glucose; (3) protein; and (4) carbon dioxide (CO_2) and water (H_2O). The latter fate means that lactic acid can be oxidized by the aerobic system. In other words, lactic acid can be used as a metabolic fuel, with its aerobic breakdown providing energy for ATP formation. Both skeletal and heart muscle and liver and kidney tissue are capable of utilizing lactic acid as a fuel. Probably the major reason for lactic acid's rapid removal during exercise-recovery is this fuel capability.

From Figure 5-14 it is easy to see that most of the accumulated lactic acid is oxidized to CO_2 and H_2O. However, regardless of the fate of lactic acid, conversion of lactic acid to any other form requires energy, and it is thought that during the immediate recovery period at least part of the energy comes from the oxygen consumed during the lactacid oxygen debt component. A relationship between the blood lactic acid removed during recovery and the lactacid oxygen debt component has been experimentally established (see Fig. 5-15). However, the amount of oxygen required to remove a given quantity of lactic acid varies considerably at different stages of recovery. Therefore, it is not known for sure whether there is a direct cause-and-effect relationship.

From Figure 5-15, it can be observed that the lactacid oxygen debt varies in size, ranging up to about 8 L. The half-time of the lactacid debt following

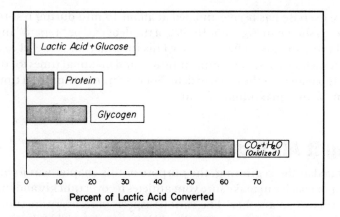

Figure 5-14 The fate of lactic acid. The lactic acid removed from blood and muscle during recovery can be converted to glucose, protein, glycogen, or CO_2 and H_2O (oxidized). Oxidation is the major fate. (Based on data from Brooks and Gaesser, 1980.)

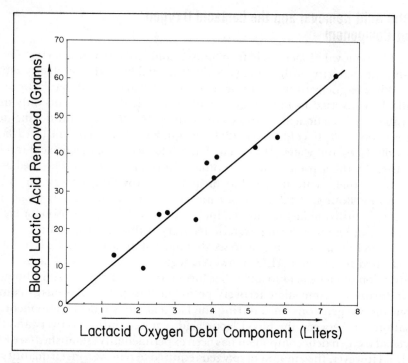

Figure 5-15 The relationship between the lactic acid removed from the blood during recovery and the lactacid debt component, as determined from experimental work. (Based on data from Fox and co-workers, 1969.)

exhaustive exercise has been estimated at about 15 min during rest-recovery. Therefore, as shown in Figure 5-16, 50% of the debt will be "repaid" in 15 min, 75% in 30 min, and about 95% in 1 hr. This information is useful to coaches and athletes who wish to determine minimal and maximal times for quick yet adequate repayment of the lactacid debt. For example, a minimum time might be 30 min, with a maximum of 1 hr.

Putting It All Together

As stated at the beginning, the purpose of this chapter was to highlight how you as a coach can make sure your athletes recover quickly and fully from one performance to another. The various aspects of recovery are summarized in Table 5-1. In reviewing them, it should be remembered that the times given for recovery are only suggested limits. You might want to modify them to better suit your specific needs. However, in so doing, remember that it is always better, in terms of performance, to allow for maximal recovery whenever possible. Chronic fatigue is the enemy of top quality performances.

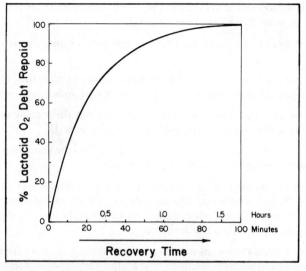

Figure 5-16 The rate of repayment of the lactacid debt following exhaustive exercise. The half-time for repayment is about 15 min, meaning that 50% of the debt will be repaid in 15 min. As you can see, 75% is repaid in 30 min and 95% in 1 hr.

Table 5-1: Recommended Recovery Times after Exhaustive Exercise

	Recommended Recovery Time	
Recovery Process	Minimum	Maximum
Restoration of muscle phosphagen (ATP and PC)	2 min	3 min
Repayment of the alactacid O_2 debt	3 min	5 min
Restoration of O_2-myoglobin	1 min	2 min
Restoration of muscle glycogen	10 hr	46 hr (after prolonged exercise)
	5 hr	24 hr (after intermittent exercise)
Removal of lactic acid from muscle and blood	30 min	1 hr (exercise-recovery)
	1 hr	2 hr (rest-recovery)
Repayment of the lactacid O_2 debt	30 min	1 hr

Summary

• The oxygen debt is defined as the amount of oxygen consumed during recovery above what would ordinarily have been consumed at rest in the same time period. The debt has two components, the alactacid that supplies the energy for phosphagen replenishment, and the lactacid that supplies energy for the removal of lactic acid from muscle and blood.

- The energy processes at work during recovery from exercise are just as important as those at work during the exercise itself.

- Replenishment of muscular stores of phosphagen is rapid, requiring only 2 to 3 min.

- During intermittent exercise, the brief relief periods provide time for some restoration of phosphagen, which can be reused during subsequent work periods.

- Energy for phosphagen restoration is derived from the aerobic system, with a possible contribution from the lactic acid system as well.

- The size of the alactacid debt is 2 to 3.5 L. It supplies the energy for phosphagen replenishment and is "repaid" in 3 to 5 min.

- Myoglobin stores oxygen (up to 0.5 L) and facilitates diffusion of oxygen into the muscle cells' mitochondria. During exercise, the O_2-myoglobin stores are decreased. During recovery, when oxygen is plentiful (alactacid O_2 debt), the stores are replenished in only a few minutes.

- Complete replenishment of muscle glycogen during recovery from prolonged, continuous exercise takes about 46 hr if a high-carbohydrate diet is eaten in the recovery period. About 60% of the stores are replenished in the first 10 hr of recovery.

- Repeated days of endurance training can reduce glycogen stores to very low levels even with dietary intake of carbohydrate. This could lead to chronic exhaustion.

- Replenishment of muscle glycogen following short-term, high-intensity, intermittent exercise is complete within 24 hr in the person with a normal carbohydrate intake. About 45% of the stores are replenished in the first 5 hr of recovery. Some glycogen replenishment takes place within 30 min of recovery without food intake.

- Glycogen replenishment in fast-twitch muscle fibers appears to be faster than in the slow-twitch fibers.

- Muscle glycogen stores can be doubled if, following exercise-induced glycogen depletion, a carbohydrate diet is consumed for three days. This is referred to as muscle glycogen loading, or supercompensation.

- The energy for glycogen resynthesis during recovery is supplied by the oxygen system. During the immediate recovery period (1 to 1½ hr) it is possible that some lactic acid is reconverted to glycogen, with the lactacid oxygen debt supplying the energy.

- Following exhaustive exercise, removal of lactic acid from muscle and blood is most rapid when light, continuous exercise is performed during recovery (exercise-recovery, or "warm-down"). The half-time for lactic acid removal is 25 min during rest-recovery but only 11 min during exercise-recovery.

- During recovery, lactic acid is converted to muscle and liver glycogen, blood glucose, protein, and particularly to CO_2 and H_2O. The latter fate means that lactic acid is used to a considerable extent as a metabolic fuel for the aerobic energy system.

- The energy required for conversion of lactic acid to any other form is supplied by the oxygen system and includes the lactacid oxygen-debt component. The lactacid debt component is larger and is repaid more slowly than the alactacid debt.

• Recommended minimal and maximal recovery times for exhausting exercise can be calculated on the basis of the depletion/repletion information given above (see also Table 5-1).

Selected References and Readings*

Bergström, J., and E. Hultman: Muscle glycogen synthesis after exercise: An enhancement factor localized to the muscle cells in man. *Nature, 210:*309–310, 1966.

Bergström, J., L. Hermansen, E. Hultman, and B. Saltin: Diet, muscle glycogen and physical performance. *Acta Physiol. Scand., 71:*140–150, 1967.

Bonen, A., and A. Belcastro: Comparison of self-selected recovery methods on lactic acid removal rates. *Med. Sci. Sports, 8:*176–178, 1976.

Brooks, G. A., and G. A. Gaesser: End points of lactate and glucose metabolism after exhausting exercise. *J. Appl. Physiol.: Respirat. Environ. Exercise Physiol. 49(6):*1057–1069, 1980.

Brooks, G. A., K. F. Brauner, and R. G. Cassens: Glycogen synthesis and metabolism of lactic acid after exercise. *Am. J. Physiol., 224:*1162–1166, 1973.

Costill, D. L., et al.: Muscle glycogen utilization during prolonged exercise on successive days. *J. Appl. Physiol., 31:*834–838, 1971.

Costill, D. L., et al.: The role of dietary carbohydrates in muscle glycogen resynthesis after strenuous running. *Am. J. Clin. Nutri. 34:*1831–1836, 1981.

diPrampero, P. E., L. Peeters, and R. Margaria: Alactic O_2 debt and lactic acid production after exhausting exercise in man. *J. Appl. Physiol., 34:*628–632, 1973.

Essén, B., L. Hagenfeldt, and L. Kaijser: Utilization of blood-borne and intramuscular substrates during continuous and intermittent exercise in man. *J. Physiol. (London), 265:*489–506, 1977.

Fox, E. L.: Measurement of the maximal alactic (phosphagen) capacity in man. *Med. Sci. Sports, 5:*66, 1973.

Fox, E. L., and D. K. Mathews: *Interval Training.* Philadelphia, W. B. Saunders Company, 1974.

Fox, E. L., S. Robinson, and D. L. Wiegman: Metabolic energy sources during continuous and interval running. *J. Appl. Physiol., 27:*174–178, 1969.

Gaesser, G. A., and G. A. Brooks: Glycogen repletion following continuous and intermittent exercise to exhaustion. *J. Appl. Physiol.: Respirat. Environ. Exercise Physiol. 49(4):*722–728, 1980.

Gisolfi, C. G., S. Robinson, and E. S. Turrell: Effects of aerobic work performed during recovery from exhaustive work. *J. Appl. Physiol., 21:*1767–1772, 1966.

Hagerman, F. C., and E. L. Fox: New records in human power. Unpublished manuscript, 1973.

Hagerman, F. C., et al.: Energy expenditure during simulated rowing. *J. Appl. Physiol.: Respirat. Environ. Exercise Physiol., 45(1):*87–93, 1978.

Harris, R. C., et al.: The effect of circulatory occlusion on isometric exercise capacity and energy metabolism of the quadriceps muscle in man. *Scand. J. Clin. Lab. Invest., 35:*87–95, 1975.

Hermansen, L., and O. Vaage: Lactate disappearance and glycogen synthesis in human muscle after maximal exercise. *Am. J. Physiol., 233(5):*E422–E429, 1977.

Hermansen, L., et al.: Lactate removal at rest and during exercise. In Howald, H., and J. R. Poortmans (eds.): *Metabolic Adaptation to Prolonged Physical Exercise.* Basel, Switzerland, Birkhauser Verlag, 1975, pp. 101–105.

*For full journal titles, see Appendix A.

Hultman, E.: Studies on muscle metabolism of glycogen and active phosphate in man with special reference to exercise and diet. *Scand. J. Clin. Lab. Invest. (Suppl. 94), 19*:1–63, 1967.

Hultman, E., and J. Bergström: Muscle glycogen synthesis in relation to diet studied in normal subjects. *Acta Med. Scand.,182*:109–117, 1967.

Hultman, E., J. Bergström, and N. McLennan Anderson: Breakdown and resynthesis of phosphorylcreatine and adenosine triphosphate in connection with muscular work in man. *Scand. J. Clin. Lab. Invest., 19*:56–66, 1967.

Karlsson, J., and B. Saltin: Oxygen deficit and muscle metabolites in intermittent exercise. *Acta Physiol. Scand., 82*:115–122, 1971.

Lesmes, G. R.: Metabolic Responses of Young Females to Different Frequencies of Sprint Versus Endurance Interval Training. Doctoral Dissertation, The Ohio State University, 1976.

MacDougall, J. D., et al.: Muscle glycogen repletion after high-intensity intermittent exercise. *J. Appl. Physiol.: Respirat. Environ. Exercise Physiol., 42*:129–132, 1977.

Margaria, R., H. T. Edwards, and D. B. Dill: The possible mechanisms of contracting and paying the oxygen debt and the role of lactic acid in muscular contraction. *Am. J. Physiol.,106*:689–715, 1933.

Margaria, R., et al.: Kinetics and mechanism of oxygen debt contraction in man. *J. Appl. Physiol., 18*:371–377, 1963.

Piehl, K.: Time course for refilling of glycogen stores in human muscle fibers following exercise-induced glycogen depletion. *Acta Physiol. Scand., 90*:297–302, 1974.

Saltin, B., and B. Essén: Muscle glycogen, lactate, ATP, and CP in intermittent exercise. *In* Pernow, B. and B. Saltin (eds.): *Muscle Metabolism During Exercise.* New York, Plenum Press, 1971, pp. 419–424.

Segal, S. S., and G. A. Brooks: Effects of glycogen depletion and work load on post-exercise oxygen consumption and blood lactate. *J. Appl. Physiol.: Respirat. Environ. Exercise Physiol. 47(3)*:514–521, 1981.

6

Neuromuscular Concepts Applied to Sports

Introduction

One of the newer and perhaps most promising areas of research in the sports sciences is that concerned with neuromuscular adaptations to exercise. Earlier, in Chapters 1 and 4, fast-twitch (FT) and slow-twitch (ST) muscle fibers were mentioned. Most human muscles contain a mixture of each fiber type. Recently it has become possible to study these fibers separately under exercising conditions (see, for instance, the study described on p. 48). This development led to many new findings, and has permitted researchers to confirm hypotheses previously drawn solely from studies of animals. For example, a correlation between muscle performance and fiber type has only recently been demonstrated in human skeletal muscle; for some time such a relationship was known to exist in animals, as determined from experiments with animal skeletal muscle.

Findings such as these are of value to the coach and athlete because they help account for variations in performance from individual to individual and from one activity to another. Obviously, if there is a relationship between muscular performance and fiber type, as described above, then variations in ST or FT distribution will affect performance. In this regard, it is important to understand such neuromuscular concepts as fiber-type distribution in athletes of different sports and recruitment patterns of fiber types during exercises of various types and intensity. On a broader scale, it is clearly necessary to understand how a motor skill is executed. Acquiring such knowledge entails at least an appreciation of the control mechanisms that precisely regulate almost every function of our body at rest and during exercise.

The term **neuromuscular** refers to both the nervous and the muscular systems. Therefore, in this chapter we will direct our attention to the structure and function of nerves and muscles as they apply to movement in general and to sports performance specifically.

Basically there are two kinds of nerves, sensory and motor. **Sensory nerves**—also called **afferent nerves**—convey information from the periphery (e.g., the skin) to the **central nervous system** (brain and spinal cord). **Motor nerves**—also called **efferent nerves**—convey information from the central nervous system to effector organs such as glands and muscles. There are three types of muscle in the human body, namely smooth, cardiac (heart), and skeletal (striated) muscle; in this section only the latter will be discussed.

Structure of Nerves

The basic functional and anatomical unit of a nerve is the **neuron**, or **nerve cell**. Its structure is shown in Figure 6-1. The neuron consists of: (1) a **cell body**, or **soma**; (2) several short nerve fibers called **dendrites**; and (3) a longer nerve fiber called an **axon**. Although technically both dendrites and axons are nerve fibers, the term "nerve fiber" is generally used in reference to an axon. The dendrites transmit nerve impulses toward the cell body, whereas the axon transmits them away from the cell body.

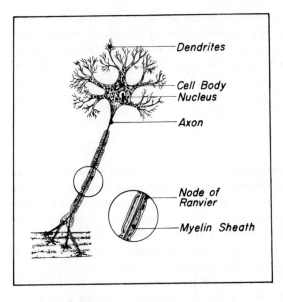

Dendrites

Cell Body
Nucleus

Axon

Node of
Ranvier

Myelin Sheath

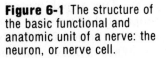

Figure 6-1 The structure of the basic functional and anatomic unit of a nerve: the neuron, or nerve cell.

In large nerve fibers, such as those innervating most skeletal muscles, the axon is surrounded by a **myelin sheath** (see Fig. 6-1). The sheath is composed mainly of lipid (fat) and protein. Nerve fibers containing a myelin sheath are referred to as **medullated fibers**, whereas those devoid of the sheath are called **nonmedullated fibers.** The myelin sheath is not continuous along the entire length of the fiber, but rather is laid down in segments with small spaces between segments. These spaces are called the **nodes of Ranvier.** We will later see that the myelin sheath and the nodes of Ranvier play important roles in how quickly the nerve impulse is transmitted along the axon.

Function of Nerves

The information sent from the periphery to the central nervous system by the afferent nerves is concerned with various kinds of sensations—heat, light, touch, smell, pressure, and so on. The connections of the sensory nerves with the central nervous system serve to supply us with the perception of these various sensations and to trigger, under certain circumstances, appropriate motor responses. An example of the latter would be the rapid reflex withdrawal of your hand from a hot stove.

To complete such a reflex response, motor nerves are required. These nerves originate in the central nervous system and terminate in effector organs such as skeletal muscles. When stimulated, the motor nerves cause the muscles in which they terminate to contract. Thus, in brief, when you accidentally place your hand on a hot stove, the heat-sensitive receptors located in the skin send information via the sensory nerve to the central nervous system. Once in the central nervous system (in this case in the spinal cord), the sensory nerve relays the information to the appropriate motor nerve, which in turn sends information to the muscles in the arm; the muscles contract, and the hand is automatically and rapidly withdrawn from the stove. Later, we will discuss another type of reflex, one involving special sense organs located within the skeletal muscles and intimately linked to the control of voluntary motor movement.

The Nerve Impulse

The information transmitted and relayed by the sensory and motor nerves is in a form of electrical energy referred to as the **nerve impulse**. A nerve impulse can be thought of mainly as an electrical disturbance at the point of stimulation of a nerve that is self-propagated along the entire length of the axon. The actual means by which a nerve impulse is generated and propagated in response to a **stimulus—a change in the environment which modifies the activity of cells**—may be summarized as follows:

When a nerve fiber is at rest, sodium ions (Na^+) are most heavily concentrated on the outside of the nerve membrane, causing it to be electrically positive while the inside of the nerve is negative (see Fig. 6-2A). Thus, a potential difference exists between the inside and outside of the nerve fiber. This is referred to as the **resting membrane potential**. When a stimulus is applied to the nerve, the nerve membrane becomes highly permeable to sodium ions, and they leak into the nerve. As a result, the outside of the nerve now becomes negative and the inside positive (Fig. 6-2B). In other words, an adequate stimulus causes a reversal of polarity of the nerve. Such a reversal in polarity is referred to as an **action potential**.

In addition to the action potential, a local flow of current is created in the membrane at the site where the stimulus was applied. This current is self-regenerating, in that it flows to adjacent areas of the nerve, causing each area to also undergo a reversal of polarity, which in turn evokes a new action potential and a local flow of current (Fig. 6-2C). This process is repeated over and over again until the action potential has been propagated the entire length of the nerve fiber.

On some nerve fibers there is a myelin sheath (mentioned earlier); this sheath insulates that part of the nerve it surrounds from electrical disturbances. Therefore, a nerve impulse can be neither generated nor propagated over that part of the fiber covered by the myelin. Instead, the nerve impulse is propagated only at the nodes of Ranvier, that is, from node to node the entire length of the fiber. This jumping from node to node, referred to as **saltatory conduction**, serves to greatly increase the conduction velocity of the nerve impulse. For example, the conduction velocity of large medullated fibers typical of those innervating skeletal muscles is 60 to 100 m per sec (135 to 225 miles per hr). In nonmedullated fibers of the same diameter, conduction velocity is only 6 to 10 m per sec (13.5 to 22.5 miles per hour).

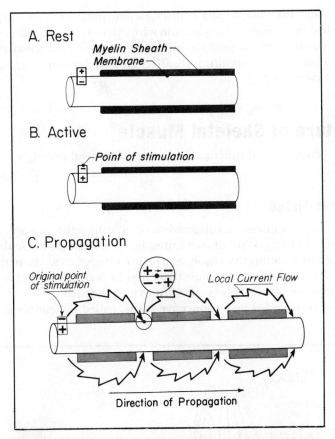

Figure 6-2 Generation and propagation of the nerve impulse. A, At rest the outside of the nerve is positive. B, A stimulus causes a reversal of polarity or action potential and a local flow of current. C, The local flow of current evokes a new action potential and flow of current in adjacent areas of the axon.

The Synapse and Neuromuscular Junction

When the nerve impulse reaches the end of the axon, it causes the release of a chemical **transmitter substance**. The transmitter substance serves to relay information either from nerve to nerve (**synapse**) or from nerve to muscle (**neuromuscular junction**). It does this by evoking a new nerve impulse in the nerve or muscle on which it is secreted. For example, a nerve impulse propagated along a motor nerve causes the transmitter substance **acetylcholine** to be released at the neuromuscular junction. In turn, the acetylcholine initiates an action potential in the muscle. The action potential is spread throughout the muscle, and the muscle contracts.

Although the synapse and neuromuscular junction have only recently been studied in animals in conjunction with exercise, it is already evident that physical training has a positive influence on their functional capacities. Whether these changes significantly affect athletic performance, however, is yet to be determined.

Structure of Skeletal Muscle

The structural and functional subunits of skeletal muscle are shown in Figure 6-3.

Connective Tissue

The entire muscle is surrounded by a connective tissue called the **epimysium**. The largest subunit of a muscle, the **bundle** (or **fasciculus**) is also surrounded by a connective tissue, a structure referred to as the **perimysium**. Contained within a muscle bundle there may be one muscle fiber or as many as hundreds of muscle fibers. The individual muscle fibers or cells are themselves surrounded by a connective tissue, called the **endomysium**.

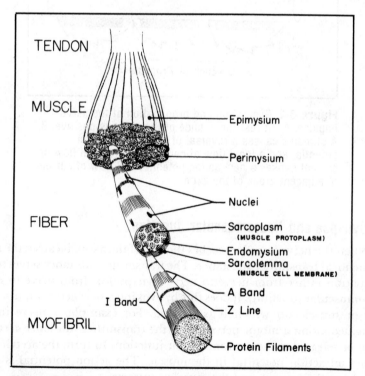

Figure 6-3 The structural and functional subunits of skeletal muscle.

The connective tissues are important, of course, in providing muscular strength and integrity. Also, as will be discussed in more detail later, the connective tissues are thought to be involved in the muscular soreness that often results during the first few days of intensive exercise.

The Myofibril

The cell membrane of a muscle fiber (or muscle cell) is called the **sarcolemma**. Inside the fiber are familiar subcellular components such as protoplasm (called **sarcoplasm** in muscle cells), nuclei, mitochondria, glycogen, ATP, and PC (to name but a few). The component of a muscle cell that distinguishes it from all other cells is the **myofibril**. A myofibril contains two basic protein filaments, a thicker one called **myosin**, and a thinner one called **actin**. These proteins are geometrically aligned throughout the muscle, as shown in Figure 6-4. Such an arrangement gives skeletal muscle its striped, or striated, appearance.

The Sarcomere

The smallest functional unit of the myofibril is the **sarcomere**. The sarcomere is defined as the distance between two Z lines (see Fig. 6-4). When stimulated, this unit will contract.

The I band of a sarcomere is composed only of actin filaments that extend from the Z lines toward the center of the sarcomere. The A band consists of both actin and myosin filaments. The tiny projections extending from the myosin filaments toward the actin filaments are called **myosin cross-bridges**. These projections are instrumental in effecting the shortening of the muscle during isotonic contraction. The area in the center of the A band where the cross-bridges are absent is called the H zone.

Function of Skeletal Muscle

Understanding the many functions of skeletal muscle entails several approaches—for example, the categorization of muscle contractions and the comparative analysis of muscle fibers. In this section we will, accordingly, cover a wide range of neuromuscular concepts, but it seems most appropriate to begin with a theory of just what happens when a muscle contracts.

The Sliding Filament Theory of Muscular Contraction

When a muscle contracts **isotonically**—that is, when it develops tension and shortens—the actin filaments slide over the myosin filaments toward the center of the sarcomere. This is shown schematically in Figure 6-5. The mechanism involved in the sliding process is not fully understood. However, it is fairly well agreed that upon stimulation of a muscle, the myosin cross-

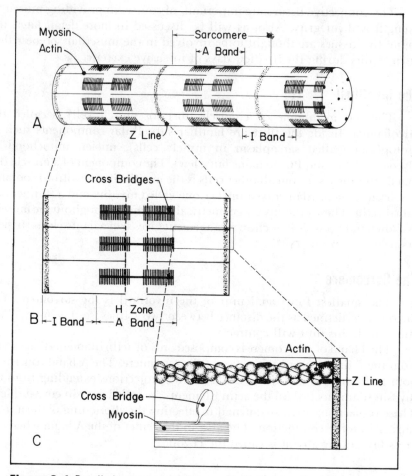

Figure 6-4 Detailed structure of the myofibril. The smallest functional unit of the myofibril is the sarcomere.

bridges form a type of bond with selected sites on the actin filaments (under resting conditions, the cross-bridges are extended toward the actin filaments but are not attached to them). This coupling process, sometimes referred to as actomyosin formation, is dependent upon the presence of calcium ions (Ca^{++}). Once attached, the cross-bridges either collapse or swivel in such a manner that the actin filaments are pulled over the myosin filaments and toward the center of the sarcomere. During this process, ATP is broken down to ADP and Pi, the muscle shortens, and tension is developed. When stimulation stops, the muscle relaxes and returns to the resting state.

A summary of some of the important events occurring during muscular contraction is given in Table 6-1.

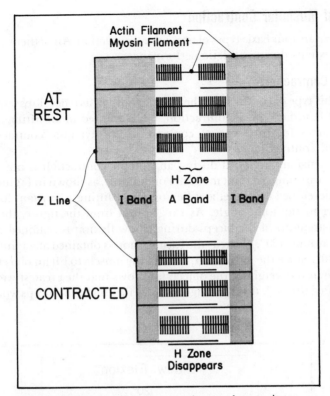

Figure 6-5 The sliding filament theory of muscular contraction. When a muscle contracts isotonically, the actin filaments slide over the myosin filaments toward the center of the sarcomere.

Table 6-1: Summary of Events during Muscular Contraction Based on the Sliding Filament Theory

Stage of Contraction	Associated Events
Rest	Cross-bridges extended toward actin Actin and myosin in uncoupled position
Stimulation	Ca^{++} released Actin and myosin coupled → actomyosin
Contraction	Cross-bridges swivel or collapse Muscle shortens → actin slides over myosin Tension developed $ATP → ADP + Pi + energy$
Relaxation	Stimulation ceases Ca^{++} removed Muscle returns to resting state

Types of Muscular Contraction

There are four basic types of muscular contraction. All of them are used to various extents during athletic performances.

Isotonic Contraction

In this type of contraction, the muscle shortens as it develops tension. It is the most familiar type of contraction, the kind used in all lifting activities. Other names for this type of contraction are dynamic contraction and concentric contraction.

The tension developed during an isotonic contraction is not maximal over the entire range of joint motion. For example, as shown in Figure 6-6, the tension developed during elbow flexion when lifting a constant load varies according to the joint angle. As can be seen from the figure, the greatest tension (strength) of the biceps during elbow flexion is obtained at a joint angle of around 120°, whereas the least tension is obtained at a joint angle of around 30°. Since the tension required of the muscle to lift an object must be greater than the weight of the object, it follows that the greatest weight that can be lifted through the full range of elbow flexion by the biceps would be no

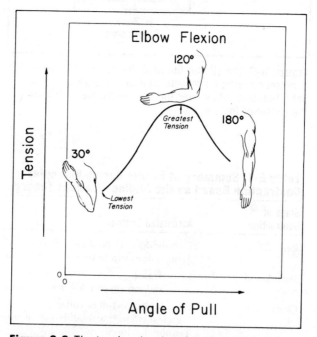

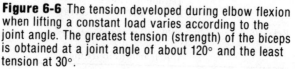

Figure 6-6 The tension developed during elbow flexion when lifting a constant load varies according to the joint angle. The greatest tension (strength) of the biceps is obtained at a joint angle of about 120° and the least tension at 30°.

greater than that weight that could be lifted at the weakest point. In other words, the muscle would be maximally contracted only at its weakest point. This is a definite disadvantage with respect to strength training programs that involve only isotonic contractions (e.g., barbells).

Isometric Contraction

The word **isometric** means same (iso) length (metric). During an isometric contraction, the muscle develops tension but does not change length. This is a familiar type of contraction. Holding a weight at arm's length or attempting to lift an immovable object are both examples of isometric contractions. Isometric contractions also occur during sports performance; wrestling is a good example. Another name for isometric contraction is static contraction.

Eccentric Contraction

This is just the opposite of an isotonic or concentric contraction. During eccentric contraction, the muscle lengthens as it develops tension. A good example of this type of contraction is during the performance of "negative work," such as when you are lowering a weight or resisting a movement or gravity. During downhill running or walking down stairs, the muscles are eccentrically contracting. It is easy to see that this type of contraction is also frequently used during various sports performances.

Isokinetic Contraction

This is a rather "new" type of contraction, at least as applied to sports performance. It is defined as a maximal contraction at constant speed (iso = same, kinetic = motion) over the full range of movement. Such contractions are common during sports performances; a good example is the arm stroke during freestyle swimming.

Although isokinetic contraction and isotonic contraction are both concentric, the two are not identical. As shown in Figure 6-7, maximal tension is developed throughout the full range of motion during isokinetic contraction but not during isotonic contractions. In addition, in an isotonic contraction, the speed of movement is not controlled and is relatively slow. This is something of a limitation, for, as mentioned in an earlier chapter, it is more and more apparent that muscular power—that is, both strength and speed of contraction—is a major success factor in many athletic performances. More about strength and speed of contraction will be presented later in this chapter.

To perform a controlled isokinetic contraction, special equipment is required, an example of which is shown in Figure 6-8.* This particular piece of equipment is a bench-press machine, but notice the absence of a weight

*For example, Cybex equipment from Lumex, Inc., Ronkonkoma, NY, 11779; and Mini-Gym equipment from Mini-Gym, Inc., Independence, MO 65051.

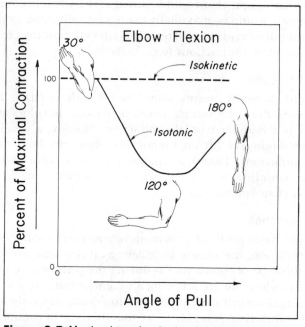

Figure 6-7 Maximal tension is developed throughout the full range of joint motion during isokinetic contractions but not during isotonic contractions.

stack, which is a characteristic of all isokinetic equipment. Basically, the equipment contains a speed governor so that the speed of movement is constant no matter how much tension is produced in the contracting muscles. Thus, if one attempts to make the movement as "fast" as possible, the tension generated by the muscles will be maximal throughout the full range of motion, but the speed of movement will be constant. The movement speed on many isokinetic devices can be pre-set, and can vary between 0 and 300° of motion per second. Many movement speeds during actual athletic performances exceed 200° per second.

Most of the isokinetic machines also have readout devices for recording muscle tension. This is a particular advantage in evaluating performance and can serve as a training monitor during actual training sessions.

From a theoretical viewpoint, isokinetic contractions—and thus isokinetic training programs—appear to be best suited for improving athletic performance. Further details of such programs and their effects will be discussed later.

A summary of the types of muscular contractions is given in Figure 6-9.

Muscle Soreness

At one time or another, all of us have experienced **muscle soreness**. From experiments specifically designed to induce such muscle soreness, it has been

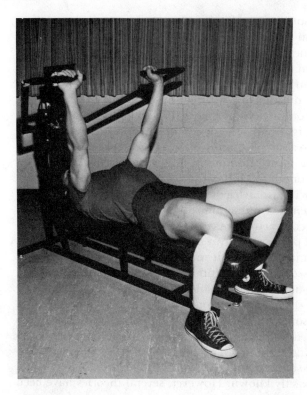

Figure 6-8 Cybex, isokinetic bench press machine. Notice the absence of a weight stack. The resistance is provided through a speed governor that allows the lever arms to move at constant speed no matter how much force is applied. (Photograph by Tom Malloy. Courtesy of the Department of Photography, The Ohio State University, Columbus, OH.)

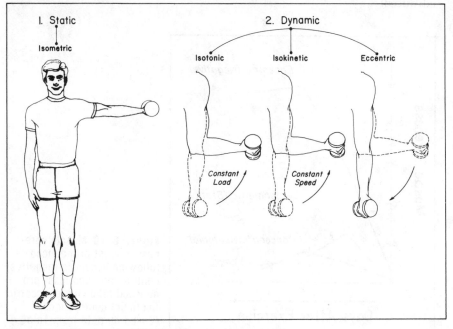

Figure 6-9 The four basic types of muscular contraction.

found that the degree of soreness is related to the type of muscle contraction performed. In one typical experiment, the results of which are shown in Figure 6-10, muscle soreness was induced with a barbell exercise. Male and female subjects performed two sets of exhaustive contractions of the elbow flexors with barbells. During eccentric contractions the barbell was only actively lowered, whereas during concentric contractions it was only actively raised; during isometric contractions, the barbell was held stationary (see the exercise illustrations in Fig. 6-10). The degree of soreness was evaluated by each subject in response to a soreness rating scale. As the figure shows, muscle soreness was found to be most pronounced following eccentric (negative) contractions and least pronounced following concentric (isotonic) contractions. The soreness following isometric (static) contractions was a bit greater than that following concentric contractions but was still considerably below that found after eccentric contractions. As can be seen, in all cases the soreness was delayed; it reached a peak one to two days after exercise.

Although not shown in the figure, it was found in this experiment that muscular strength decreased appreciably following eccentric contractions and remained depressed throughout the duration of the soreness period. No significant decrease in strength was noted during the soreness period following concentric or isometric contractions. In a separate study, little or no muscle soreness was noted following exercise involving isokinetic contractions, nor was there any decrease in strength.

What causes muscle soreness and how can it be avoided? The cause of muscle soreness is not exactly known. However, several theories have been advanced:

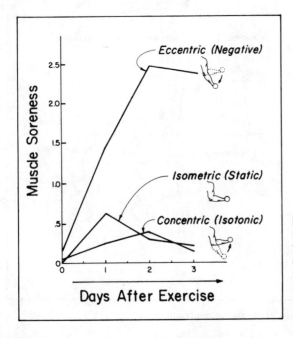

Figure 6-10 Muscle soreness is most pronounced following eccentric (negative) contractions and least pronounced following concentric (isotonic) contractions. (Based on data from Talag, 1973.)

Muscle Soreness Theories

Tissue damage such as the tearing of muscle fibers could explain muscle soreness.

Muscle soreness is possibly caused by local muscular spasms (these reduce muscle blood flow, resulting in pain). This explanation of muscle soreness is called the "spasm theory."

Overstretching could damage the connective tissues that surround the muscle fibers and the tendons, producing muscle soreness.

In a recent study designed specifically to investigate these theories, it was concluded that muscle soreness is most likely related to disruption of the connective tissue elements in the muscles and tendons.

The "connective tissue theory" appears to be consistent with the finding of greatest soreness following eccentric contractions. You will recall, for instance, that during eccentric contractions the muscle lengthens under tension, thus stretching the connective tissue components associated with both the tendons and the muscle fibers. In contrast, during concentric contractions (isotonic and isokinetic), only the connective tissues associated with tendons are stretched. The tension developed during maximal eccentric contractions is, after all, greater than that possible during other types of contractions, and this tension affects the connective tissue.

As far as prevention of muscle soreness is concerned, the following suggestions have been made:

Prevention of Muscle Soreness

Stretching appears to help not only the prevention of soreness but also the relief of it when present. Stretching exercises should be performed, however, without bouncing or jerking, since this may further damage the connective tissues. More about stretching exercises will be presented in a later chapter.

It has been proposed that ingestion of 100 mg per day of vitamin C (about twice the daily recommended dosage) for a period of 30 days will prevent or at least reduce subsequent muscle soreness. The value of consuming such a quantity of vitamin C (ascorbic acid) has not been entirely established through scientific experimentation.

Unfortunately, for a definite solution to the problem of muscle soreness, more research is needed.

The Motor Unit

Most single motor nerves (or motoneurons, as they are also called) have many branches and thus in entering a muscle supply or innervate many muscle fibers. However, a given muscle fiber is innervated by only one motor nerve. A motor nerve plus all the muscle fibers it innervates is called a **motor unit**. The motor unit is the basic functional unit of skeletal muscle. When the motoneuron of a motor unit is stimulated, all the muscle fibers within that unit contract more or less synchronously. If there are many muscle fibers in the unit the contraction will be strong. However, if there are only a few muscle fibers within a unit, the contraction will be weak. The response of the muscle can thus be graded depending upon the size and number of motor units stimulated. Such an arrangement allows for fine, delicate movements as well as for gross, large-scale movements.

Although all skeletal muscle motor units function in the same general manner described above, there is also a degree of specialization among the units. There are two basic—and hence very important—motor units whose specific functions are quite different, a factor of obvious significance with respect to various sports performances. These are the **fast-twitch (FT)** and **slow-twitch (ST)** units or fibers. These units or fiber types were briefly discussed earlier and will be examined in greater detail here.

It should be mentioned at this time that the fast-twitch fibers can be further subdivided in both human and animal muscles. However, for our purposes we will need to understand only the differences between the two basic types, slow- and fast-twitch.

Method of Classifying Fiber Types

The classification of fiber types is done by histochemical analysis of a sample of muscle tissue obtained by a needle biopsy procedure. The analysis involves chemically staining the tissue for the presence of various aerobic and anaerobic enzymes. The variations in the intensity of the stain reflect the variations in the enzyme concentrations.

When the stained muscle sample is viewed in cross-section with a light microscope, it looks like the one shown in Figure 6–11. It should be pointed out at this time that all muscle fibers within any given motor unit are of the same type. For example, FT motor units contain only FT fibers and ST units only ST fibers. Also, as indicated in Figure 6–11, the fibers of FT and ST motor units are mixed together in the muscle giving a checkerboard appearance.

Aerobic and Anaerobic Potential of FT and ST Units

The anaerobic capacity of FT units is much greater than that of ST units. For example, while both units contain enzymes involved in facilitating the reactions of the ATP-PC system, the enzymes in FT fibers are about three times as active as those in ST fibers (an enzyme is more "active" when it has greater functional capabilities than another enzyme). Similarly, some of the

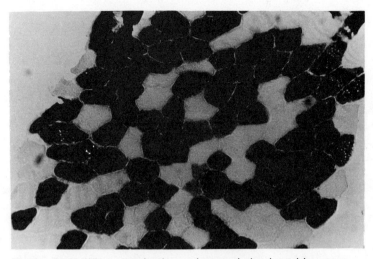

Figure 6-11 When a stained muscle sample is viewed in cross section, it has a checkerboard appearance, because the fibers of fast-twitch (FT) and slow-twitch (ST) motor units are mixed together in the muscle. In this human muscle sample from the vastus lateralis, the darkly stained fibers are ST and the lightly stained fibers are FT.

more important glycolytic (lactic acid system) enzymes are found in both units, but the enzymes in FT fibers are up to two times more active than those in ST fibers. In other words, the FT fibers are best suited, biochemically, for "sprint-like" activities.

On the other hand, the aerobic capacity of ST fibers is much greater than that of FT fibers. The enzymes involved in the reactions of the aerobic system have higher activities in ST fibers. In addition, the number and size of the mitochondria, where the aerobic reactions occur, as well as the number of capillaries per fiber, are much greater in ST fibers. Also contributing to the greater aerobic capacity of ST fibers is their much higher myoglobin content. The ST units are therefore biochemically best suited for "endurance-type" activities.

The amount of stored glycogen is the same in the two fiber types. However, ST fibers have nearly three times the triglyceride (fat) store of FT fibers.

Speed of Contraction of FT and ST Units

As shown in Figure 6-12A, the time required for FT fibers to generate maximal tension is about one third that required by ST fibers. As might be suspected, one of the reasons for the faster contraction time in FT units is their greater anaerobic capacity. Another important factor is the size of the motoneuron (motor nerve) that innervates the fast-twitch unit. As can be seen

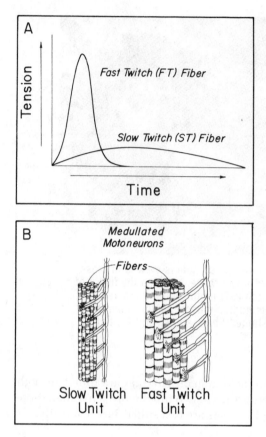

Figure 6-12 The time required by FT fibers to generate maximal tension is about one third that required by ST fibers (A). One of the reasons for this is that the motoneuron innervating the FT unit is larger than the motoneuron in the ST unit (B) and, thus, can propagate the nerve impulse more quickly.

from Figure 6-12B, the motoneuron innervating the FT unit is larger than the motoneuron in the ST unit. This means that the nerve impulse that causes the motor unit to contract is transmitted along the axon faster.

What the above information implies is that individuals with higher percentages of FT fibers should be able to contract their muscles faster. In recent experiments, this has been shown to be true for one of the knee extensor muscles (the vastus lateralis), as indicated in Figure 6-13A. The experiments were conducted with 15 male subjects, whose maximal knee extension velocity was measured without load. The percentage of FT fibers in the vastus of the subjects was determined through the needle biopsy technique. The discovery of faster contraction times in the subjects with the higher percentage of fast-twitch fibers provided the first direct evidence in humans of a relationship that had long been observed in animals.

From a practical viewpoint two questions arise:

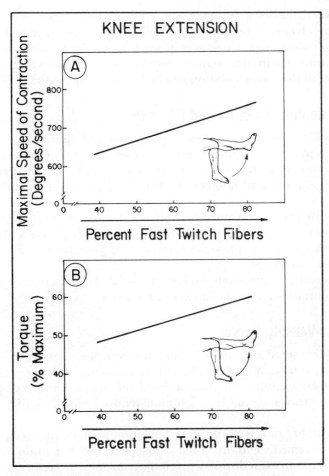

Figure 6-13 The relationship between the percentage distribution of fast-twitch fibers and maximal speed of contraction (A) and torque (B) in man. As the percentage of fast-twitch fibers increases, torque increases, as does the maximal speed of contraction (the muscles contract more quickly). (Based on data from Thorstensson and co-workers, 1976.)

Do athletes whose sport requires high speeds of motion (e.g., sprinters, high-jumpers, shot-putters) have higher than normal percentages of FT units in the muscles involved in the motion?

If so, are these higher percentages a result of training for and participation in these specific kinds of activities?

The answer to the first question is "yes," and will be discussed in greater depth later in this chapter. A definite "yes or no" answer to the second question is as yet unavailable. However, it would appear that heredity is an important factor in determining the final percentage distribution of FT and ST fibers. Further discussion of this latter question can be found on pages 108 to 109.

Force of Contraction of FT and ST Units

From Figure 6-12A, it is evident that the force of contraction (tension) in FT units is much greater than that in ST units. The greater force is related to the size of individual fibers and to the number of fibers making up the motor unit. Both the size and number of fibers are greater in FT units (see Fig. 6-12B).

As with speed of contraction, this information implies that those individuals with higher percentages of FT motor units should be able to exert greater muscular forces. This too has recently been confirmed in humans, as is shown in Figure 6-13B.

The preceding questions concerning speed of contraction apply also to force of contraction, and the answers are similar.

The Force-Velocity Curve

While the speed and force of contraction separately are important factors influencing muscular performance, their combined effects are even more important. For example, the application of muscular force through a range of motion at various speeds is a common requirement of nearly all sports activities.

Look at the "force-velocity curve" in Figure 6-14. What exactly does such a curve represent? Essentially, it relates the peak force or tension that a given muscle group can exert during a given movement to the performance of that movement at a given speed (velocity). For the data shown in the figure, the muscle group that was used was the vastus lateralis, one of the quadriceps, and the movement tested was knee extension. The peak force was recorded on an isokinetic machine during knee extensions performed at speeds ranging from 0 to 180° per sec (see Fig. 6-15). Since the full range of motion included only 90° (see the illustration at the top of the figure), the fastest speed corresponded to extending the knee in half a second. As for the speed of 0° per sec, this occurred when the muscular force that was exerted, although maximal, was not great enough to overcome the external resistance of the machine (thus no movement was possible). This represented the maximal isometric force of the muscle group. As can be seen, the force exerted by a muscle decreases as the speed of movement increases.

Incidentally, in studying the force-velocity curve, the terms force, torque, and even tension are sometimes used more or less interchangeably as a measure of muscular strength. While for our general purposes this is permissible, technically speaking, **torque** is defined as the product of force and

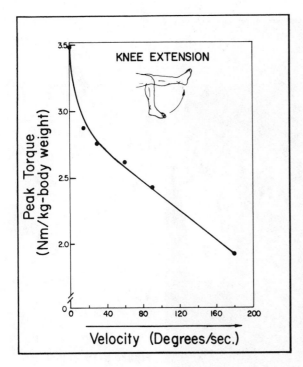

Figure 6-14 The force-velocity curve, relating the peak torque or force that a given muscle can exert during a given movement to the speed of that movement. The curve shown here is for knee extension. (Based on data from Thorstensson and co-workers, 1976.)

the lever-arm or moment-arm distance. Because the isokinetic machines used to measure force-velocity curves have lever arms, torque is the more correct term. The common metric unit of measure for torque is a **Newton-meter**, abbreviated **Nm**. The English counterpart to Nm is the foot-pound (ft-lb). (1 ft-lb = 1.356 Nm and 1 Nm = 0.7375 ft-lb).

Intuitively, we might suspect that because force and speed of contraction are independently related to the percentage of FT units present in muscle (see Fig. 6-13), the force-velocity curve would be shifted upward and to the right in those individuals who have relatively greater percentages of FT fibers. In other words, these individuals should be capable of exerting a greater force at the same velocity of movement and a greater velocity of movement while exerting the same force.

Only recently have such presumed relationships been experimentally verified in human subjects. Figure 6-16A shows the force-velocity curves for subjects who have a large percentage of FT fibers (greater than 60%) and for those who have a small percentage (less than 50%). Notice, as we suspected, that the curve for the subjects with higher percentages of FT fibers is indeed shifted upward and to the right. When this curve is compared with that of subjects with lower percentages of FT fibers, the magnitude of the shift is quite impressive. Calculations based on the complete data (the figure is only a summary) showed that the force exerted at the same velocity of movement was around 15% greater in the group with the high percentage of FT fibers.

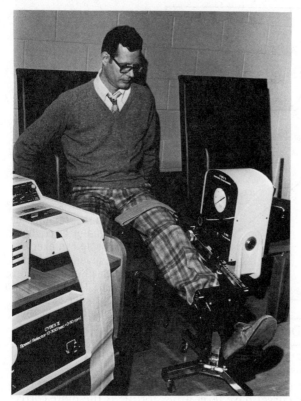

Figure 6-15 Author performing knee extension exercises on the Cybex II isokinetic machine.

Perhaps even more impressive, at the same force, the velocity of movement was 85% greater in the high FT group!

The above information can, of course, be applied to athletes. The force-velocity curves for athletes who have high percentages of FT fibers are in fact shifted upward from and to the right of the curves for athletes with fewer FT fibers. A "family of curves" for various athletes is shown in Figure 6–16B. Notice that athletes who train for and participate in high-power events (sprinters and jumpers) are capable of exerting much greater forces at much higher velocities of movement than are the other athletes. Note also that the curve for the endurance athletes (orienteers*), who have the lowest percentage of FT fibers, is lower than that for the untrained group.

Although the shift in the curve for power athletes is related to their higher percentages of FT fibers, it should be pointed out that the untrained subjects—who had a much lower curve—had only a slightly lower percentage of FT fibers than the sprinters and jumpers (61% vs. 56%). Since interconversion of fast- and slow-twitch fibers through training does not occur to any

---

*Orienteering is a European sport that combines long distance running and land navigational skills.

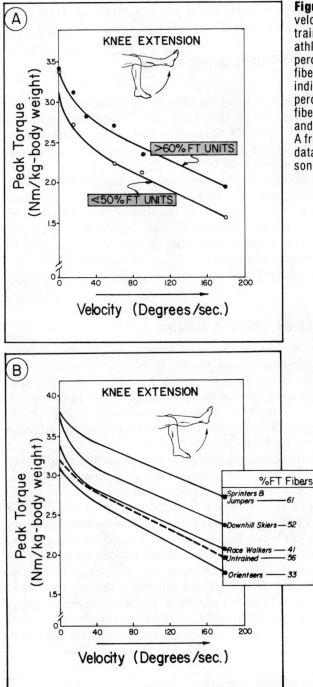

Figure 6-16 The force-velocity curves for untrained subjects (A) and athletes (B) with various percentages of fast-twitch fibers. The curves for individuals with higher percentages of fast-twitch fibers are shifted upward and to the right. (Data in A from Thorstensson, 1977; data in B from Thorstensson and co-workers, 1977.)

extent in humans, this suggests that training per se can significantly influence the force-velocity curve. (For more on training, see Chapters 7 and 9).

Recruitment of FT and ST Units during Sports Performance

Although both FT and ST units are probably called upon during most sports activities, ST units are preferentially used during performance of endurance activities. Conversely, FT fibers are preferentially recruited during the performance of sprint-like activities. Other examples of recruitment patterns were given in Chapter 4 (p. 50).

One of the most important applications of this information to sports is in the area of training. It is very clear that in order to increase the metabolic potential of FT fibers, the activity during training must consist of high-intensity exercise. This will ensure that the FT fibers will be active during the training sessions. By the same token, to increase the metabolic potential of ST fibers, the training activity must consist of lower intensity, longer duration exercises. Under these conditions, ST fibers will be preferentially used during the training sessions.

Distribution of FT and ST Fibers in Athletes

It was previously mentioned that most muscles in humans contain a mixture of fast- and slow-twitch units. In this regard, it was pointed out that athletes who participate in and train for sports that involve short-duration, high-intensity efforts tend to have greater percentages of FT fibers than do nonathletes and endurance athletes. In contrast, endurance athletes tend to have greater percentages of ST fibers than do nonathletes and nonendurance athletes. This holds true for both men and women.

An analysis of the distribution of fiber types in male and female athletes is shown in Figure 6–17. In many cases, the percentages represent findings in world class competitors (particularly males). Although one can readily discern from the mean values that FT fibers tend to predominate in nonendurance athletes, and that ST fibers predominate in endurance athletes, notice how large the variation is in each group. For example, the group of elite marathon runners had 82% ST fibers on the average, but one marathoner had only 50%. At the other end of the spectrum, the group of sprinters/jumpers had 62% FT fibers on the average, but one athlete had only 48%. In other words, a marathon runner and a sprinter had approximately the same percentages of ST and FT fibers. This suggests that fiber distribution is only one of many factors that contributes to successful performances, and that successful performances can be achieved without such fiber-type preference.

Heritability of Neuromuscular Factors

Earlier the questions of the influence of physical training and heredity on fiber-type distribution were mentioned (p. 104). The majority of studies have shown that the percentage distribution of fiber types in humans does not change following endurance, sprint, or weight resistance training (see pp. 153 and 227). Only one study is available showing some interconversion of FT and ST fibers following training in humans.

Additionally, recent evidence has strongly suggested that fiber-type distribution in humans is determined solely by heredity. Hereditary information of this kind is obtainable by comparing the intrapair variability of identical (monozygous) twins and fraternal (dizygous) twins, as is shown in Figure 6-18. In the left half of the figure, the percentage of ST fibers in identical twin A (vertical axis) is plotted against that in identical twin B (horizontal axis). The diagonal line represents the "line of identity"; if the percentage of ST fibers in twin A were the same as in twin B, then all of the points would fall on this line. The same kind of plot for fraternal twins is shown in the right half of Figure 6-18. Notice how much more the points scatter about the line of identity for the fraternal twins. The variability in identical twins is clearly much smaller. From such variances, it has been estimated that the heritability of fiber-type distribution is 99.5% for males and 92.2% for females. These figures indicate a very strong genetic component.

It can be concluded from heritability studies that the distribution pattern of FT and ST fibers in athletes (see Fig. 6-17) is most likely due to "natural selection." That is to say, those athletes who are genetically endowed with a preponderance of ST fibers select endurance activities because they are successful in those activities whereas athletes who are genetically endowed with a greater percentage of FT fibers select sprint-like activities because they are successful in those kinds of exercises.

Other neuromuscular factors that have been studied in males and females with respect to heritability are: (1) maximal muscular power; (2) patellar reflex time; (3) reaction time; (4) nerve conduction velocity; and (5) maximal isometric, eccentric, and concentric muscular strength. It has been found that patellar reflex time, reaction time, and muscular power have substantial genetic components but only in males. None of the factors studied in females shows significant heritability tendencies. This means that these neuromuscular factors are perhaps more susceptible to environmental modification in females than in males. As yet, no satisfactory explanation can be given for these sex differences.

Whatever the case, the fact that reflex time, reaction time, fiber type, and muscular power have substantial genetic components suggests that speed and agility might also be highly genetic. The old saying, "Sprinters are born, not made" may have some truth after all!

Fatigue of FT and ST Fibers

Experimental work with animals—and, more recently, humans—has shown that FT motor units are more easily fatigued than are ST units. The comparative degrees of fatiguability in FT and ST units in humans can be seen in Figure 6-19. Figure 6-19A shows the results of an experiment in which

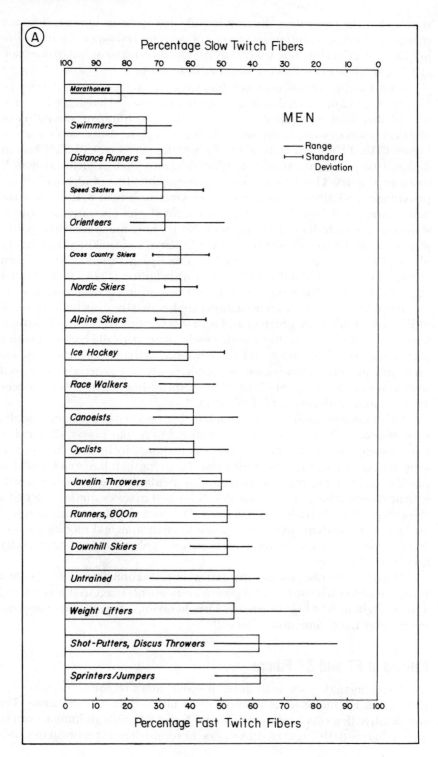

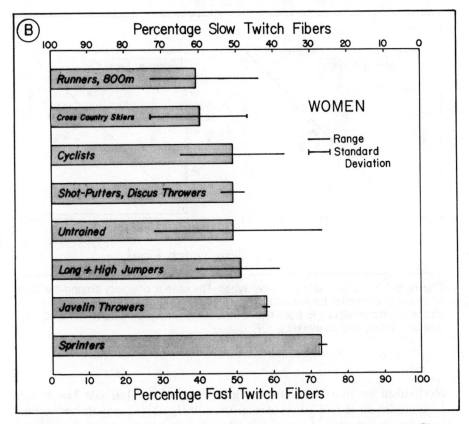

Figure 6-17 Fiber type distribution in male athletes (A) and female athletes (B). In general, endurance athletes, whether male or female, have a predominance of slow-twitch fibers, whereas nonendurance athletes have a predominance of fast-twitch fibers. However, note the large variation within each group of athletes. (Based on data from Burke and co-workers, 1977; Costill and co-workers, 1976; Gollnick and co-workers, 1972; Komi and co-workers, 1977; and Thorstensson and co-workers, 1977.)

two subjects, one with 61% and the other with 38% FT fibers in the vastus lateralis, performed repeated maximal knee extensions at a speed of 180° per sec. Two points should be noticed: first, the peak force generated by the vastus lateralis was much greater in the subject with 61% FT fibers; and second, the decrease in force during repeated contractions was less in the subject with only 38% FT fiber distribution. This means that while the FT units are capable of generating greater forces, they fatigue more rapidly. This greater fatiguability of FT fibers compared to ST fibers is also illustrated in Figure 6-19B.

Local Muscular Fatigue

With respect to athletic performance, local muscular fatigue appears to be confined to the contractile mechanism (as opposed, for instance, to the neuromuscular junction). As we know, the FT fibers of the contractile

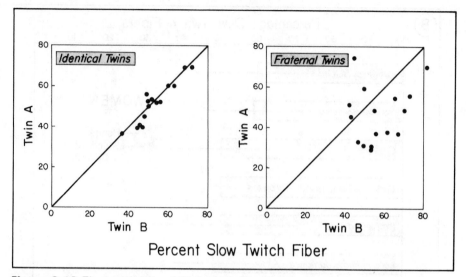

Figure 6-18 The heritability of fiber types. The scatter of points around the "line of identity" is smaller for identical twins than for fraternal twins, indicating a strong genetic tendency in fiber-type distribution. (Based on data from Komi, Vitasalo, Havu, and co-workers, 1977.)

mechanism are more subject to fatigue than are the ST fibers. The greater fatiguability of the FT fibers is more than likely related to their low aerobic capacity. As mentioned earlier, FT fibers have a low aerobic capacity but a high glycolytic capacity. Thus, the majority of energy they generate is by anaerobic glycolysis. This leads to large accumulations of lactic acid. In fact, experimental studies with animals have shown that during high-intensity, exhaustive running, the majority of lactic acid that is accumulated is produced by FT fibers.

This also appears to be the case in human muscle as shown in Fig. 6-20. In the figure, lactic acid accumulation is represented as the ratio of lactic acid concentration in FT and ST fibers (plotted on the horizontal axis). This means that as the ratio increases, more lactic acid is being produced in FT fibers in comparison to ST fibers. Notice how the tension in the muscle (measured here as torque) declines as the FT/ST lactic acid ratio increases. This decline in torque is a measure of fatiguability of the muscle.

It would appear, then, that local muscular fatigue following short-term, high-intensity exercise is caused by lactic acid accumulation in the blood and muscles.

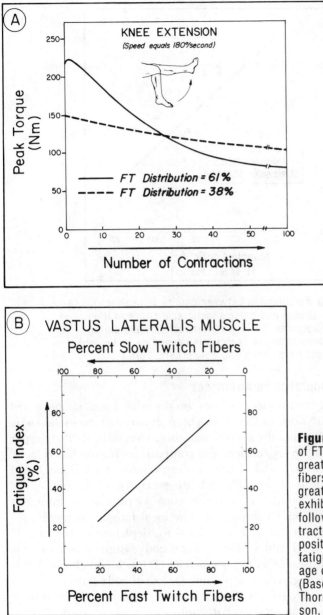

Figure 6-19 Fatiguability of FT and ST fibers. The greater fatiguability of FT fibers is indicated by the greater decrease in torque exhibited by these fibers following repeated contractions (A) and by the positive relationship of fatiguability and percentage of FT fibers (B). (Based on data from Thorstensson and Karlsson, 1976.)

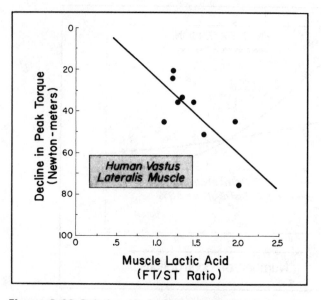

Figure 6-20 Relationship between decline in peak torque (a measure of fatigue) and muscle lactic acid concentration. This finding supports the idea that muscle fatigue during short-term, high-intensity exercise is caused by lactic acid. (Based on data from Tesch and co-workers, 1978.)

Fatigue Following Endurance Performances

Fatigue following endurance exercises, on the other hand, is not caused by lactic acid accumulation. In fact, it has been shown that the blood lactic acid concentration following the Boston marathon averaged only 19.3 mg per 100 ml of blood (mg%) on six runners. For comparison, resting blood lactic acid values range between 5 and 15 mg% (to cause muscular fatigue, blood lactic acid concentrations of over 100 mg% are generally required).

Fatigue following endurance exercise consists of a local muscular component and a total body component. The local fatigue, as mentioned before, is probably due to, or at least related to, depletion of the muscle glycogen stores in both FT and ST fibers. Total body fatigue would include local muscular fatigue plus other factors such as: (1) low blood glucose levels (hypoglycemia); (2) liver glycogen depletion; (3) loss of body water (dehydration); (4) loss of body electrolytes (e.g., salt and potassium); (5) high body temperature (hyperthermia); and (6) boredom.

A summary of the differences between fast-twitch and slow-twitch motor units is presented in Table 6-2.

Fatigue and Sports Performance

The possibility of delaying or preventing both local muscular and total body fatigue during performance has intrigued many researchers. Note, though, that prevention of fatigue during athletic performance should not be

Table 6-2: A Summary of Differences Between Fast-Twitch (FT) and Slow-Twitch (ST) Motor Units

Characteristic	Fast-Twitch (FT)	Slow-Twitch (ST)
Aerobic Capacity	Low	High
Anaerobic Capacity	High	Low
Capillary Density	Low	High
Contraction Time	Fast	Slow
Force of Contraction	High	Low
Recruitment Pattern	Sprint-like activities	Endurance-like activities
Distribution in Athletes	High (nonendurance athletes)	High (endurance athletes)
Fatiguability	Rapid	Slow

a major concern of the athlete. After all, an athlete who is not fatigued at the end of a performance probably has not given an all-out effort. Delaying fatigue is more desirable. For example, delaying fatigue will allow the athlete to finish the race, game, match, or event with greater effort. At the same time the athlete's efforts during the start and middle portions of the performance will not be compromised. Ideally, delaying fatigue should allow an athlete to maintain or improve his or her performance in the early and middle portions of a particular contest and still provide for a greater "kick" or effort at the finish. We all know that it is at the finish where many contests are won or lost.

Physical training produces physiological changes that are instrumental in delaying fatigue. For example, the athlete can work harder but not produce as much lactic acid following training. Additionally, there is a "glycogen sparing" effect in the trained athlete—he or she uses more fat, rather than glycogen, as fuel. As a result, muscle and liver glycogen stores are not so readily depleted, and thus fatigue is delayed. Certain other effects of training involve adaptation to the environment. Increased acclimatization to environmental heat, for instance, helps to reduce hyperthermia, dehydration, and excessive loss of electrolytes during performance. These training changes are discussed in more detail in a later chapter (see p. 322).

Muscle Sense Organs

Two important muscle sense organs are the **muscle spindles** and the **Golgi tendon organs**. Both of these organs are concerned with what is generally referred to as kinesthetic sense—that is, awareness of body position. However, they are also involved in the control of voluntary and reflex movements.

The Muscle Spindles

The muscle spindles are located within special muscle fibers called **intrafusal fibers** (regular muscle fibers are called **extrafusal fibers**). A sensory nerve is wrapped around the center portion of the spindle. When the spindle is stretched, nerve impulses are generated in the sensory nerve, and information relative to both the rate and magnitude of stretch is sent to the central nervous system. Automatically, information concerning how many motor units should be contracted in order to effect a smooth movement is sent back via the motor nerves to the muscles. In a way, then, the spindles act as scales. For example, when you first attempt to lift an object, the muscle stretches. If the load is heavy, the stretch is heavy, and many motor units are recruited in lifting the object. If the load is light, the stretch is light, and only a few motor units are called into play.

The spindles also play important roles during the performance of motor skills. Under the control of the motor cortex in the brain, the ends of the spindles can contract (just as extrafusual fibers contract). When this happens, the center portion of the spindle is stretched. In other words, when a motor skill is voluntarily initiated, the ends of the spindles within the muscles involved in that particular skill will contract, thus stretching the center portion of the spindles. The information relayed to the central nervous system is, of course, the same as before—that is, information regarding recruitment of appropriate numbers of motor units. A smooth, coordinated movement is produced. The involvement of the muscle spindles in voluntary motor movements is referred to as the **gamma loop** or **gamma system**.

The Golgi Tendon Organs

The Golgi tendon organs, located within the tendons, are also sensitive to stretch. However, since they lie in the tendon rather than in the muscle itself, they are stretched when the muscle in whose tendon they lie contracts. The information that the Golgi tendon organs sends to the central nervous system is concerned with the strength of contraction. When the contraction is so strong that injury may result, the information returned from the central nervous system causes the muscle to relax. The importance of such a reflex is obvious; not only does it guard against potential muscle injury but it also provides further information concerning the status of muscular activity. In the latter capacity, the tendon organs complement the muscle spindles and in so doing facilitate efficient and effective movement patterns.

Higher Centers and Control of Movement

As already indicated, simple movements, such as removing your hand from a hot stove, are controlled reflexively at the level of the spinal cord without involvement of higher centers such as the brain. More complicated movement patterns, such as those involved in many sports skills, are controlled by higher centers (i.e., by the brain and higher levels of the spinal cord). Generally speaking, the motor neurons located in the spinal cord (**lower**

motor neurons) affect the actual contraction of muscles, whereas the **upper motor neurons** in the higher centers (brain) program the sequences of contractions.

Motor Areas of the Brain (Cortex)

Located within the cerebral cortex of the brain are two areas containing specialized neurons that cause motor movement when stimulated. Each area gives rise to its own kinds of movement patterns.

Primary Motor Area and the Pyramidal Tract

The primary motor area, or motor cortex, of the brain contains groups of motor neurons, some of which are referred to as **Betz cells**. The motor cortex is divided into subareas according to body areas involving specific movement patterns. For example, subareas are localized for movement patterns involving the feet, hands, thighs, shoulders, tongue, fingers, and so on. Most of the voluntary movement patterns initiated by the motor cortex are highly specific, being delicate and discrete in nature. It is important to emphasize that subareas in the motor cortex are localized according to movement patterns, not the contraction of individual muscles. The practical aspects of this arrangement are obvious. If we had to initiate movements according to individual muscles, we all would have to be expert kinesiologists and functional anatomists, knowing every muscle by name and action!

As shown schematically in Figure 6-21, the axons of the upper motor neurons located in the motor cortex descend, via the **pyramidal tract**, to lower motor neurons that lie in the spinal cord. The axons of the pyramidal tract synapse with these lower motor neurons. In turn, the axons from the lower motor neurons exit from the ventral root of the spinal cord and terminate within specific muscles.

Premotor Area and Extrapyramidal Tracts

In front of the primary motor area is a region called the **premotor area**, where another group of motor neurons is located. (The motor area and the premotor area are neurally connected by what are called association fibers.) Stimulation of the motor cells within the premotor area causes movement patterns that are grosser and more complex than those controlled by the motor cortex.

The axons from the neurons located in the premotor area descend to the lower motor neurons via a complicated and indirect series of tracts, collectively referred to as the **extrapyramidal tract**. This is shown to the right in Figure 6-21. Notice that one of the relay stations in the extrapyramidal tract is the **cerebellum**. This part of the brain is responsible for the coordination of movement patterns involving large groups of muscles. In other words, it is responsible for the synchronous and orderly activity of groups of muscles.

Obviously, cerebellar control would be greatly aided by sensory input, and sensory information is in fact relayed from the muscle sense organs

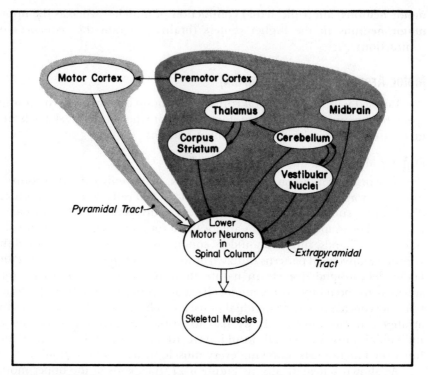

Figure 6-21 The neural pathways of the pyramidal and extrapyramidal tracts. (Modified and redrawn from Gatz, 1966.)

(proprioceptors) to the cerebellum. This type of information, you will recall, is associated with the exact location in space of the parts of the body and the amount of tension that exists in the muscles and tendons. With this additional information, a more precise and exacting movement is effected by the cerebellum through its coordinating and synchronous functions. It is easily seen that such information is of vital importance in the execution of the involved and detailed movements associated with sports activities. The cerebellum is very important indeed to the athlete, and to any one interested in sports activities.

Execution of a Voluntary Movement

By way of summary, let's take a sports skill, such as a forehand stroke in tennis, and outline the neural pathways involved in its execution. If the skill is new (i.e., if you are just learning it), the movement will be initiated in the subarea of the motor cortex dealing with those body areas involved in the movement. From there a series of responses will be relayed via the pyramidal tracts to the lower motor neurons of the spinal cord, proceeding from there to the specific muscles necessary to execute the skill. To this flow is added the proprioceptor input—the information from the muscle sense organs. Relayed by way of the cerebellum, this input effects smoothness (in terms, for instance, of the exact number of motor units to be recruited) and precision (e.g., the location of body parts in space). Once the skill is "learned," the movement pattern becomes less conscious. It is at this point, when the movement becomes more general, that the initiation of the movement is shifted to the premotor area. As you can see, there is every reason for the premotor area to be referred to as the "sport skills" area.

Summary

- The basic functional unit of a nerve is the neuron, or nerve cell. It consists of a cell body, dendrites, and an axon. The axon can be either medullated or nonmedullated.

- Sensory nerves convey information from the periphery to the central nervous system (brain and spinal cord), whereas motor nerves convey information from the central nervous system to effector organs such as glands and muscles. The reflex is an example of sensory and motor nerves and the central nervous system working together.

- The nerve impulse is information in the form of electrical energy (action potential) that is self-propagated along the entire length of the axon. Conduction of the nerve impulse along a medullated axon is fast and is referred to as saltatory conduction. Conduction along nonmedullated axons is slow.

- A synapse is a junction between nerves, whereas the neuromuscular junction is a point of connection between nerve and muscle. Chemical transmitter substances help relay information at the synapse and neuromuscular junction.

- Connective tissues surround the skeletal muscle. Surrounding the entire muscle is epimysium; around the muscle bundles, or fasciculi, is the perimysium; around the muscle fibers (cells) is the endomysium. The sarcolemma is the muscle cell membrane.

- Myofibrils, components of the muscle fiber, contain two protein filaments, myosin and actin. Cross-bridges that project toward actin are part of the myosin filament. The smallest functional unit of the myofibril is the sarcomere (distance between two Z lines).

- It is thought that when a muscle shortens, the actin filaments slide over the myosin filaments toward the center of the sarcomere. (This is referred to as the sliding filament theory of muscular contraction.)

- Muscular contractions have been classified as:

   Isotonic—muscle shortens while developing tension
   Isometric—muscle develops tension but does not change length
   Isokinetic—muscle shortens while developing maximal tension throughout the full range of movement at constant speed
   Eccentric—muscle lengthens while developing tension

- Muscle soreness is most pronounced one to two days after eccentric contractions. A lesser degree of soreness usually results from isotonic and isometric contractions, and isokinetic contractions produce the least amount of soreness. Muscle soreness is probably caused by damage to the connective tissues.

- A motor nerve and all the muscle fibers it innervates are called a motor unit. There are basically two types of motor units (or muscle fibers) in human muscle, fast-twitch (FT) and slow-twitch (ST).

- As their name suggests, fast-twitch units are fast to contract. Preferentially used during sprint-like activities, FT units are also characterized by:

Low aerobic capacity
High glycolytic (lactic acid) capacity
Low capillary density
Large force of contraction
High fatiguability
Large distribution in nonendurance athletes

- ST units, which are slow to contract, are preferentially used during activities requiring endurance. Slow-twitch units are also characterized by:

High aerobic capacity
Low glycolytic (lactic acid) capacity
High capillary density
Small force of contraction
Low fatiguability
Large distribution in endurance athletes

- The force-velocity curve represents the muscular force generated during movement performed at various speeds. Power athletes, in comparison to nonathletes and endurance athletes, are capable of exerting greater forces at similar velocities of movement and achieving greater velocities of movement while exerting similar forces. This capability is positively related to the percentage distribution of FT units and to physical training.

- Fiber-type distribution, maximal muscular power, patellar reflex time, and reaction time have substantial genetic components, suggesting that they are highly heritable.

- Local muscular fatigue following short-term, high-intensity exercise is most likely caused by lactic acid accumulation in the blood and muscles.

- Fatigue following endurance exercises is not caused by lactic acid accumulation, but rather by such factors as depletion of muscle and liver glycogen, low blood glucose, loss of body water and electrolytes, high body temperature, and boredom.

- Muscle spindles and Golgi tendon organs provide sensory information relative to the status of muscular activity, thereby providing for smooth, coordinated movement patterns.

- The motor area of the brain (cortex) causes motor movement when stimulated. The primary motor area, which is divided into subareas according to body areas, is responsible for specific movement patterns, whereas the premotor area is responsible for more complex and grosser patterns. The premotor area is also called the "sports skills" area.

Selected References and Readings*

Abraham, W.: Factors in delayed muscle soreness. *Med Sci. Sports, 9*:11-20, 1977.

Assmussen, E.: Observations on experimental muscle soreness. *Acta Rheumatologica Scand., 1*: 109-116, 1956.

Baldwin, K. M., P. J. Campbell, and D. A. Cooke: Glycogen, lactate, and alanine changes in muscle fiber types during graded exercise. *J. Appl. Physiol.: Respirat. Environ. Exercise Physiol., 43(2)*:288-291, 1977.

Burke, E., F. Cerny, D. Costill, and W. Fink: Characteristics of skeletal muscle in competitive cyclists. *Med. Sci. Sports, 9*:109-112, 1977.

Burke, R., and V. Edgerton: Motor unit properties and selective involvement in movement. *In* Wilmore, J., and J. Keogh (eds.): *Exercise and Sport Sciences Reviews.* Vol. 3. New York, Academic Press, 1975, pp. 31-81.

Costill, D., et al.: Skeletal muscle enzymes and fiber composition in male and female track athletes. *J. Appl. Physiol., 40*:149-154, 1976.

Costill, D. L., and E. L. Fox: Energetics of marathon running. *Med. Sci. Sports, 1(2)*:81-86, 1969.

Costill, D., W. Fink, and M. Pollock: Muscle fiber composition and enzyme activities of elite distance runners. *Med. Sci. Sports, 8*:96-100, 1976.

DeVries, H.: Quantitative electromyographic investigation of the spasm theory of muscle pain. *Am. J. Phys. Med., 45*:119-134, 1966.

Essén, B., et al.: Metabolic characteristics of fiber types in human skeletal muscle. *Acta Physiol. Scand., 95*:153-165, 1975.

Fox, E. L., and D. K. Mathews: *The Physiological Basis of Physical Education and Athletics.* 3rd ed. Philadelphia, Saunders College Publishing, 1981, pp. 81-114.

Gatz, A.: *Manter's Essentials of Clinical Neuroanatomy and Neurophysiology.* 3rd ed. Philadelphia, F. A. Davis Company, 1966, p. 121.

Gollnick, P., et al.: Enzyme activity and fiber composition in skeletal muscle of untrained and trained men. *J. Appl. Physiol., 33*:312-319, 1972.

Hough, T.: Ergographic studies in muscular soreness. *Am. J. Physiol., 7*:76-92, 1902.

Jansson, E., B. Sjödin, and P. Tesch: Changes in muscle fibre type distribution in man after physical training. *Acta Physiol. Scand., 104*:235-237, 1978.

Karlsson, J., et al.: Relevance of muscle fibre type to fatigue in short intense and prolonged exercise in man. *In Human Muscle Fatigue: Physiological Mechanisms.* Pitman Medical, London (Ciba Foundation Symposium 82), pp. 59-74, 1981.

Komi, P., and E. Buskirk: The effect of eccentric and concentric muscle activity on tension and electrical activity of human muscle. *Ergonomics, 15*:417-434, 1972.

Komi, P., V. Klissouras, and E. Karvinen: Genetic variation in neuromuscular performance. *Int. Z. Angew. Physiol., 31*:289-304, 1973.

Komi, P., et al.: Anaerobic performance capacity in athletes. *Acta Physiol. Scand., 100*:107-114, 1977.

Komi, P., et al.: Skeletal muscle fibers and muscle enzyme activities in monozygous and dizygous twins of both sexes. *Acta Physiol. Scand., 100*:385-392, 1977.

Pipes, T., and J. Wilmore: Isokinetic vs. isotonic strength training in adult men. *Med. Sci. Sports, 7*:262-274, 1975.

Schwane, J. A., et al.: Delayed-onset muscular soreness and plasma CPK and LDH activities after downhill running. *Med. Sci. Sports Exercise, 15(1)*:51-56, 1983.

Staton, W.: The influence of ascorbic acid in minimizing post-exercise soreness in young men. *Res. Quart., 23*:356-360, 1952.

---

*For full journal titles, see Appendix A.

Talag, T.: Residual muscular soreness as influenced by concentric, eccentric and static contractions. *Res. Quart., 44:*458–469, 1973.

Tesch, P., et al.: Muscle fatigue and its relation to lactate accumulation and LDH activity in man. *Acta Physiol. Scand., 103:*413–420, 1978.

Thorstensson, A., G. Grimby, and J. Karlsson: Force-velocity relations and fiber composition in human knee extensor muscles. *J. Appl. Physiol., 40:*12–16, 1976.

Thorstensson, A., and J. Karlsson: Fatiguability and fiber composition of human skeletal muscle. *Acta Physiol. Scand., 98:*318–322, 1976.

Thorstensson, A., et al.: Muscle strength and fiber composition in athletes and sedentary men. *Med. Sci. Sports, 9:*26–30, 1977.

Thorstensson, A.: Muscle strength, fiber types and enzyme activities in man. *Acta Physiol. Scand.* [*Suppl. 443*]:1977.

7

Weight-Resistance Training: Methods and Effects

Introduction

Not too long ago, weight-resistance programs designed to develop muscular strength were thought to render the user incapable of successfully carrying out most sports activities. Trainees were described with such terms as

123

"muscle-bound," "stiff," and "inflexible." Furthermore, if the trainees were women, it was thought that they would almost certainly develop all of the male characteristics, including large, "bulging" muscles, deep voices, and even beards given enough time!

Of course, none of the above is true. However, it is true that weight-resistance training has been one of the most misunderstood concepts in athletics. It is the general purpose of this chapter, therefore, to clear up some of the misconceptions associated with weight-resistance training, particularly as they apply to athletic programs and sports performance. More specifically, the following areas will be discussed: the basic principles associated with weight-training programs; the construction of weight-resistance programs for various sports; the physiological changes in the neuromuscular system resulting from weight-resistance training; the effects of weight-resistance training on sports performance; and the effects of steroid consumption on muscular size and strength during weight-resistance training.

Basic Principles Associated with Weight-Training Programs

There are four principles that should form the basis of most weight-resistance programs. It is best for training to involve **overload** and **progressive resistance**, with careful attention going to the **arrangement** of the program and the **specificity** of its effects.

The Overload Principle

Muscular strength is most effectively developed when the muscle or muscle group is **overloaded**—that is, exercised against resistances exceeding those normally encountered. The use of resistances that overload the muscle stimulates the physiological adaptations that lead to increased muscular strength. The strength of an **underloaded** muscle—a muscle exercising against resistances that are normally encountered—will be maintained at its present level but will not increase (see Fig. 7-1).

The Principle of Progressive Resistance

Since an overloaded muscle gains in strength during the course of a weight-training program, the initial overload (resistance) will, sometime later in the program, no longer provide adequate overload for continued gains in strength. In other words, the original overload eventually becomes an underload as strength is gained. For this reason, the resistance against which the muscle is exercised must be increased periodically throughout the course of the weight-training program. One way to judge when a new overload should be introduced is to count the number of times a given weight can be

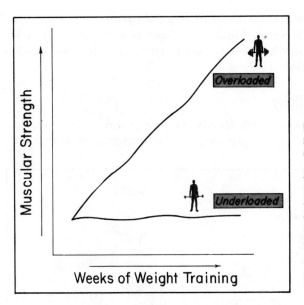

Figure 7-1 Muscular strength is most effectively developed when the muscle is overloaded—that is, exercised against resistances that exceed those normally encountered. The strength of an under-loaded muscle—one that is exercised against normally encountered resistance—will be maintained but not increased.

lifted before fatigue sets in. For example, suppose an athlete, at the beginning of a program, can curl 80 lb eight times before fatigue sets in. That amount of overload may be used until the athlete can make perhaps 12 lifts before becoming fatigued. At that time, the load should be increased to such a degree that the number of repetitions to the point of fatigue is once again reduced to eight. This pattern should be repeated as often as required throughout the duration of the program. In this manner, the muscle will always work in the overload zone. Strength programs that follow this principle are called **progressive-resistance exercises.**

The Principle of Arrangement of Exercises

The exercises in a weight-resistance program should be arranged so that the larger muscle groups are exercised before the smaller ones. The reason for this arrangement is that smaller muscles tend to fatigue sooner and more easily than do larger groups. Therefore, in order to ensure proper overload of the larger muscles, they should be exercised first, before the smaller ones fatigue. The larger leg and hip muscle groups should, for instance, be exercised before the smaller arm muscles.

Training programs should also be so arranged that no two successive exercises involve the same muscle groups. This ensures adequate recovery time after each lift. For example, the bench press and overhead or standing press should not be performed one after the other, since they both involve similar muscle groups. Instead, several exercises involving other muscle groups should intervene. The stiff-legged dead lift, for the back and the posterior muscles of the legs, and heel (toe) raises, for the lower legs and ankles, would be appropriate. The order in which the major muscle groups should be exercised is shown in Figure 7-2. Note how the larger muscle groups are exercised first and how no two exercises involving the same muscle groups follow in succession.

The Principle of Specificity

Weight-training programs are specific in several ways. For example, strength development is specific not only to the muscle groups that are

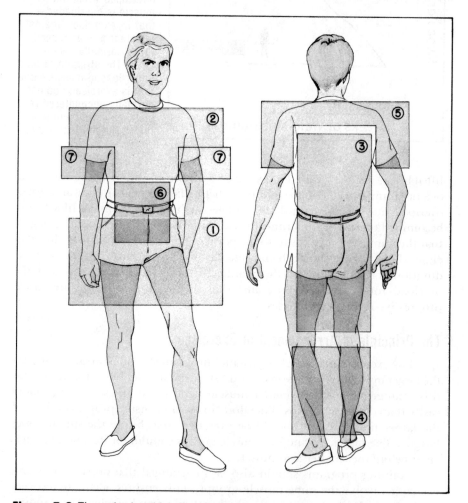

Figure 7-2 The order in which the major muscle groups should be exercised. The larger muscle groups should be exercised first, and no two exercises involving the same muscle groups should follow in succession. Code: 1, upper legs and hips; 2, chest and upper arms; 3, back and posterior aspect of legs; 4, lower legs and ankles; 5, shoulders and posterior aspect of upper arms; 6, abdomen; and 7, anterior aspect of upper arms.

exercised but also to the movement patterns they produce. In other words, weight-resistance training appears to be motor-skill specific. This means that exercising the muscle groups involved in a particular movement in order to develop strength that may be directly applied during the execution of the movement will be most effective if the **pattern** of the movement is simulated as closely as possible. Thus, if you wish to increase your strength for purposes of improving your skill in the soccer kick, the weight-training program must involve those muscles working through the movement patterns associated with the soccer kick.

Motor-skill specificity is perhaps most apparent in athletes who participate in back-to-back seasonal sports. Although in most cases the same muscle groups are used in both sports, the movement patterns they produce are quite different. Thus, frequently, the football player who is in excellent condition to play football is in poor condition to play basketball. This type of specificity is even seen within a single sport. For example, the Olympic sprinter who is in excellent condition to sprint would be considered in poor condition to run the marathon (and vice versa). Yet, both activities involve the same general muscle groups and movement patterns.

Motor-skill specificity may be attributed at least in part to the force-velocity relationships that govern the functioning of the skeletal muscles. That is, as was pointed out in the last chapter (p. 104), the amount of muscular force exerted during the execution of a particular movement pattern is related to the speed at which the movement is performed (see Fig. 7-3). In most sports

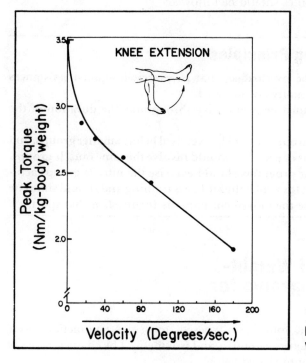

Figure 7-3 The force-velocity curve.

activities, even though similar muscle groups are active, the performance of a specific motor skill requires a specific force-velocity relationship.

The physiological mechanisms underlying this kind of specificity are not completely understood. Recent evidence supports the idea that neuromuscular factors such as improved coordination of different muscles and even of different motor units within the same muscle are involved. If this is the case, there must be changes not only in the muscle itself but within the central nervous system as well (more will be said about these changes later—see p. 156).

Besides being motor-skill specific, strength development from training is specific to the joint angles at which the muscle groups are exercised and the type of contraction the muscles perform. Joint-angle specificity is particularly evident following isometric-training programs, in which the exercises are generally performed at a single joint angle. In this case, the increase in strength is usually greatest at the "training" angle, with little carry-over to other joint angles. As for strength development specific to the type of muscular contraction, it has been found (for example) that isotonic weight-training programs will increase isotonic strength more than isometric strength, and vice versa. Although the same applies to isokinetic programs, recent information suggests that strength gains resulting from isokinetic training at fast speeds are more general, in that there is a carry-over to isotonic strength. This is not true for isokinetic training at slow speeds.

In order to ensure the greatest benefits from any weight-training program, several guidelines should be followed:

Weight-Training Principles

Muscles must be overloaded, that is, exercised against resistances exceeding those normally encountered.

The overload must be progressive throughout the duration of the program.

Larger muscle groups should be exercised before smaller groups, and no two successive lifts or exercises should involve the same muscle groups.

Weight-training programs should exercise the muscle groups actually used in the sport for which the athlete is training and should simulate as closely as possible the movement patterns involved in that sport.

Construction of Weight-Resistance Programs for Various Sports

In the last chapter, four basic types of muscular contractions were analyzed: isotonic, isometric, eccentric, and isokinetic. The characteristics of these contractions are summarized below:

1. Isotonic (dynamic, concentric)—muscle shortens as tension is developed
2. Isometric (static)—muscle develops tension but does not change length
3. Eccentric—muscle lengthens as tension develops
4. Isokinetic—muscle shortens as tension is developed through a full range of motion performed at constant speed

Since each kind of contraction is used (to various extents) in most sports activities, weight-training programs designed around each type of contraction will be discussed.

Isotonic Programs

An isotonic program involves exercises performed against resistance, typified by lifting either free weights (barbells) or weight stacks such as used on the Universal Gym, Nautilus, and other similar equipment.

One of the first systematic isotonic weight training programs was developed by DeLorme and Watkins over 35 years ago. Although their program was developed mainly for rehabilitation purposes, their basic concepts are still used today for athletic programs. One of their most important concepts was the **repetition maximum** (**RM**). A repetition maximum is defined as the maximal load a muscle or muscle group can lift a given number of times before fatiguing. For example, if a person can lift a particular weight eight times and no more before fatiguing, that weight is an eight-RM load. Obviously, the same weight could be a ten-RM load for another person or for the same individual under different circumstances.

For each muscle group to be trained, DeLorme and Watkins' original isotonic program is as follows:

Set 1   10 repetitions at a ½ 10-RM load
Set 2   10 repetitions at a ¾ 10-RM load
Set 3   10 repetitions at a 10-RM load

The structure of this program is worth examining. The program requires the performance of three sets. A **set** is the number of repetitions done consecutively without resting. As you can see, the first two sets are not maximal but are only one half and three quarter loads. Specifically, Set 1 calls for ten repetitions performed against a load that is only one half of the maximum for that number of repetitions. Thus, if the full ten-RM load were 80 lb, a one half ten-RM load would equal 40 lb. Lifting the 40-lb load ten times without resting would meet the requirements of Set 1. Set 2 calls for ten repetitions with a three quarter ten-RM load. Again taking 80 lb as the full ten-RM load, the requirement in Set 2 is to lift 60 lb ten times. Whatever the actual poundage of the ten-RM load, you can see that the first two sets are designed as warm-ups. The third set is designed to satisfy the overload principle. (In keeping with the **progressive** overload principle, a new overload was to be established when 15 repetitions of each ten-RM load could be performed.)

The majority of today's isotonic programs follow the general principles set forth by DeLorme and Watkins. However, several questions have been raised. What, for instance, are the optimal numbers of sets and RM loads with regard to development of strength and muscular endurance? How many training days per week and how many weeks are necessary for optimal strength and endurance gains? Can strength and muscular endurance be optimally obtained from a single program?

Sets and Repetitions

It is not possible to claim with absolute confidence that a certain number of sets performed at a certain RM load is, in all cases, the one combination that will increase strength and muscular endurance more than any other combination. Consider the comparative data in Figure 7–4, which shows the results of a study using isotonic programs that varied widely in sets and RM loads. Note first that significant isotonic strength gains were made in programs consisting of as few as one set at two-RM loads and as many as three sets at ten-RM loads. Secondly, it may be seen that three quite different combinations produced equivalent strength gains: three sets at two-RM loads, two sets at six-RM loads, and one set at a ten-RM load all yielded a 25% gain. As for the greatest strength gains, in this study a program consisting of three sets at six-RM loads appeared to be most productive. However, in a study specifically comparing programs involving three sets, it was found that RM loads of two to three, five to six, and nine to ten produced equivalent strength gains. To further complicate the issue, in a study involving only **one** set it was concluded that the optimal RM load was somewhere between three and nine. And, in yet another study, programs consisting of six sets at two-RM loads, three sets at six-RM loads, and three sets at ten-RM loads all produced significant and equivalent gains in strength.

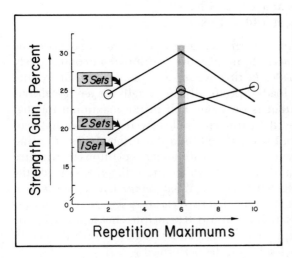

Figure 7-4 Significant isotonic strength gains may be made from programs ranging in requirements from one set at a 2-RM load to three sets of 10-RM loads. Notice that equivalent strength gains may be made from programs of three sets at 2-RM loads, two sets at 6-RM loads, and one set at a 10-RM load. Note also that a program of three sets at 6-RM loads appears to produce the greatest strength gains. (Based on data from Berger, 1962b.)

It may be concluded from the above findings that significant isotonic strength gains may be made from programs consisting of as few as one set and as many as six sets, with the load varying from two-RM to ten-RM. From a practical viewpoint, it is recommended that isotonic strength programs consist of between one and three sets and two- and ten-RM loads. Six sets at most RM loads would require a considerable amount of time.

Frequency and Duration

In DeLorme and Watkins' original program, a training frequency of four days per week was the maximum that could be tolerated consistently over a relatively long period of time. Among today's weight-training coaches, it is generally agreed that an isotonic weight-training program of three days per week will produce significant gains in strength without risking the possibility of chronic fatigue. It should be stressed at this time that chronic fatigue due to inadequate day-to-day recovery from heavy weight resistance programs is the enemy of training. Adequate recovery, not only from day to day but also between sets, should always be emphasized.

Provided the frequency of exercise is within the proper bounds just cited, significant strength gains may be expected to occur following weight training programs of six weeks or longer.

Strength versus Muscular Endurance

Isotonic **strength** is defined as the maximal pulling force of a muscle, whereas isotonic **muscular endurance** is the ability of a muscle group to repeatedly lift a load over an extended period of time. Traditionally, the development of muscular strength through isotonic weight resistance training was thought to be best accomplished with programs consisting of low repetitions and high resistance. Muscular endurance, on the other hand, was thought to be best developed through programs of high repetition and low resistance. Although many authorities still differentiate between "strength" and "endurance" programs, scientific evidence for such a distinction is not consistent. Although the idea may be valid, it needs first to be clarified, and second to be extended.

Clarification involves the term "low resistance." We must remember that the progressive overload principle is also a requisite for improvement of muscular endurance. Prolonged repetitions of "underloaded" muscles have little effect on endurance.

Extension of the rule is based on the fact that both strength and endurance have been shown to be equally developed from either a low-repetition and high-load program or a high-repetition and low-load program. This can be seen in Figure 7–5. In this case, both the so-called endurance and strength programs consisted of three training sessions per week for six or seven weeks. Each training session of the "endurance" program consisted of elbow flexion at a rate of 40 repetitions per min with a load of 11 lb until exhaustion was reached. The "strength" program consisted of arm curls performed according to the DeLorme-Watkins progression outlined on page 129. It should be

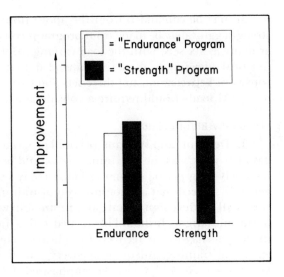

Figure 7-5 Isotonic strength and muscular endurance have been shown to be equally developed by programs of low repetitions and high resistance ("strength" programs) and high repetitions and low resistance ("endurance" programs). (Based on data from Clarke and Stull, 1970, and Stull and Clarke, 1970.)

noted, however, that this progression involves a total of 30 repetitions and as such may not be considered as a low-repetition program. For example, in a more recent study, it was found that isotonic strength could be improved significantly more with a weight-training program involving 12 repetitions of an 80% maximum load than with 20 repetitions of a 50% maximum load. Isotonic endurance, on the other hand, increased significantly more in the latter program.

In another recent study, three types of isotonic programs were compared for strength and endurance gains. One program consisted of performing three sets of a six to eight repetition-maximum load (RM). This was designated as a high-resistance, low-repetition program. A second program consisted of performing two sets of a 30 to 40 RM load. This was called a medium-resistance, medium-repetition program. The third program tested was a low-resistance, high-repetition program in which the subjects lifted one set of a 100 to 150 RM load. The frequency of each program was three days per week; the duration was nine weeks. Both isotonic strength and endurance were measured before and after training, the results of which are shown in Figure 7-6. Notice that strength gains were significantly greater following the high-resistance, low-repetition program. However, the gain in endurance, although greater in the medium- and low-resistance programs, was not **statistically different*** from that gained in the high-resistance program. These findings again point to a high-resistance, low-repetition program as most effective in increasing both strength and endurance.

---

*If differences are not statistically significant, it means that the difference could be due to chance.

Despite these conflicting results, one of the implications of these findings is that the same strength and endurance gains may be achieved in a more economical way by higher-intensity, lower-repetition techniques. Programs involving a very high number of repetitions with a very low resistance require more time. If time is a factor, the overload technique heretofore considered characteristic of strength training would be preferable.

Since most sports activities involve the major muscle groups of the body, a basic isotonic program should consist of a core of exercises that develops these groups. Examples of core programs are given in Table 7-1, and a description of which muscle groups are involved and how to perform the various weight exercises is given in Appendix C. Remember, the number of sets should be between one and three, and the RM loads should be between two and ten. At the beginning of the program, lighter loads and more repetitions are recommended, for example, two sets of ten-RM loads. Later in the program, three sets of six-RM loads might be used, since this combination has been shown to yield substantial strength gains (see Fig. 7-4).

When beginning an isotonic program, there is always the question of how to determine the starting loads for the various exercises. Ultimately, the best way is by trial and error. If, for instance, a ten-RM load is desired, then the athlete must lift several loads over a period of time in order to pinpoint the load that can be lifted just ten times to exhaustion. For some weight exercises, rough estimates of the starting load (for two sets at ten-RM loads) may be made if one knows either the trainee's body weight or the maximum amount of

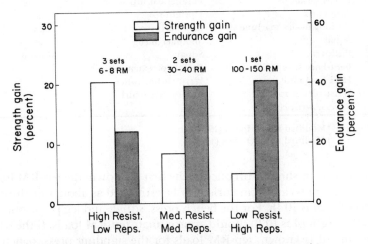

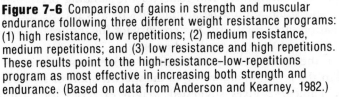

Figure 7-6 Comparison of gains in strength and muscular endurance following three different weight resistance programs: (1) high resistance, low repetitions; (2) medium resistance, medium repetitions; and (3) low resistance and high repetitions. These results point to the high-resistance–low-repetitions program as most effective in increasing both strength and endurance. (Based on data from Anderson and Kearney, 1982.)

Table 7-1: Examples of Basic Isotonic Weight-Training Programs for Athletes

Frequency	3 days per week
Duration	6 weeks or more
Repetitions and Load	First 2 weeks = 2 × 10-RM (sit-ups = 2 × 25). Remaining weeks = 3 × 6-RM (sit-ups = 1 × 25 + 1 × maximum)
Rest between sets of exercise	5-10 min

Program A*

Monday	Wednesday	Friday
Squats		
Bench press		
Stiff-legged dead lift		
Heel (toe) raises	Same	Same
Standing press	as	as
Bent-knee sit-ups	Monday	Monday
Arm curls		
Wrist curl or roller		
Reverse wrist curl		

Program B†

Monday	Wednesday	Friday
Bench press	Incline press	
Power clean	Parallel bar dip	
Arm curls	Upright row	
Pulldown—lat machine	Arm curls	Same
Squat	Shoulder shrug	as
Pullover	Squat	Monday
Bent-knee sit-up	Back hyperextension	
Heel (toe) raise	Wrist curl or roller	
Wrist curl or roller	Reverse wrist curl	
Reverse wrist curl		

*Modified from Hooks (1974).
†Modified from O'Shea (1969).

weight that he or she can lift once. If the first is known, the ten-RM loads for the clean and press and arm curls may be estimated as about one third of the body weight plus 10 lb. For the bench press, squat, and leg press, one half of the body weight plus 10 lb should approximate ten-RM loads. If the trainee's maximum lift is known, ten-RM loads for the standing press, bench press, arm curl, and squat should be around 40% of this lift. As useful as these approximations are, it will still be necessary for the trainee to find his or her **exact** starting load through trial and error.

Using the basic principles outlined above, more exercises may be included in the program according to the specific sport or sports activity in question. Table 7-2 gives suggested weight exercises for various sports activities. Remember, descriptions of these exercises are given in Appendix C.

Isometric Programs

Isometrics involve muscular contractions performed against fixed, immovable resistances. This type of muscular training became very popular in the United States when two German scientists, Hettinger and Müller, reported that strength could be increased an average of 5% per week when isometric tension was held for just 6 sec at two thirds of maximum strength once a day for five days per week.

As would be expected, the above findings revolutionized the entire concept of strength training and triggered many new studies involving the isometric technique. Interestingly, most of these new studies failed to support the original contention that strength could be improved at a rate of 5% per week. However, they did confirm that strength could be significantly increased when isometric tension is held for 6 sec at two thirds of maximum strength once a day for five days per week.

Number and Intensity of Contractions

Several studies dealing with the effects of the number and intensity of isometric contractions on strength gains have been conducted. Researchers have specifically sought to determine if one or more contractions performed at higher than the two thirds maximum reported by Hettinger and Müller would produce greater gains in strength. The results so far have been mixed. For example, in one study it was found that strength gains in subjects using the once-per-day, two thirds maximum contraction equaled those in subjects using an 80% maximum contraction performed five times per day. In another study, one contraction per day was used, with different groups of high school students (boys and girls) performing the contraction at 25, 50, 75, or 100% of their maximum strength. The results, shown in Figure 7-7, revealed that all groups, with the exception of the subjects who trained with 25% maximum resistance, significantly increased their strength. Other studies have produced results that differ still further. In fact, in one study conducted by Müller himself, it was found that maximal isometric strength could best be developed if training sessions were scheduled for five days per week and consisted of five to ten maximal contractions held for 5 sec each.

It would appear that this last program—Müller's newly suggested five to ten maximal contractions held for 5 sec—is the best from a practical viewpoint. The practicality stems from the use of maximal contractions; if a fraction of maximum is used, it is difficult if not impossible to accurately judge the true percentage of one's exertion without proper equipment. Thus, although strength may be increased with contractions as low as 50% of maximum (as pointed out above), the best choice would seem to be contraction at an absolute (maximum) level.

In terms of isometric muscular endurance, isometric training has been shown to increase one's ability to sustain an isometric contraction; however,

Table 7-2: Suggested Weight Exercises for Various Sports Activities*

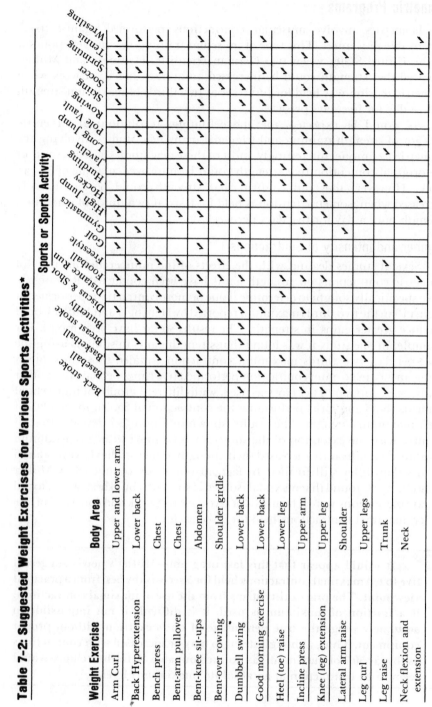

Weight Exercise	Body Area	Back stroke	Baseball	Basketball	Breast stroke	Butterfly	Discus & Shot	Distance Run	Football	Freestyle	Golf	Gymnastics	High Jump	Hockey	Hurdling	Javelin	Long Jump	Pole Vault	Rowing	Skiing	Soccer	Sprinting	Tennis	Wrestling
Arm Curl	Upper and lower arm	✓	✓	✓			✓		✓		✓	✓		✓		✓		✓	✓	✓			✓	✓
Back Hyperextension	Lower back						✓		✓			✓				✓		✓	✓	✓	✓	✓		
Bench press	Chest	✓		✓	✓	✓	✓		✓	✓	✓	✓		✓		✓		✓	✓	✓	✓	✓		
Bent-arm pullover	Chest	✓		✓	✓	✓	✓		✓	✓									✓	✓				
Bent-knee sit-ups	Abdomen	✓	✓	✓	✓	✓	✓	✓	✓	✓	✓	✓	✓	✓	✓	✓	✓	✓	✓	✓	✓	✓	✓	✓
Bent-over rowing	Shoulder girdle	✓		✓	✓	✓	✓		✓	✓		✓		✓		✓		✓	✓	✓				
Dumbbell swing	Lower back	✓	✓	✓	✓	✓	✓	✓	✓	✓	✓	✓	✓	✓	✓	✓	✓	✓	✓	✓	✓	✓	✓	✓
Good morning exercise	Lower back	✓	✓		✓		✓		✓		✓			✓		✓		✓	✓	✓		✓		
Heel (toe) raise	Lower leg	✓		✓			✓	✓	✓			✓	✓	✓	✓	✓	✓	✓		✓	✓	✓		
Incline press	Upper arm	✓	✓	✓		✓	✓		✓		✓	✓		✓		✓		✓	✓	✓			✓	✓
Knee (leg) extension	Upper leg	✓	✓	✓		✓	✓	✓	✓		✓	✓	✓	✓	✓	✓	✓	✓		✓	✓	✓	✓	
Lateral arm raise	Shoulder	✓	✓	✓	✓	✓					✓	✓				✓				✓		✓		
Leg curl	Upper legs		✓	✓			✓	✓	✓			✓	✓	✓	✓	✓	✓	✓		✓	✓	✓		
Leg raise	Trunk	✓	✓	✓			✓	✓	✓			✓				✓			✓	✓	✓			
Neck flexion and extension	Neck						✓		✓		✓			✓										✓

Exercise	Muscle group
Parallel bar dip	Shoulder, upper and lower arm
Power clean	Trunk, shoulder girdle
Power snatch	Trunk, shoulder girdle
Press behind neck	Shoulder
Pulldown—lat machine	Shoulder girdle
Reverse curl	Lower arm
Reverse wrist curl	Forearm
Shoulder shrug	Shoulder
Squat	Lower and upper back, upper legs
Standing press	Shoulder, upper arms
Stiff-legged dead lift	Lower back
Straight-arm pullover	Chest
Triceps extension	Shoulder, upper arm
Upright rowing	Shoulder
Wrist curl or wrist roller	Forearm

*Modified from O'Shea (1969) and Hooks (1974).

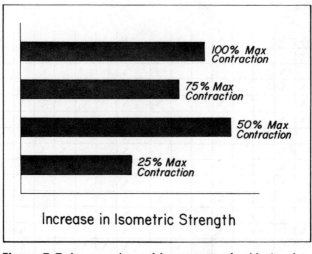

Figure 7-7 A comparison of four groups of subjects who isometrically trained using one contraction per day at 25%, 50%, 75%, or 100% of maximum strength. All groups, with the exception of the 25% group, significantly increased their strength. (Based on data from Cotten, 1967.)

the programs that produce this increased isometric muscular endurance vary considerably.

Duration and Frequency

The early isometric programs generally had a training frequency of five days per week. Successful though such a schedule may be, substantial gains in both strength and muscular endurance have been observed in programs with a training frequency of three days per week. Whatever the frequency, the duration of the training program should be at least four to six weeks, with greater gains being made with longer durations.

Joint-Angle Specificity

As mentioned earlier, strength development in isometric training tends to be greatest at the joint angle at which the exercise is performed. Figure 7-8 shows the results of a study establishing this specificity. In the study, the isometric program consisted of three maximum pulls (contractions) in elbow flexion held for 6 sec. The angle of pull was 170°. As is clearly shown, the increase in isometric strength was much greater at the training angle than at 90°. This information serves to point out that if isometric strength over the full range of motion is desired, then exercises must be performed at several angles rather than just one. In most cases, this is a definite disadvantage of isometric training.

Functional, or Power Rack, Isometrics

Functional isometrics involve isometric contractions performed with weights. Such training actually combines isotonic and isometric exercises, in that the athlete performs a rapid and explosive isotonic movement, then isometrically sustains the movement for several seconds. Thus, the benefits of both types of contractions are gained. The exercises are performed with a piece of equipment referred to as a power rack. As shown in Figure 7-9, this apparatus is basically a rack for supporting a barbell at different levels. Stops or pins are positioned a few inches (usually 2 in) above the pins on which the barbell is resting. Both the resting and stop pins are adjustable. The exercises are performed by rapidly lifting the barbell against the upper stops, then holding it there for between 3 and 7 sec. In the figure, the standing or overhead press is being performed.

Isometric Programs for Athletes

Many sports require isometric strength and endurance. In wrestling, for example, some isometric endurance and strength will be needed by the wrestler who resists or attempts to position his opponent. In gymnastics, isometric strength and endurance are obviously required in balancing or sustaining certain body positions.

A basic isometric program for athletes is given in Table 7-3. The exercises that are listed may be performed with either regular isometrics or with the power rack (functional isometrics). Notice that the exercise angle is also given if only one angle is used. However, remember that for strength gains over a greater range of joint motion, at least two other angles, one lower and one higher, should be used. Also, remember that five to ten maximal contractions held for 5 to 7 sec should be performed at each joint angle that is used.

If an isotonic program is used along with an isometric program, then the training sessions should be scheduled so that the isotonic program is performed on Monday and Thursday and the isometric program on Tuesday and Friday, with Wednesday, Saturday, and Sunday as days of rest. Also, since

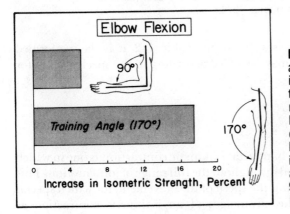

Figure 7-8 Isometric training and joint-angle specificity. The isometric program used in this study consisted of three maximum contractions in elbow flexion at an angle of pull of 170°, with each contraction held for 6 sec. The increase in isometric strength was greater at the training angle than at 90°. (Based on data from Meyers, 1967.)

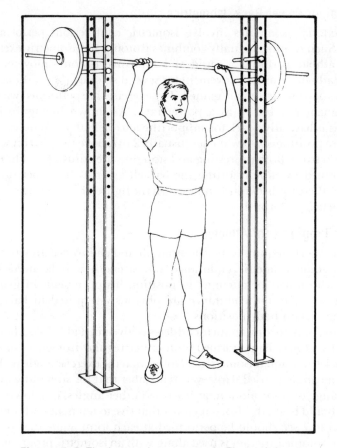

Figure 7-9 The isometric power rack. The rack has two sets of adjustable pins. The lower pins support a barbell with weights; the upper pins act as stops for the barbell. The exercise in this case (the standing or overhead press) is performed by rapidly lifting the barbell against the upper pins, where it is held for 3 to 7 sec. (Modified and redrawn from Hooks, 1974.)

most of the isotonic exercises listed in Table 7-2 may be performed isometrically as well, these may be added according to the specific sport for which the athlete is training.

Isokinetic Programs

As discussed in the last chapter, an isokinetic contraction is one in which maximal tension is developed throughout the full range of joint motion. This is accomplished by controlling the speed of the movement, for which special equipment is required. The advantages of an isokinetic contraction as

Table 7-3: An Example of a Basic Isometric Program for Athletes

Type	Regular Isometrics or Functional Isometrics
Frequency	3-5 days per week
Duration	4 weeks or more
Number of repetitions	5-10
Intensity	Maximum
Duration of contraction	5-7 seconds

Core Exercises*	Exercise Angle
Bench press	90°—Elbow joint
Dead lift	135°—Knee joint
Heel (toe) raises	135°—Foot angle
Standing press	90°—Elbow joint
Bent-knee sit-ups	90°—Knee joint
Arm curls	90°—Elbow joint
Upright rowing	135°—Elbow joint

*Modified from Hooks (1974).

compared to an isotonic contraction were discussed in the last chapter (see p. 95).

Isokinetic training is relatively new and has therefore not been the subject of a great many studies. However, based on the studies that have been conducted so far, it is clear that substantial strength gains from isokinetic training are possible. For example, following a three-day-per-week, eight-week program of isokinetic training, it was found that isokinetic strength increased nearly 30%.

Speed Specificity

As mentioned earlier, one of the unique features of isokinetic training is that the speed of movement may be controlled during the exercise. This is perhaps the most important feature of isokinetic training as related to sports training, since, in most sports activities, muscular force is applied during movement at various speeds. The relationship between muscular force and speed of movement was discussed earlier (see p. 104). It was pointed out then that the force-velocity curve is shifted upward and to the right in athletes, particularly those whose muscles contain a high percentage of fast-twitch fibers. In view of the fact that fiber-type distribution probably does not change through training, the question arises, "Can the force-velocity curve be shifted upward and to the right following isokinetic weight training?"

Several studies have recently been conducted in an attempt to answer this question, with research proceeding along many lines. In one study, the changes in isokinetic strength and endurance of the quadriceps muscle group were determined in two groups of subjects who trained three days per week for six weeks. The training consisted of a 2-min bout of maximal extension and flexion exercises at the knee joint. One group of subjects trained at a slow speed of movement (36° per sec) while the other group trained at a fast speed of movement (108° per sec). The effects on strength are shown in Figure 7-10. It

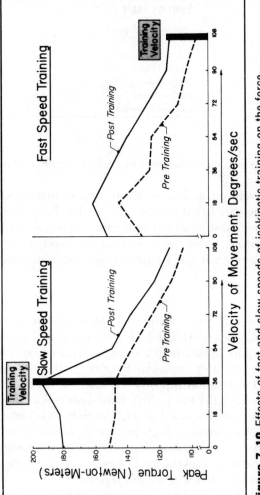

Figure 7-10 Effects of fast and slow speeds of isokinetic training on the force-velocity curve. Training at a slow speed produced the greatest increase in strength only at slow speeds of movement. However, with fast isokinetic training, the entire force-velocity curve is shifted upward and to the right. (Based on data from Moffroid and Whipple, 1970.)

is apparent that training at a slow speed produced the greatest increase in strength **only** at slow speeds of movement. On the other hand, training at a fast speed produced increases in strength at all speeds of contraction at and below the training speed. In other words, the entire force-velocity curve was indeed shifted upward and to the right following the fast-speed isokinetic training.

Although not shown in the figure, it was also found that training at a fast speed increased muscular endurance at fast speeds more than slow speed training increased endurance at slow speeds.

In another study, two different training speeds were again investigated. Once again the training program consisted of maximal knee extensions. In one group of subjects, training consisted of performing five sets of six maximal knee extensions at a speed of 60° per sec. This was designated as the slow-speed training program. In a second group of subjects, training consisted of performing five sets of 12 maximal knee extensions at a speed of 300° per sec. This constituted the fast-speed training program. Each of the groups performed the same amount of total work during the training sessions, and each trained three days per week for six weeks. Force-velocity curves were measured before and after the respective training programs. Strength gains at various velocities of movement are shown in Figure 7-11. Notice the speed specificity. For example, training at a fast speed (300° per sec) increased strength equally at both fast and slow speeds of movement whereas training at

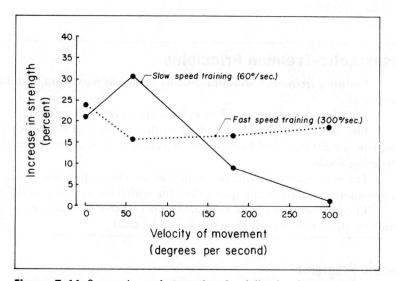

Figure 7-11 Comparison of strength gains following fast- and slow-speed isokinetic training. Training at a fast speed of movement (300°/sec) increased strength equally at both fast and slow speeds of movement, whereas training at a slow speed (60°/sec) produced increases in strength only at the slower speeds of movement. (Based on data from Coyle and co-workers, 1981.)

a slow speed (60° per sec) produced increases in strength only at the slower speeds of movement.

The following may be concluded from the above findings:

Isokinetic training at slow speeds produces substantial increases in strength only at slow movement speeds.

Isokinetic training at fast speeds produces increases in strength at all speeds of movement (i.e., at rates at and below the training speed).

Isokinetic training at fast speeds increases muscular endurance at fast speeds more than slow-speed training increases endurance at slow speeds of movement.

Getting back to the original question—"Can the force-velocity curve be shifted upward and to the right following isokinetic strength training?"—the answer is yes. However, remember that in order to shift the entire curve, fast-speed isokinetic training must be used.

Isokinetic Programs for Athletes

Since very little research has been conducted using isokinetic training, it is not possible at this time to suggest a specific isokinetic program for athletes. However, in attempts to set up such a program, the following guidelines should be useful:

Isokinetic-Training Principles

Training frequency should probably be between two and four days per week.

Training duration should be at least six weeks or longer.

The movement pattern involved in the sports skill for which the athlete is training should be simulated as closely as possible during the training sessions.

Training speed should be as fast as or faster than the speed of movement involved in the sports skill for which the athlete is training.

The number of maximal contractions per set should be between eight and 15; three sets of each exercise should be used.

Eccentric Programs

Not much popular interest in eccentric weight-training programs for athletes has been generated over the years. However, academic researchers have been intrigued by the fact that a muscle can maximally produce nearly 40% more tension eccentrically than concentrically. Indeed, at one time it was theorized that with greater tension possible, greater strength could be developed with eccentric programs. When several studies were conducted in order to test this hypothesis, the results showed that training with maximal eccentric contractions produced no greater increases in strength than did training with maximal concentric (isotonic) contractions. In fact, as shown in Figure 7-12, programs involving either concentric or eccentric contractions resulted in identical concentric strength gains.

As pointed out in the last chapter (p. 96), muscular soreness during the first few days of weight training is much greater with eccentric contractions than with any other type of contraction. Therefore, it may be concluded that the use of eccentric contractions for purposes of increasing strength does not appear to be advantageous and, in fact, may lead to excessive muscular soreness.

Which Program Is the Best?

By now, it should be obvious that each of the training programs we have discussed has certain advantages and disadvantages. The question of which program is the best is not really appropriate. Furthermore, in comparing programs, complications arise around research design problems. For example, there are problems associated with equating the various programs in such a way that the only differing factor is the type of contraction. Even further complications result because of specificity. Nevertheless, several studies have been conducted comparing the different types of weight-training programs. Let's see what they have to say.

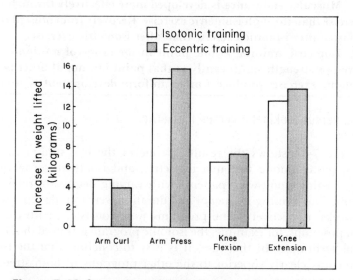

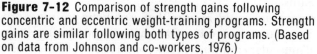

Figure 7-12 Comparison of strength gains following concentric and eccentric weight-training programs. Strength gains are similar following both types of programs. (Based on data from Johnson and co-workers, 1976.)

Isotonic versus Isometric Programs

Figure 7-13 presents a comparison of strength gains resulting from various isotonic programs and one type of isometric (static) program. The exact designs of the isotonic programs are given in the figure. The isometric program consisted of two maximal contractions held for 6 to 8 sec; each contraction was at a different joint angle. The subjects were college-aged men; the training frequency and duration were three days per week and 12 weeks, respectively, for all programs. Only one isotonic program was superior to the isometric program. By the same token, the isometric program was superior to only one isotonic program. In other words, the two types of programs are quite comparable in this case.

A survey of studies comparing isotonic and isometric programs has been conducted by Clarke (1974a) and is summarized below:

Isotonic vs. Isometric Training

Motivation is generally superior with isotonic exercises because they are self-testing. However, isometrics may be performed anywhere, whereas some isotonics may place considerable demands on available space and may require special equipment.

Both isometric and isotonic forms of exercise improve muscular strength. Most studies do not favor one method over another; however, some investigators have reported greater gains for trainees using the isotonic form.

Muscular endurance is developed more effectively through isotonic exercise than through isometric exercise. Recovery from muscular fatigue is faster after isotonic exercise than after isometric exercise.

Isometric training at one point in the range of motion of a joint develops strength significantly at that point but not at other positions. Isotonic exercises produce a more uniform development of strength.

Isotonic versus Isokinetic versus Isometric Programs

Figure 7-14 shows the results of one of the few studies comparing strength gains among isotonic, isometric, and isokinetic programs. The subjects in this study were patients with varying degrees of rehabilitative problems. The training frequency and duration were four days per week and eight weeks, respectively. The programs were consistent with the normal clinical programs, for example, the isotonic program followed the DeLorme-Watkins technique. In this case, it is easy to conclude that the isokinetic program was clearly superior to the other programs in both strength and endurance gains.

In summary, it would appear that isokinetic training programs are somewhat better than the other programs in promoting both muscular strength and muscular endurance. However, it should be pointed out that the

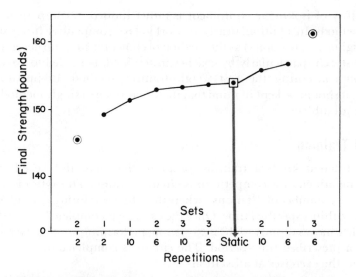

Figure 7-13 Comparison of strength gains resulting from various isotonic programs and one isometric (static) program. All programs were performed 3 days per week for 12 weeks. Only one isotonic program (circled dot to the right) was superior to the isometric program, and the isometric program was superior to only one isotonic program (circled dot at left). (Based on data from Berger, 1962z.)

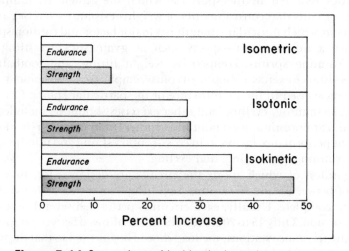

Figure 7-14 Comparison of isokinetic, isotonic, and isometric programs. All programs were performed four days per week for eight weeks. The isokinetic program was superior to the other programs in both strength and endurance gains. (Based on data from Thistle and co-workers, 1967.)

availability of isokinetic equipment is rather limited in comparison to the other methods. In addition, nearly all world-class, competitive lifters still use free weights (i.e., isotonics) as the method of choice for strength development. More research, particularly by coaches in the field, is needed to answer the question concerning the best weight-training method. In pursuing the answer, it should be kept in mind that there may not be a single method that is best for all athletes.

Circuit Training

A different kind of training program that may also be effective in preparing athletes for competition is **circuit training**. This type of program consists of a number of "stations" where the athlete performs a given exercise, usually within a specified time. Once the exercise is completed at one station, the athlete moves rapidly to the next station, performing another exercise also within a prescribed time period. The circuit is completed once the athlete performs the exercises at all stations.

The exercises at the various stations consist mainly of weight-resistance exercises, but running, swimming, cycling, calisthenics, and stretching exercises may also be included. Circuit training, therefore, may be designed to increase muscular endurance, flexibility, and if running, swimming, or cycling is involved, cardiorespiratory endurance as well.

Designing the Circuit

The circuit should include exercises that will develop the particular capabilities required in the sport for which the athlete is training. For example, circuits that consist mainly of weight-resistance exercises are good for sports in which muscular strength is a major factor and cardiorespiratory endurance a minor factor—sports such as gymnastics, wrestling, swim sprints, running sprints, competitive weight lifting, and football. (The weight-resistance exercises should, of course, emphasize development of those muscles most used in the performance of the particular sport.) Conversely, running, swimming, cycling, and other exercises should be included in the circuit if cardiorespiratory endurance rather than strength is the more important performance factor, as in cross-country skiing and middle- or long-distance running, swimming, and cycling.

Regardless of which sports the circuits are designed for, they should consist of between 6 and 15 stations, requiring a total time of between 5 and 20 min to complete. Usually, each circuit is performed several times in one training session. Only 15 to 20 sec rest should be allowed between stations. For the weight-resistance stations, the load should be adjusted so that the working muscles are noticeably fatigued after performing as many repetitions as possible within a designated time period (e.g., 30 sec). This load should be increased periodically in order to ensure progressive overload. In addition, the sequence of exercises should be arranged so that no two consecutive stations consist of exercises involving the same muscle groups. Training frequency should be three days per week, with a duration of at least six weeks.

Examples of Circuits

Examples of typical circuits are shown in Table 7–4. Note that circuits A and C involve only weight resistance exercises, whereas circuit B includes both weight-resistance and cardiorespiratory activities. Thus circuits A and C are designed primarily for those sports mentioned earlier in which muscular strength is a primary performance factor; circuit B is designed for those sports in which cardiorespiratory endurance is involved. Other circuits based on the general principles outlined above are also possible.

Table 7-4: Examples of Circuit-Training Programs

Duration	10–12 weeks
Frequency	3 days per week
Circuits/Session	Circuit A = 3, Circuit B = 2
Time/Circuit	Circuit A = 7½ min, Circuit B = 15 min
Total Time/Session	Circuits A & C = 22½ min, Circuit B = 30 min
Load	40 to 55% of 1-RM load
Repetitions	As many as possible in 30 sec for Circuits A & B; 12–15 in 30 sec for Circuit C
Rest	15 sec between stations

Circuit A*		Circuit B	
Station	Exercise	Station	Exercise
1	Bench press	1	Running (440 yd)
2	Bent-knee sit-up	2	Push-ups or pull-ups
3	Knee (leg) extension	3	Bent-knee sit-ups
4	Pulldown—lat machine	4	Vertical jumps
5	Back hyperextension	5	Standing (overhead) press
6	Standing (overhead) press	6	Bicycling (3 min)
7	Dead lift	7	Hip stretch
8	Arm curl	8	Rope jumping (1 min)
9	Leg curl (knee flexion)	9	Bent-over rowing
10	Upright rowing	10	Hamstring stretch
		11	Upright rowing
		12	Running (660 yd)

Circuit C†	
Station	Exercise
1	Squat
2	Shoulder press
3	Knee flexion
4	Bench press
5	Leg press
6	Elbow flexion
7	Back hyperextension
8	Elbow extension
9	Sit-ups
10	Vertical fly (horizontal swing forward of the arm with the elbow bent at 90°)

*Modified from Wilmore and co-workers (1978).
†From Gettman and co-workers (1982).

Effects of Circuit Training

As previously mentioned, circuit training may be designed to increase muscular strength and power, muscular endurance, flexibility, and cardio-respiratory endurance. However, it should be emphasized that the physiological effects are to a large extent dependent upon the type of circuit that is set up. For example, it has been shown that some circuits consisting only of weight-resistance exercises produce substantial gains in strength but only minimal gains in cardiorespiratory endurance (the latter is affected least of all if the circuits have only five or six stations). Although an increase in cardiorespiratory endurance can and does result from circuit training especially when endurance activities are included in the stations, the magnitude of the increase is generally not as great as that from endurance programs consisting entirely of running, swimming, or cycling.

From the rather limited research thus far available, it may be concluded that circuit training appears to be an effective training technique for altering muscular strength and endurance, and, to a limited extent, flexibility and cardiorespiratory endurance. The use of circuit training, particularly for off-season programs, therefore, may be recommended for athletes whose sports require high levels of muscular strength, power, and endurance and lower levels of cardiorespiratory endurance.

Weight-Training Programs for Women

Like men, women respond to weight-resistance programs with increases in strength and muscular endurance. Therefore, the construction of weight-resistance programs for male and female athletes should follow the same general principles.

An example of strength gains in normal college-aged men and women is shown in Figure 7-15. The percent increase in strength for the women in all but one muscle group (the arms) was the same or better than in the men. Although part of this greater relative strength gain can be explained on the basis of the lower initial strength levels of the women, these results indicate that the women can make substantial gains in strength through weight-lifting activities. This is an important point, since earlier information indicated that women were less trainable than men with respect to muscular strength. The strength gains shown here were made over a ten-week period, two days per week, using the progressive resistance principle. For example, the initial weights were chosen so that the subjects could perform only seven to nine repetitions. When the subjects increased in strength to the point where the same weights could be lifted 14 to 16 times, additional weight was added so that only seven to nine repetitions could again be performed.

Figure 7-16 also shows the effects of a weight-training program on strength gains, but this time for women athletes. The women were nationally

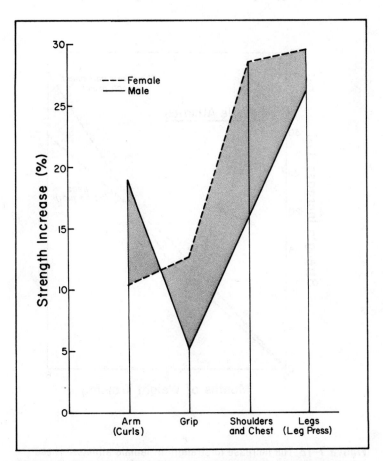

Figure 7-15 Both men and women increase in muscular strength following a weight-training program. The percent increase in strength for females in most muscle groups is the same or even better than for males. (Based on data from Wilmore, 1974.)

prominent track-and-field and throwing-event athletes between the ages of 16 and 23. The important point here is that these women are much stronger than normal women but their strength gains are still very substantial, particularly after six months of training. This information suggests that weight-training programs can and should be used by women who wish to improve their performance in those activities demanding a great deal of strength.

Weight Training the Year Round

The question often arises as to whether athletes should weight-train the entire year. The general answer is yes, but it needs some clarification. The most concentrated weight-resistance program should take place during the off-season. Such a program should emphasize increasing strength, power, and muscular endurance in those muscle groups most directly involved in the

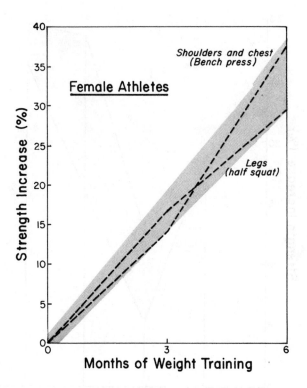

Figure 7-16 The increase in strength in female athletes. These females are much stronger than nonathletic females, yet their strength gains are still very substantial. (Based on data from Brown and Wilmore, 1974.)

specific sports event for which the athlete is training. Guidelines presented earlier for the various types of programs should be used in constructing the program.

During the preseason, athletes may continue to weight-train, but probably at a reduced frequency. For example, the frequency should be two days per week rather than three to four days per week (the schedule used during the off-season). Provided the off-season program has been successful, the major concern during the preseason should be maintaining the strength gained during the off-season.

Another question often raised by coaches is whether athletes should weight-train **during** the season. The answer depends on whether or not the athletes are losing strength or need to gain more strength during the season. Under these conditions, weight-training sessions at least twice per week are probably in order. However, if the desired strength level has already been attained through the off-season and preseason programs, then maintenance of strength might require only one workout per week. In this case, the once-per-week sessions may be alternated on a weekly basis between upper body and lower body workouts (i.e., one week, upper body; the next, lower body).

Effects of Weight-Resistance Programs

The most obvious effects of weight-resistance programs are increases in strength and muscular endurance, as just discussed. What causes these increases? What other changes occur as a result of weight-resistance training? The answers to these questions are provided below.

Muscular Hypertrophy

Gains in strength and muscular endurance are usually accompanied by an increase in the size of individual muscle fibers. This is referred to as **muscular hypertrophy**. Scientific evidence that muscular hypertrophy can occur as a result of weight-resistance training has been gathered for almost two centuries. As for the mechanics of such hypertrophy, in a classic study conducted over 80 years ago it was concluded that the increased size is due entirely to increases in the diameters of already existing fibers. In other words, no new fibers are developed.

This conclusion has recently been challenged in studies with animals. An increase in the number of muscle fibers has, for instance, been shown to occur in rats put through a weight-training program. The increased number of fibers results from what is referred to as **longitudinal fiber splitting**. An example of this kind of splitting is shown in Figure 7-17. The thing to notice is that the splitting occurred in both fast-twitch fibers (dark) and slow-twitch fibers (light).

In another study, this time involving cats, a 20% increase in the number of fibers was found following a five-day-per-week, 34-week program of weight lifting (see Fig. 7-18). Note that fiber splitting in this case was related to intensity, occurring after a high-resistance program, but not following a low-resistance program.

Occasionally, longitudinal fiber splitting is seen in diseased or pathological muscle. However, since the split fibers resulting from weight-training programs have been shown to demonstrate normal enzyme function and adequate capillary blood and motor-nerve supply, muscle-fiber splitting should be thought of as representing a physiological rather than pathological response to weight training.

It must be pointed out that although fiber splitting has been shown to occur in animals (rats and cats), it has not as yet been demonstrated to occur in humans following weight-training programs. It is also fair to add that only limited research has been conducted along these lines in humans. Therefore, much more research is needed before the importance of such a change (at least in humans) can be estimated.

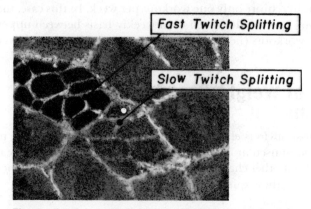

Fast Twitch Splitting

Slow Twitch Splitting

Figure 7-17 Longitudinal fiber splitting in rat muscle as a result of chronic weight-resistance exercise. Notice that splitting occurred in both fast-twitch fibers (dark) and slow-twitch fibers (light). (Based on data from Ho and co-workers, 1980.)

It would appear that the major factor contributing to increases in skeletal muscle size in humans following weight-training programs is an increased diameter of existing fibers, which is itself due to a greater number of myofibrils per fiber, more total protein, and hypertrophy of connective, tendinous, and ligamentous tissues.

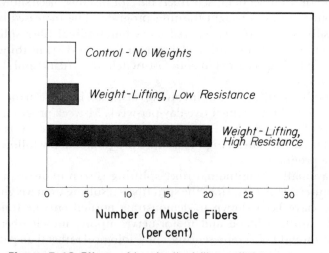

Control - No Weights

Weight-Lifting, Low Resistance

Weight - Lifting, High Resistance

Number of Muscle Fibers (per cent)

Figure 7-18 Effects of longitudinal fiber splitting on number of muscle fibers. A 20% increase in the number of muscle fibers was found in cats following a 5-day-per-week, 34-week-long program of weight lifting. Note that the fiber splitting is apparently intensity related in that it occurred only after a high-resistance program. (Based on data from Gonyea, 1980.)

It should also be mentioned that some evidence points to a selective hypertrophy of fast-twitch (FT) units in conjunction with weight training. For example, the area of FT fibers has been observed to increase after eight weeks of weight training. Moreover, it is known that the percent area of FT fibers in muscle is generally larger in weight lifters than in untrained subjects and endurance athletes. No evidence of interconversion of fast-twitch and slow-twitch fibers has been found in participants in weight-training programs.

It should be emphasized at this time that muscular hypertrophy is generally not as great in women as in men even when they make the same relative gains in strength. Comparative measurements such as shown in Figure 7–19 bear this out. In the study that produced the findings presented in the figure, increases in girth (circumference) were in every case greater in men than in women. In addition, the largest increase in muscular size exhibited by the women was 0.6 cm, or less than a quarter of an inch. Such small increases in girth clearly demonstrate that muscular hypertrophy in women as a result of weight-training programs will certainly not lead to excessive muscular bulk or produce a "masculinizing" effect. Muscular hypertrophy is regulated mainly by the hormone testosterone, which is found in much higher levels in normal men than in normal women. Thus, regardless of strength gains, there is less muscular hypertrophy in women than in men.

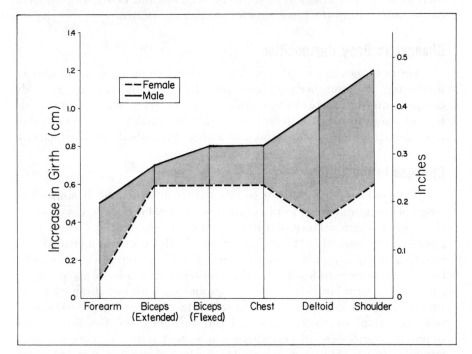

Figure 7-19 Muscular hypertrophy in women is generally not as great as that in men, even when the same relative gains in strength have been made. (Based on data from Wilmore, 1974.)

Biochemical Changes

Findings in recent studies dealing with the biochemical changes resulting from weight-resistance training can be summarized as follows:

No changes have been noted in the enzymes involved in the ATP-PC system. Similarly, enzymes involved in anaerobic glycolysis have been shown to be unchanged in weight lifters' muscles. Substantially reduced activities of enzymes involved in the aerobic system have been found, however (on the average, the drop is 30%).

The volume (density) of mitochondria has been shown to decrease owing to increases in size of the myofibrils and sarcoplasmic volume.

Increases have been noted in the concentrations of ATP (18%), PC (22%), and glycogen (66%).

The above findings suggest that improvements in muscular strength and endurance resulting from weight-training exercises are due, in part, to metabolic alterations within the muscle. However, neuromuscular factors such as better coordination of different muscles (and perhaps of different motor units within the same muscle) are also implicated.

Changes in Body Composition

For most men and women, weight-resistance training produces little or no change in total body weight, but there will be changes in body composition—i.e., there can be significant losses of relative and absolute body fat **and** a significant gain in fat-free weight (presumably muscle mass). (For more details on body composition, in athletes and others, see Chapter 11.)

Changes in Flexibility

Two kinds of flexibility may be recognized: **static** and **dynamic**. The range of motion about a joint is called static flexibility, whereas dynamic flexibility is the resistance of a joint to motion. The first of these is most commonly thought of as "flexibility." Static flexibility may be increased with weight-training programs and also with stretching exercises (the fact that flexibility improves following weight-training programs is reason enough to consider the term "muscle-bound" a misnomer). With stretching exercises, significant gains in flexibility may be realized with a two-day-per-week, five-week program. In most sports and physical activities, flexibility is an important component of performance and often serves to prevent serious muscular injury. However, it should also be pointed out that too much flexibility may lead to muscular trauma as well as joint injury, particularly in contact sports. More about flexibility is presented in Chapter 9.

Effects on Motor and Athletic Performances

Research involving weight-resistance training and changes in motor and athletic performances has demonstrated that specific skills such as speed in swimming, throwing, and running (e.g., the 40-yd dash) can be significantly improved through weight-training programs.

In a recent review of research into strength development and motor and/or sports improvement, Clarke (1974b) reached the following conclusions:

Both isometric and isotonic forms of strength training can produce improvements in many motor sports performances. Although the evidence is at times conflicting,* it is generally accepted that progressive weight-training programs (isotonic) are superior.

In general, exercises confined to single static contractions of short duration or isotonic efforts limited to a single bout have not been effective in developing either strength or motor skills. Strenuous resistance exercises of either the isotonic or the isometric form are needed for best results.

Fears of "muscle-bound" effects from weight training should be laid to rest. Most studies show that speed of movement may be enhanced rather than retarded as a consequence of strength development.

As supplements to regular practice, exercise programs designed to strengthen muscles primarily involved in a particular sport can be effective in improving the athlete's skills and motor fitness.

A summary of the effects of weight-training programs is presented in Table 7–5.

Effects of Steroid Consumption during Weight Training

Among athletes in certain sports (e.g., competitive weight lifting), it is a fairly common practice to use anabolic-androgenic steroids. A **steroid** is a derivative of the male sex hormone testosterone, secreted by the testicles. The term "**anabolic**" refers to tissue-building, and "**androgenic**" denotes the development of the male secondary sex characteristics. Steroids are taken with the idea of gaining exceptional muscular mass and muscular strength, which will ultimately lead to increased performance. However, such a practice is extremely dangerous from a medical standpoint and should never be sanctioned by any individual or athletic organization.

The American College of Sports Medicine conducted a comprehensive survey of the world literature and carefully analyzed the claims made for and

---

*Some studies did not provide adequate overload in applying both isometric and isotonic strength training.

Table 7-5: Summary of Effects of Weight-Training Programs

Changes in Muscle Function

> increased muscular strength
> increased muscular endurance
> right-upward shift of force-velocity curve

Changes in Muscle Size

> hypertrophy, attributable to:
>> increased diameters of existing fibers
>> increased numbers of fibers due to longitudinal fiber splitting

Biochemical Changes

> no change in enzyme activities of ATP-PC system
> decreased aerobic enzyme activity
> no change in glycolytic enzyme activity
> decreased volume (density) of mitochondria
> increased concentrations of ATP, PC, and glycogen

Changes in Muscle and Joint Motion

> increased flexibility

Changes in Body Composition

> decreased total and relative body fat
> increased fat-free weight (muscle mass)

Changes in Motor and Sports Skills

> improved performance of some skills

---

against the efficacy of anabolic-androgenic steroids in improving human physical performance. The following is their position statement:

"The administration of anabolic-androgenic steroids to healthy humans below age 50 in medically approved therapeutic doses often does not of itself bring about any significant improvements in strength, aerobic endurance, lean body mass, or body weight.

"There is no conclusive scientific evidence that extremely large doses of anabolic-androgenic steroids either aid or hinder athletic performance.

"The prolonged use of oral anabolic-androgenic steroids (C_{17}-alkylated derivatives of testosterone) has resulted in liver disorders in some persons. Some of these disorders are apparently reversible with the cessation of drug usage, but others are not.

"The administration of anabolic-androgenic steroids to male humans may result in a decrease in testicular size and function and a decrease in sperm production. Although these effects appear to be reversible when small doses of steroids are used for short periods of time, the reversibility of the effects of large doses over extended periods of time is unclear.

"Serious and continuing efforts should be made to educate male and female athletes, coaches, physical educators, physicians, trainers, and the general public regarding the inconsistent effects of anabolic-androgenic steroids on improvement of human physical performance and the potential dangers of taking certain forms of these substances, especially in large doses, for prolonged periods."

Summary

- In order to ensure maximal training benefits from weight-resistance programs, several principles must be followed:

  Muscles must be overloaded, that is, exercised against resistances exceeding those normally encountered.

  The overload must be progressive throughout the program.

  Larger muscle groups should be exercised before smaller groups, and no two consecutive exercises should involve the same muscle groups.

  Weight-training exercises should simulate the movement patterns involved in the sport for which the athlete is training.

- Weight-training programs may be constructed around isotonic, isometric, isokinetic, and/or eccentric types of contractions.

- Isotonic programs calculate work in terms of repetition maximums and sets. A repetition maximum (RM) is the maximal load a muscle group can lift a given number of times before fatiguing. A set is the number of repetitions performed consecutively without resting.

- Isotonic programs for athletes should be six weeks or longer in duration, with the exercises performed three days per week and consisting first of 2×10-RM loads and then of 3×6-RM loads.

- Both muscular endurance and strength may be gained from isotonic programs designed either for low repetitions and high resistance or for high repetitions and low resistance.

- Isometric programs for athletes should be four weeks or longer in duration, with the training to be scheduled for three to five days per week and the exercises to consist of five to ten maximal contractions held for 5 to 7 sec each.

- Isometric programs have angle-specific effects—that is, they increase strength only at the joint angle that is exercised. Therefore, for strength gains over a range of joint angles, isometric exercises should be performed at three joint angles or more.

- Functional isometrics involve isometric contractions performed with weights.

- Isokinetic programs for athletes should be six weeks or longer in duration, with training exercises performed between two and four days per week. Training speed should be as fast as or faster than the speed of movement involved in the sports skill for which the athlete is training. The number of maximal contractions per set should be between eight and fifteen; three sets should be used.

- Isokinetic training at slow speeds produces gains in strength only at slow movement speeds, whereas training at fast speeds produces strength gains at all speeds at and below the training speed.

- The force-velocity curve for a muscle exercised in fast-speed isokinetic training will be shifted upward and to the right.

- Training programs based on eccentric contractions produce no greater gains in strength than do programs based on concentric (isotonic) contractions. Muscular soreness is greatest following eccentric programs.

- Theoretically, isokinetic-training programs should be better than other programs in promoting muscular strength and endurance. However, it is likely that no single method is best for all athletes. Each has its advantages and disadvantages.

- Athletes may need to weight-train the entire year. In such cases, the most concentrated program should take place during the off-season and the least concentrated during the actual playing season.

- Circuit training consists of a number of exercise stations where the athlete performs a given activity, usually within a specified time period. Circuit training is recommended as an off-season program for those sports that require high levels of muscular strength, power, and endurance and lower levels of cardiorespiratory endurance.

- Like men, women respond to weight-resistance training with increases in strength and muscular endurance. Therefore, the construction of weight-resistance programs for women should follow the same general principles as for men.

- The effects of weight-resistance programs include:

  Muscular hypertrophy

  Biochemical changes in skeletal muscle

  Decrease in body fat, increase in fat-free weight, and little change in total body weight

  Increased flexibility

  Increases in many motor and athletic performances

- The practice of taking anabolic-androgenic steroids does not always lead to increased muscular mass and strength, and these drugs may in fact constitute a serious health hazard for the user. The use of steroids for the sole purpose of improving athletic performance should never be sanctioned by any individual or athletic organization.

Selected References and Readings*

Anderson, T., and J. T. Kearney: Effects of three resistance training programs on muscular strength and absolute and relative endurance. *Res. Quart. Exercise Sport, 53(1)*:1-7, 1982.

Allen, T. E., R. J. Byrd, and D. P. Smith: Hemodynamic consequences of circuit weight training. *Res. Quart., 47(3)*:299-306, 1976.

American College of Sports Medicine. Position statement on the use and abuse of anabolic-androgenic steroids in sports. *Med. Sci. Sports, 9(4)*:xi-xii, 1977.

Berger, R. A.: Comparison of static and dynamic strength increases. *Res. Quart., 33*:329-333, 1962a.

Berger, R. A.: Effect of varied weight training programs on strength. *Res. Quart., 33*:168-181, 1962b.

Brown, C., and J. Wilmore: The effects of maximal resistance training on the strength and body composition of women athletes. *Med. Sci. Sports, 6*:174-177, 1974.

Clarke, D. H.: Adaptations in strength and muscular endurance resulting from exercise. *In* Wilmore, J. H. (ed.): *Exercise and Sport Sciences Reviews.* Vol. 1. New York, Academic Press, 1973, pp. 73-102.

Clarke, D. H., and G. A. Stull: Endurance training as a determinant of strength and fatigability. *Res. Quart., 41*:19-26, 1970.

Clarke, H. H. (ed.): Development of muscular strength and endurance. *Physical Fitness Research Digest.* President's Council on Physical Fitness and Sports. Washington, D.C., U.S. Government Printing Office, Series 4, No. 1, January, 1974a.

Clarke, H. H. (ed.): Strength development and motor-sports improvements. *Physical Fitness Research Digest.* President's Council on Physical Fitness and Sports. Washington, D.C., U.S. Government Printing Office, Series 4, No. 4, October, 1974b.

Cotten D.: Relationship of the duration of sustained voluntary isometric contraction to changes in endurance and strength. *Res. Quart., 38*:366-374, 1967.

Coyle, E. F., et al. Specificity of power improvements through slow and fast isokinetic training. *J. Appl. Physiol.: Respirat. Environ, Exercise Physiol., 51(6)*:1437-1442, 1981.

DeLorme, T., and A. Watkins: Techniques of progressive resistance exercise. *Arch. Phys. Med. Rehabil., 29*:263-273, 1948.

Edgerton, V. R.: Morphology and histochemistry of the soleus muscle from normal and exercised rats. *Am. J. Anat., 127*:81-88, 1970.

Fox, E. L., and D. K. Mathews: *The Physiological Basis of Physical Education and Athletics.* 3rd ed. Philadelphia, Saunders College Publishing, 1981.

Gettman, L. R., P. Ward, and R. D. Hagan: A comparison of combined running and weight training with circuit weight training. *Med. Sci. Sports Exercise, 14(3)*:229-234, 1982.

Girandola, R. N., and V. Katch: Effects of nine weeks of physical training on aerobic capacity and body composition in college men. *Arch. Phys. Med. Rehabil. 54*:521-524, 1973.

Gollnick, P., et al.: Enzyme activity and fiber composition in skeletal muscle of untrained and trained men. *J. Appl. Physiol., 33*:312-319, 1972.

Gonyea, W. J.: The role of exercise in inducing skeletal muscle fiber number. *J. Appl. Physiol., 48(3)*:426-431, 1980.

Hettinger, T., and E. Müller: Muskelleistung und Muskeltraining. *Arbeitsphysiol., 15*:111-126, 1953.

Ho, K., et al.: Skeletal muscle fiber splitting with weight-lifting exercise in rats. *Am. J. Anat., 157(4)*:433-440, 1980.

---

*For full journal titles, see Appendix A.

Hooks, G.: *Weight Training in Athletics and Physical Education.* Englewood Cliffs, NJ, Prentice-Hall, Inc., 1974.

Johnson, B. L.: Eccentric vs. concentric muscle training for strength development. *Med. Sci. Sports, 4(2)*:111–115, 1972.

Johnson, B. L., et al.: A comparison of concentric and eccentric muscle training. *Med. Sci. Sports, 8(1)*:35–38, 1976.

Larsson, L.: Physical training effects on muscle morphology in sedentary males at different ages. *Med. Sci. Sports Exercise, 14(3)*:203–206, 1982.

MacDougall, J. D., et al.: Mitochondrial volume density in human skeletal muscle following heavy resistance training. *Med. Sci. Sports, 10(1)*:56, 1978.

MacDougall, J. D., et al.: Biochemical adaptation of human skeletal muscle to heavy resistance training and immobilization. *J. Appl. Physiol.: Respirat. Environ. Exercise Physiol., 43(4)*: 700–702, 1977.

Meyers, C. R.: Effects of two isometric routines on strength, size, and endurance in exercised and nonexercised arms. *Res. Quart., 38*:430–440, 1967.

Moffroid, M. T., and R. H. Whipple: Specificity of speed of exercise. *J. Amer. Phys. Therapy Assoc., 50*:1699–1704, 1970.

Müller, E., and W. Röhmert: Die Geschwindigkeit der Muskelkraft—Zunahme bei isometrischem training. *Arbeits Physiol., 19*:403–419, 1963.

O'Shea, J. P.: *Scientific Principles and Methods of Strength Fitness,* 2nd ed. Reading, MA, Addison-Wesley Publishing Co., 1976.

Riley, D. P.: *Strength Training: By the Experts.* West Point, NY, Leisure Press, 1977.

Seaborne, D., and A. W. Taylor: The effects of isokinetic exercise on vastus lateralis fibre morphology and biochemistry. *J. Sports Med., 21*:365–370, 1981.

Stull, G. A., and D. H. Clarke: High-resistance, low-repetition training as a determiner of strength and fatigability. *Res. Quart., 41*:189–193, 1970.

Thistle, H., et al.: Isokinetic contraction: a new concept of resistive exercise. *Arch. Phys. Med. Rehab., 48*:279–282, 1967.

Thorstensson, A., et al.: Effect of strength training on enzyme activities and fiber characteristics in human skeletal muscle. *Acta Physiol. Scand., 96*:392–398, 1976.

Wilmore, J. H.: Alterations in strength, body composition and anthropometric measurements consequent to a 10-week weight training program. *Med. Sci. Sports, 6*:133–138, 1974.

Wilmore, J. H., et al.: Physiological alterations consequent to circuit weight training. *Med. Sci. Sports, 10(2)*:79–84, 1978.

8

The Oxygen Transport System—Respiration and Circulation

Introduction

In Chapter 2, we discussed the importance of oxygen with respect to the production of ATP energy. For this function, oxygen must be transported from the environment to the muscles, where it is then consumed by the mitochondria. The transport of oxygen (and the removal of carbon dioxide) necessarily involves the respiratory and circulatory systems. It is in the respiratory system that movement of air into and out of the lungs takes place, along with the exchange of oxygen and carbon dioxide between lungs and blood. In the circulatory system, the transport of oxygen and carbon dioxide by the blood occurs, as does gas exchange between blood and muscle. Figure 8-1 shows all these relationships.

The major purpose of this chapter will be to discuss the circulatory and respiratory processes as they relate to athletic performance.

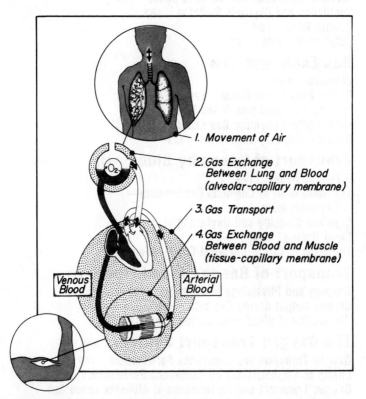

1. Movement of Air

2. Gas Exchange Between Lung and Blood (alveolar-capillary membrane)

3. Gas Transport

4. Gas Exchange Between Blood and Muscle (tissue-capillary membrane)

Venous Blood

Arterial Blood

Figure 8-1 The functional relationships between the respiratory and circulatory systems in the transport of oxygen to and the removal of carbon dioxide from the muscle.

Movement of Air: Pulmonary Ventilation

The rhythmic movement of air into and out of the lungs is called **pulmonary ventilation.** The amount of air ventilated by the lungs in one minute is referred to as **minute ventilation.**

Minute Ventilation

Respiratory physiologists denote minute ventilation in this form: $\dot{V}_E$. The V means volume, the E stands for "expired," and the dot over the V refers to 1 min; thus, $\dot{V}_E$ = the amount of air expired in 1 min. The $\dot{V}_E$ is a function of the volume of air ventilated per breath, referred to as the tidal volume (TV) and the number of breaths taken per minute (f). Again using respiratory physiologist's symbols,

$$\underset{\substack{\text{minute} \\ \text{ventilation}}}{\dot{V}_E} \quad = \quad \underset{\text{tidal volume}}{TV} \quad \times \quad \underset{\text{frequency}}{f}$$

If you expired 0.5 L of air per breath and took 15 breaths per minute, your $\dot{V}_E$ would equal $0.5 \times 15 = 7.5$ L per min. This would be a normal value under resting conditions. During exercise, ventilation increases, with values reaching as high as 180 L per min for trained endurance athletes (males).

Ventilation during Exercise

Ventilation changes before, during, and after exercise, as shown in Figure 8-2. The slight increase in ventilation before exercise begins is referred to as the **anticipatory rise**, since it is a result of the anticipation of the ensuing exercise. When exercise begins, there is an immediate large increase in ventilation. The rapidity of the rise has led researchers to believe that it is the result of nervous influences generated from receptors located in the working muscles and joints. After several minutes of submaximal exercise, ventilation continues to rise, but at a much slower rate, finally leveling off until the end of exercise. If the exercise is maximal, then ventilation continues to rise slowly until exhaustion. After exercise is terminated, ventilation returns toward resting values, rapidly at first, then more slowly.

Ventilation as a Limit to Performance

It is generally agreed that physical performance is not limited by pulmonary ventilation in healthy individuals. This is evident in Figure 8-3. Notice how ventilation increases out of proportion to work load at moderate to heavy loads (shaded area). This means that ventilation at these work loads is greater than required for the amount of oxygen being consumed. This is

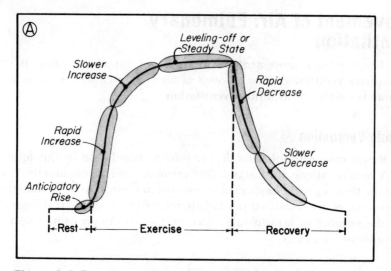

Figure 8-2 Exercise and changes in ventilation. Before exercise, there is an anticipatory rise in ventilation. During exercise, there are greater rises (first rapid, then continuing slow) until a leveling-off is reached (steady state). After exercise, there are decreases in ventilation (first rapid, then continuing slow).

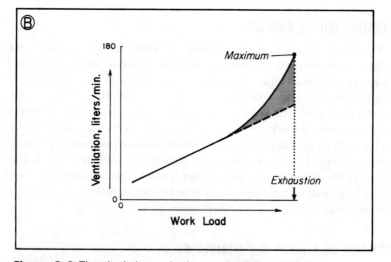

Figure 8-3 The shaded area in the graph of the relationship between steady-state ventilation and work load indicates that ventilation increases out of proportion to work loads (hyperventilation) at moderate to heavy loads. It is generally agreed that physical performance is not limited by pulmonary ventilation in healthy individuals.

called **hyperventilation** ("hyper" means "over" or "greater"). The cause of hyperventilation under these conditions is related to the large increases in carbon dioxide and lactic acid that accompany heavy exercise.

Alveolar Ventilation versus Dead Space

In order to eventually supply the muscles with adequate oxygen and remove excess carbon dioxide, a large portion of the ventilated air must reach the **alveoli**, the tiny terminal air sacs deep in the lung that are in intimate contact with the blood in the pulmonary capillaries. It is here that gas exchange between air and blood occurs. The ventilation of these alveoli (singular: alveolus) is called **alveolar ventilation**. Air that does not enter the alveoli remains in what is referred to as **dead space**, "dead" because no gas exchange with the blood can take place there. Examples of dead space areas are the nose, mouth, and other respiratory passages, such as the bronchi.

Normally, in a person at rest, the respiratory dead space volume is around 150 ml. Out of a 500-ml tidal volume, then, only 350 ml ventilate the alveolar spaces (this is only 70% of the tidal volume). Thus, it is important to breathe at a sufficient depth to ensure adequate alveolar ventilation. If one's breaths are shallow, it will not matter how rapid they are, for most of the air will remain in the dead spaces and be ineffective in terms of gas exchange. A good example of inadequate ventilation may be seen in a dog panting on a hot day. Rather than ventilating the alveoli, the air is rapidly passed in and out over the respiratory passages (dead space) for purposes of thermal regulation through evaporative cooling. Fortunately, the proper rate and depth of breathing are automatically regulated both at rest and during exercise without conscious effort on our part.

Ventilation and Cigarette Smoking

Most of us who have participated in physical activity and sport are familiar with the phrase, "Smoking makes you short of breath." There is some truth in this statement. Chronic cigarette smoking causes, among other things, an increased airway resistance, making it harder to move air into and out of the lungs. In other words, the respiratory muscles (the diaphragm, the intercostals, scaleni, sternocleidomastoids, and abdominals) have to work harder in order for the lungs to ventilate a given volume of air. This means that, in turn, the respiratory muscles will require more oxygen, thus leaving less for the skeletal muscles performing the work. As shown in Figure 8-4, during heavy exercise, airway resistance in chronic smokers can be up to twice that in nonsmokers. Notice that persons who do not smoke for 24 hr prior to exercise reduce their airway resistance, but it still is much greater than that of nonsmokers. In this respect, it should be mentioned that in studies in which respiratory resistance approaching that of chronic smokers was experimentally imposed during endurance exercise, there were significant reductions in

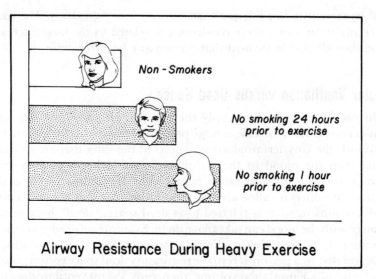

Figure 8-4 Chronic cigarette smoking causes, among other things, an increased airway resistance, making it harder to move air into and out of the lungs. (Based on data from Rode and Shephard, 1971.)

pulmonary ventilation, maximal oxygen consumption, and endurance time. The following conclusions concerning cigarette smoking and sports performance are warranted:

Cigarette Smoking and Performance

Added resistance to ventilation caused by chronic cigarette smoking can lead to significant decreases in the oxygen available to the working muscles. As a consequence, endurance performance, pulmonary ventilation, and maximal oxygen consumption may be significantly decreased.

Some of the added resistance to ventilation can be noticeably reduced by abstinence from cigarette smoking 24 hr prior to performance. Thus, endurance athletes who cannot or will not "kick the habit" may aid their performance by not smoking on the day of competition.

Other effects of cigarette smoking are discussed later in this chapter (see p. 174).

Second Wind

All of you have no doubt heard of, and perhaps even experienced, a phenomenon called **second wind**. Second wind is usually described as a sudden transition from an ill-defined feeling of distress or fatigue during the early portions of prolonged exercise to a more comfortable, less stressful feeling later in the exercise. As the term itself suggests, second wind is often associated with more comfortable breathing, although other factors, such as relief from muscular fatigue, may also be involved. The following are possible causes of second wind:

Causes of Second Wind

Relief from breathlessness caused by slow ventilatory adjustments early in exercise.

Removal (oxidation) of lactic acid accumulated early in the exercise as a result of delayed blood flow changes in the working muscles.

Adequate warm-up.

Relief from local muscle fatigue, particularly of the diaphragm.

Psychological factors.

Stitch in the Side

This phenomenon is also very familiar to most athletes. A **stitch in the side** is usually described as a sharp pain in the side or rib cage. Like second wind, it occurs early during exercise (generally during running and swimming), subsiding as exercise continues. However, for some, the pain is so great that they must either slow down or stop exercising altogether. While the cause of such pain is not known for sure, it has been suggested that lack of oxygen (hypoxia) in the diaphragm and intercostal muscles due to insufficient blood flow is involved. Unfortunately, there is no simple remedy.

Gas Exchange

Once fresh air is in the alveoli, the exchange of oxygen and carbon dioxide between air and blood can take place. The site of this exchange is the **alveolar-capillary membrane**, the thin layer of tissue separating the air in the alveoli from the blood in the pulmonary capillaries. A second gas exchange occurs between blood and tissue (e.g., skeletal muscle) at what is referred to as the **tissue-capillary membrane**. Although these two gas exchanges take place at different sites, they both involve the physical process of diffusion and thus will be discussed together.

Diffusion

Diffusion results from the random movement of molecules, in this case gas molecules. The random motion is itself due to the kinetic energy of the gas molecules. Gases diffuse from areas of greater molecular motion, a characteristic of high concentrations, to areas of lesser molecular motion (low concentrations). The pattern is easily summarized: gases move by diffusion from higher to lower concentrations.

Partial Pressure of Gases

Because of their constant state of motion, gas molecules occasionally collide with each other and with the walls of their container. The number of such collisions is proportional to the concentration of the gas, since with greater concentrations there are more molecules and more collisions possible. The number of collisions is also proportional to the **partial pressure** exerted by a gas. The partial pressure of a gas may be defined as the pressure exerted in relation to the percentage or concentration of the gas within a volume. For example, in dry air,* the concentration of oxygen is approximately 21% (0.21 as a decimal fraction), and that of nitrogen is 79% (0.79). The total (barometric) pressure (P_B) exerted by both gases at sea level is 760 mm of mercury (Hg). By definition, then, the partial pressure of oxygen (P_{O_2}) is equal to $760 \times 0.21 = 159.6$ mm Hg, and that of nitrogen (P_{N_2}) is $760 \times 0.79 = 600.4$ mm Hg. Mathematically, the partial pressure of any gas may be calculated as follows:

$$P_X \qquad = \qquad P_B \qquad \times \qquad F_X$$

partial pressure of gas   barometric pressure   fractional concentration of gas

---

Gas partial pressure is the single most important factor determining gaseous exchange at the alveolar-capillary and tissue-capillary membranes.

P_{O_2} and P_{CO_2} Gradients in the Body

In order for oxygen to diffuse from the air in the alveoli to the pulmonary capillary blood, the P_{O_2} in the alveoli must be higher than the P_{O_2} in the blood. Just the opposite is true for carbon dioxide: the P_{CO_2} in the blood must be higher than in the alveoli since carbon dioxide diffuses from the blood to the alveoli. The diffusion rules for exchange at the alveolar-capillary membrane also hold true for exchange at the tissue-capillary membrane. The partial pressures and gradients for oxygen and carbon dioxide at the membranes are given in Table 8-1.

Other Factors Affecting Gas Exchange

Although the partial pressure gradients of oxygen and carbon dioxide are the most important factors in the process of diffusion, there are other

---

*Moist air contains water vapor, which also exerts a partial pressure.

Table 8-1: Partial Pressures and Gradients for Oxygen and Carbon Dioxide at the Alveolar-Capillary and Tissue-Capillary Membranes

Diffusion Site	Partial Pressure (mm Hg)	
	O_2	CO_2
Alveolar-Capillary Membrane		
alveoli	100	40
	↓	↑
venous blood (pulmonary capillaries)	40	47
DIFFUSION GRADIENT =	60	7
Tissue-Capillary Membrane		
arterial blood	100	40
	↓	↓
muscle venous blood	30	50
(rest)	↓	↓
muscle venous blood	10	70
(exercise)		
DIFFUSION GRADIENT =	70–90	10–30

influences on the rate and amount of gaseous exchange. Some of these additional factors are:

Factors Affecting Gas Exchange

Gas partial pressure.

The length of the diffusion path—i.e., the thickness of the membranes across which the diffusion occurs.

The number of red blood cells (the major gas-transporting vehicles) and the amount of myoglobin (muscle hemoglobin).

The surface area available for diffusion.

The latter factor, the area of the diffusion surface, is related to body size and is dependent upon the number of open capillaries that are in direct contact with ventilated alveoli and/or muscle fibers. Exercise increases the number of ventilated alveoli and open capillaries, thus promoting diffusion of gases.

Diffusion Capacity of Athletes

The diffusion capacity at the alveolar-capillary membrane of various male athletes during maximal exercise is shown in Figure 8-5. The diffusion capacity is measured as the amount of oxygen diffused per minute and per mm Hg pressure gradient between the alveolar air and pulmonary capillary blood

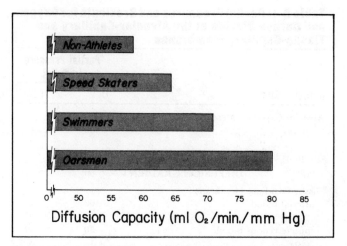

Figure 8-5 The diffusion capacity at the alveolar-capillary membrane during maximal exercise is greater in athletes (particularly endurance athletes) than in nonathletes. (Based on data from Magel and Lange-Anderson, 1969; Maksud and co-workers, 1971; and Reuschlein and co-workers, 1968.)

(ml O_2 per min per mm Hg). Notice that all the athletes, particularly the endurance athletes (swimmers and oarsmen), have much greater diffusion capacities than nonathletes. This same pattern applies to female athletes, although their absolute values are somewhat lower. The greater diffusion capacity of athletes is thought to be related (in part) to a greater alveolar-capillary surface area. The latter is related to body size, as indicated earlier. In this respect it should be pointed out that oarsmen, who have the largest diffusion capacity, also have the largest body size among the groups compared in the figure. (On this basis, the lower absolute diffusion for women may be attributed, at least in part, to their smaller body size.)

Transport of Gases by Blood

Oxygen and carbon dioxide are carried in the blood in two forms: they may be **dissolved** in the blood or **chemically combined with the blood**.

Dissolved Gases

When oxygen and carbon dioxide are exposed to blood **plasma**, the liquid portion of the blood, their molecules dissolve or mix in solution but do not chemically combine with the liquid molecules making up the plasma. (This is similar to what happens in carbonated drinks. Basically, carbon dioxide is dissolved in the drink under pressure, and then the drink is capped. When the bottle or can is opened, the pressure decreases and carbon dioxide "bubbles out" of solution.) The amount of gas dissolved in blood is dependent upon the solubility, or dissolving power, of the gas and its partial pressure. Under normal partial pressures (see Table 8-1) the amount of dissolved oxygen is very small, representing only 1.5% of the total amount transported. The amount of dissolved CO_2 is also small, representing only 5% of the total CO_2 carried in the blood.

Transport of O_2 in Chemical Combination—Oxyhemoglobin

The greatest portion of oxygen is carried by the red blood cells in chemical combination with **hemoglobin (Hb)**. Hemoglobin is a complex compound housed within the red blood cell and made up of two basic units, a heme unit, which contains iron, and a globin unit, which is a protein. Oxygen chemically combines with the heme, or iron, portion, to form **oxyhemoglobin**:

$$Hb \; + \; O_2 \xrightarrow{\hspace{2cm}} HbO_2$$
hemoglobin   oxygen $\longleftarrow$ oxyhemoglobin

As you might guess, the amount of O_2 that combines with Hb is determined by the Po_2. Each gram of Hb is capable of combining with at most 1.34 ml of oxygen. The hemoglobin concentration is normally about 15 g per 100 ml of blood.* Since each gram of Hb can maximally combine with 1.34 ml of O_2, then each 100 ml of blood can transport up to $1.34 \times 15 = 20.1$ ml of oxygen.

The relationship between the amount of oxygen chemically combined with Hb and the partial pressure of O_2 is shown in Figure 8-6. Each curve in

*Note: The hemoglobin concentration in women is normally lower than that in men.

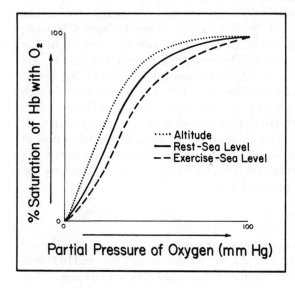

Figure 8-6 The relationship between the amount of oxygen chemically combined with hemoglobin (Hb) and the partial pressure of oxygen (oxyhemoglobin curve). Note that Hb is nearly 100% saturated with O_2 at a Po_2 around 100 mm Hg, which is the normal Po_2 found in the alveoli at sea level. Note also that the position of the curve is not fixed.

the figure is called an **oxyhemoglobin curve**. From these curves, you can see that as the P_{O_2} increases, so does the amount of oxygen combined with Hb. Several other features of the curves should be noticed:

The Oxyhemoglobin Curve

Hemoglobin is nearly 100% saturated with oxygen at a P_{O_2} of around 100 mm Hg, the normal P_{O_2} found in the alveoli at sea level. This means that very little O_2 can be further combined with Hb at higher partial pressures of oxygen. One practical aspect of this fact relates to the breathing of pure O_2 at sea level: it is obvious that only an insignificant amount of O_2 will be further added to the blood under these conditions. How many of you have seen professional football and hockey teams provide their players with pure oxygen during time-out periods? Would you recommend this at sea level?

The "exercise" curve is shifted to the right of the "rest"curve. The shift of the curve to the right represents an enhanced release of oxygen to the working muscles, which occurs when exercise increases the body temperature as well as the levels of carbon dioxide and lactic acid.

The "altitude" curve is shifted to the left of the "rest" curve. The shift of the curve to the left represents enhanced loading of oxygen at the alveolar-capillary membrane, which helps to offset the decreased availability of oxygen caused by the lower partial pressure of oxygen in the inspired air. More will be said about altitude later in this chapter.

Cigarette Smoking and Oxyhemoglobin

Earlier, the effect of cigarette smoking on airway resistance was mentioned. Cigarette smoking also affects the amount of oxygen that can be carried by hemoglobin. One of the by-products of smoke from a burning cigarette is carbon monoxide (CO). Carbon monoxide has a much higher affinity for Hb than does oxygen. Therefore, when both CO and O_2 are present, such as would be the case when a smoker inhales after taking a puff, carbon monoxide is quicker to combine with Hb. This is true even though carbon monoxide may be present in only trace amounts. Once carbon monoxide has combined with Hb, it is not possible for oxyhemoglobin to be formed, because carbon monoxide combines with the same chemical unit of Hb (heme) that ordinarily would be linked to the oxygen. As a result, the oxygen-carrying capacity of blood is reduced. In heavy, chronic smokers, the reduction can amount to as much as 10%.

Blood Doping

In 1976, the Finnish long-distance runner Lasse Viren was said by the press to be "blood doping," since he placed first both in the 5,000- and 10,000-m races and fifth in the marathon. Such a performance was indeed spectacular;

no wonder an "excuse" was sought! Blood doping, the removal and subsequent reinfusion of blood, is done to temporarily increase blood volume and, most importantly, raise the number of red blood cells. As just discussed, red blood cells contain hemoglobin. Thus, overloading the blood with hemoglobin would increase the oxygen-carrying capacity of the blood and, theoretically at least, lead to an increased endurance performance.

Scientific studies of blood doping and endurance performance have produced conflicting results. Several studies have shown that blood doping increases endurance performance between 15 and 35% (measured by a treadmill run to exhaustion) and maximal oxygen consumption between 5 and 13% in both nonathletic subjects and trained endurance athletes.

The results of one such study are shown in Figure 8-7. In this study, the

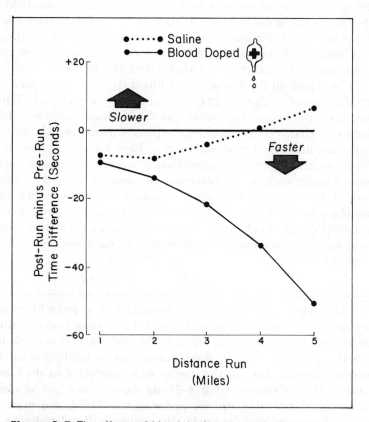

Figure 8-7 The effects of blood doping on treadmill running performance (5-mi run). It is clear that the runners were able to run the 5 mi much faster (51 sec faster on the average) after blood doping. Also notice that saline infusion had no significant effect on running performance. This means that the increased performance after blood doping was due to red-blood-cell infusion and not just an increase in blood volume. (Based on data from Williams and co-workers, 1980.)

effects of blood doping on treadmill running performance was investigated using experienced runners as subjects. Each subject performed four 5-mile runs on the laboratory treadmill. On one occasion, the subjects ran under normal conditions, that is, without blood either withdrawn or infused. This was called the "prerun." On another occasion, the subjects ran two days after having received 920 ml of their own red blood cells (previously withdrawn) diluted with normal saline. (Saline is a slightly salty fluid that has the consistency of blood water.) This was called the "postrun." For a control and for comparison to the blood-doped performance, the subjects performed two other runs, one before (prerun) and another after (postrun) the infusion of 920 ml of saline. The study was "double blind," meaning that neither the subjects nor the researchers knew during the experiment whether the subjects received red blood cells or pure saline. This was done to offset any possible psychological effects on running performance due to the runners knowing that they either did or did not receive red cells. In the figure, the vertical axis represents the time difference in seconds between the postrun and the prerun of each condition, that is, before and after blood doping and before and after saline infusion. It is clear that the runners were able to run the 5 miles much faster (51 sec faster on the average) after blood doping. Also notice that the saline infusion had no significant effect on running performance. This latter finding, of course, means that the increased performance after blood doping was due to red blood cell infusion and not just to an increase in blood volume.

An equal number of studies, however, have found no effects of blood doping on endurance performance, maximal oxygen consumption, heart rate responses during exercise, or perceived exertion. (Perceived exertion is a measure of how difficult the subjects think the exercise is that they are performing.) Some of the reasons for this inconsistency stem from poor experimental design, inadequate reinfusion volumes, premature reinfusion of blood following withdrawal, and storage of the blood by refrigeration rather than by freezing.

Although research suggests a beneficial effect from blood doping, several points should be kept in mind. First, most studies either used untrained subjects or good, but not elite athletes. It is possible that the beneficial effects of blood doping may not be applicable to the best athletes. Second, most of the studies were conducted in the laboratory (such as the one shown in Fig. 8-7) and therefore may not be applicable to actual, competitive athletic performance. Third, and most importantly, the use of blood doping by elite runners is illegal under the current Olympic Committee doping rules. Doping is defined, in part, as the use of physiological substances in abnormal amounts and with abnormal methods with the exclusive aim of improving competitive performance. Blood doping should never be sanctioned by any individual or athletic organization.

Transport of CO_2 in Chemical Combination

Carbon dioxide is carried in chemical combination in the blood in two different forms. One form is the **bicarbonate ion**. In the red blood cell, an enzyme called **carbonic anhydrase** (CA) speeds up the reaction of CO_2 and water (H_2O) to form carbonic acid (H_2CO_3):

$$\underset{\text{water}}{H_2O} + \underset{\text{carbon dioxide}}{CO_2} \xrightleftharpoons{CA} \underset{\text{carbonic acid}}{H_2CO_3}$$

The carbonic acid breaks down or dissociates into hydrogen ions (H^+) and bicarbonate ions (HCO_3^-):

$$\underset{\text{carbonic acid}}{H_2CO_3} \rightleftharpoons \underset{\text{hydrogen ion}}{H^+} + \underset{\text{bicarbonate ion}}{HCO_3^-}$$

About 65% of the CO_2 transported by the blood is in the form of the bicarbonate ion.

The other chemical form of CO_2 is called a **carbamino compound**. A carbamino compound is a chemical combination of CO_2 and a protein. One such protein is the globin of hemoglobin; others are the proteins found in plasma, collectively called **plasma proteins**. About 30% of the total CO_2 transported in the blood is in the carbamino form.

Transport of Gases— Blood Flow

Two major aspects of the circulatory system's relationship to the physiology of sport and physical activity are **cardiac output** and the **distribution of blood flow**. In discussing these important concepts, we will start with a review of the anatomy and physiology of the heart.

Anatomy and Physiology of the Heart

Figure 8-8 is an illustration of a human heart. It consists of four chambers, the left and right **atria** (singular = **atrium**) and the left and right **ventricles**. Usually, the heart is considered to be two pumps, the left heart consisting of the left atrium and ventricle and the right heart consisting of the right atrium and ventricle. The left heart pumps blood through the systemic circuit to the body tissues, such as the skeletal muscles; the right heart pumps blood to the lungs via the pulmonary circuit.

Heart Valves and Direction of Blood Flow

The direction of blood flow is shown by arrows in Figure 8-8. Its direction is controlled by unidirectional valves that are strategically located

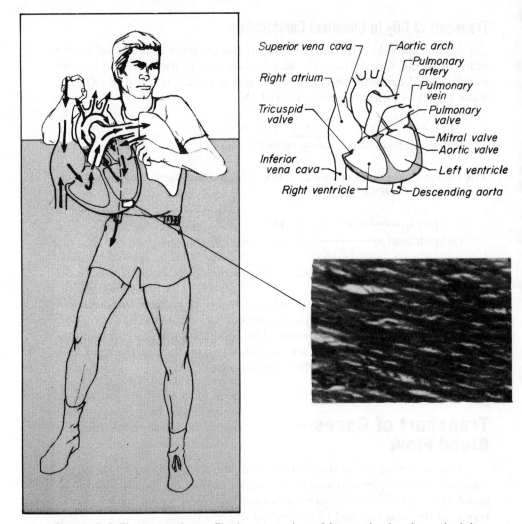

Superior vena cava — ┌Aortic arch
┌Pulmonary artery
Right atrium — ┌Pulmonary vein
Tricuspid valve — ┌Pulmonary valve
— Mitral valve
— Aortic valve
Inferior vena cava —
— Left ventricle
Right ventricle — └Descending aorta

Figure 8-8 The human heart. The heart consists of four main chambers, the left atrium and left ventricle (left heart) and the right atrium and right ventricle (right heart). The flow of blood is indicated by arrows. The left heart pumps blood to the body tissues and the right heart to the lungs. Inset, Microscopic structure of the heart muscle (myocardium) showing the intercalated discs and syncytial arrangement of fibers. (Inset courtesy of Dr. Julianne Chase, The Ohio State University, Columbus, OH.)

throughout the heart. Blood from the head and upper extremities and from the trunk and lower extremities returns via the superior and inferior **vena cava**, respectively, to the right atrium. From there it goes to the right ventricle. As the right ventricle contracts, the **tricuspid valve** closes, preventing blood from backflowing to the atrium. At the same time, the **pulmonary valve** opens, channeling the blood out the pulmonary arteries toward the lungs. On returning from the lungs (by the pulmonary veins), the blood empties into the left atrium and then into the left ventricle. The valve arrangement here is the same as in the right ventricle, except that the names are different: the **mitral valve** closes to prevent backflow into the atrium, and the **aortic valve** opens, directing the blood to the body tissues. Incidentally, if a valve is damaged or does not close properly, blood regurgitates, causing a noise. This type of noise is referred to as a "heart murmur."

Microscopic Structure of Heart Muscle

A closer look at the heart muscle, called the myocardium, is shown in the inset of Figure 8-8. In some ways, heart muscle is similar to skeletal muscle. For example, it is striated, containing myofibrils and actin and myosin protein filaments. In fact, the actual contraction of the myocardium is thought to occur according to the sliding filament theory of muscular contraction as outlined in Chapter 6.

However, in other ways, the heart muscle is quite different from skeletal muscle. In cardiac muscle, all of the individual fibers or cells are anatomically interconnected. This is shown in the inset of Figure 8-8. Notice that the myocardial fibers are connected end-to-end by what are referred to as **intercalated discs.** These discs are actually nothing more than cell membranes. Because all of the fibers of heart muscle are interconnected, the heart acts as if it were one large fiber. This means that when one fiber contracts, all fibers within the heart contract. In skeletal muscle, when one fiber contracts, only those fibers in that particular motor unit contract, not all of the fibers in the muscle. Such an arrangement is referred to as a **functional syncytium,** functional in the sense that when one fiber contracts, all fibers contract, and a syncytium by the fact that all the cells interconnect. Actually, there are two functional syncytia, one for the atria and one for the ventricles. What this means is that first the atria contract together and then the ventricles. It is easy to see that this type of arrangement is most effective in producing the pumping action required of the heart.

Conduction System of the Heart

The heart has an inherent contractile rhythm. That is to say, if all nerves supplying the heart are severed, the heart still continues to generate nervous impulses causing it to contract in a rhythmical fashion. Usually, this autorhythm originates in a specialized area of tissue referred to as the **sinoatrial node (S-A node)**; however, all heart tissue has this property. The S-A node is located in the posterior wall of the right atrium, as illustrated in Figure 8-9. Because the normal heartbeat is initiated in the S-A node, it is sometimes referred to as the **pacemaker** of the heart.

From the S-A node, the cardiac or nervous impulse spreads throughout the atria. Therefore, the atria contract first, emptying their contents into the ventricles. Next the impulse from the atria activates another specialized area of the heart referred to as the **atrioventricular node (A-V node).** It is located also in the right atrium at the atrioventricular junction (Fig. 8-9). From the A-V

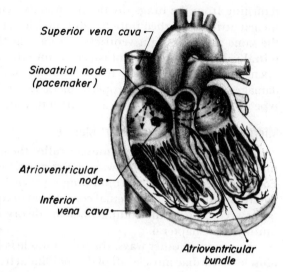

Superior vena cava

Sinoatrial node
(pacemaker)

Figure 8-9 The electrical
conduction system of the
heart. The S-A node is
considered the pacemaker of
the heart since the cardiac
impulse is normally initiated
there. (Modified and redrawn
from Landau, 1976.)

Atrioventricular
node

Inferior
vena cava

Atrioventricular
bundle

node extends a bundle of this same type of special tissue, called the
atrioventricular bundle (A-V bundle), into the right (right bundle branch) and
left (left bundle branch) ventricles. These bundles give off many branches that
eventually reach throughout the entire ventricular myocardium, causing it to
contract.

Blood Supply to the Heart

Like any living tissue, the cardiac muscle also requires a blood supply to
provide it with oxygen and to remove waste products. The blood supply to the
heart is referred to as the **coronary circulation** and is shown in Figure 8-10.
The heart muscle is supplied by two major arteries, the **left coronary artery**
and the **right coronary artery**. They originate from the aorta, just beyond
(above) the aortic valve, and encircle the heart. They **anastomose**, that is, join
together, on the posterior (back) surface of the heart (Fig. 8-10B). All along the
way, branches are given off such that the entire myocardium is supplied with a
rich network of vascular tissue. The major branch of the left coronary artery is
called the **circumflex branch**, whereas that of the right coronary artery is
simply referred to as the branch of the right coronary artery.

The coronary veins run alongside the arteries (Fig. 8-10). They eventually all drain into a very large vein referred to as the **coronary sinus**, which in
turn deposits the venous blood directly into the right atrium of the heart.

Figure 8-10 The coronary circulation. A, The heart muscle is supplied by two
major arteries—the left and right coronary arteries. B, The arteries give off many
branches as they encircle the heart, eventually anastomosing (joining) on the
posterior surface of the heart. (Modified and redrawn from Landau, 1976.)

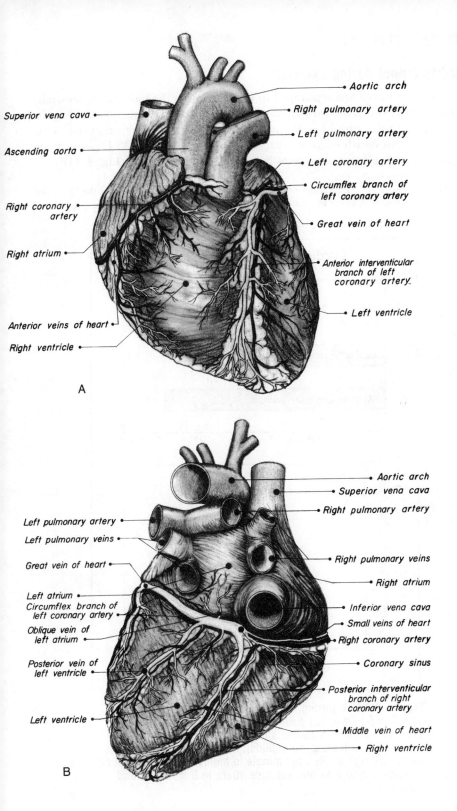

Superior vena cava

Ascending aorta

Right coronary artery

Right atrium

Anterior veins of heart

Right ventricle

A

Aortic arch

Right pulmonary artery

Left pulmonary artery

Left coronary artery

Circumflex branch of left coronary artery

Great vein of heart

Anterior interventicular branch of left coronary artery

Left ventricle

Left pulmonary artery

Left pulmonary veins

Great vein of heart

Left atrium

Circumflex branch of left coronary artery

Oblique vein of left atrium

Posterior vein of left ventricle

Left ventricle

B

Aortic arch

Superior vena cava

Right pulmonary artery

Right pulmonary veins

Right atrium

Inferior vena cava

Small veins of heart

Right coronary artery

Coronary sinus

Posterior interventicular branch of right coronary artery

Middle vein of heart

Right ventricle

Cardiac Output during Exercise

The amount of blood pumped in 1 min by either the right or left ventricle of the heart is called the **cardiac output**, denoted by $\dot{Q}$.* As shown in Figure 8-11A, the cardiac output is about 5 to 6 L per min in a person at rest. The output increases with exercise, reaching values as high as 35 L per min in highly trained endurance athletes during maximal exercise (Fig. 8-11B).

---

*The Q stands for the quantity of blood that is pumped, and the dot over the Q for per minute; $\dot{Q}$ = amount of blood pumped by the heart in 1 min.

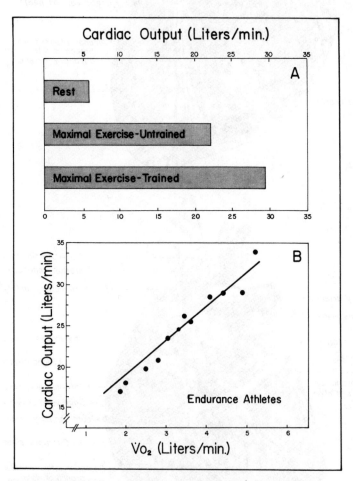

Figure 8-11 A, During resting conditions, cardiac output is only 5 to 6 L/min, but during working conditions—maximal exercise—cardiac output is substantially greater (in both trained and untrained individuals). B, Cardiac output reaches values as high as 35 L per minute in highly trained endurance athletes during maximal exercise. (Data in B from Fox and Costill, 1972.)

The cardiac output has two components, the **stroke volume (SV)** and the **heart rate (HR)**. These components are related as follows:

$$\dot{Q} \quad = \quad SV \quad \times \quad HR$$
cardiac output   stroke volume   heart rate

For example, in a person with a stroke volume of 75 ml per beat and a heart rate of 70 beats per min (both values taken at rest), the cardiac output will be $75 \times 70 = 5250$ ml per min, or 5.25 L per min.

Stroke Volume during Exercise

The stroke volume is defined as the amount of blood pumped by the heart per beat. In untrained men at rest and in the upright position,* the stroke volume is between 70 and 80 ml per beat; in highly trained male endurance athletes at rest and in the upright position, the SV is 100 to 110 ml per beat. The stroke volume increases to its highest values during **submaximal** exercise and does not increase further during maximal work (see Fig. 8-12A). Maximal stroke volumes for untrained men reach values of between 110 and 120 ml per beat, whereas in highly trained male endurance athletes the average values range from 150 to 170 ml, with individual values as high as 200 ml per beat (Fig. 8-12B).

The stroke volume in women shows the same pattern seen in men (low in untrained individuals and high in endurance athletes). However, the absolute stroke volume is smaller in women, mainly because of their smaller heart size.

Heart Rate during Exercise

The heart rate is the number of times the heart beats per minute. Usually the heart beats between 60 and 80 times per min in untrained men and women, but the rate is generally much lower (40 to 55 beats per min) in highly trained endurance athletes. As shown in Figure 8-13, the heart rate increases during exercise; it is directly related to the intensity of the work performed. The increase in heart rate during exercise is normally **lower** in men and women who are trained athletes than in those who are nonathletes, even during maximal effort. However, as previously indicated, because the stroke volume is much higher in athletes, the cardiac output is also much higher during maximal exercise. The heart is more efficient—that is, it requires less oxygen—when the same amount of blood is pumped with a relatively high stroke volume and a relatively low heart rate. Thus the heart of the athlete is more efficient—at rest and during all levels of exercise.

Unlike the cardiac output and stroke volume, the heart rate is easily measured, either by an electrocardiograph or by self-testing (placing the hand directly over the left breast or palpating the radial artery at the wrist or the temporal artery in front of the ear). Because of the ease of measurement, the

---

*Stroke volume is larger when one is lying down.

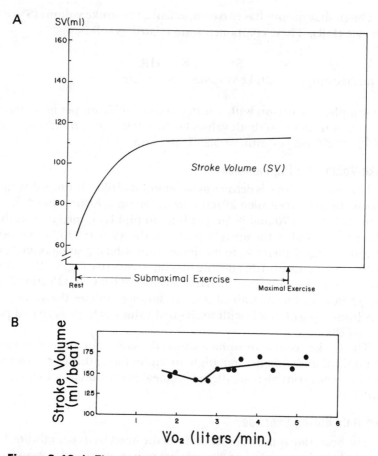

Figure 8-12 A, The stroke volume increases to maximal values during submaximal exercise and does not increase further during maximal work. B, Stroke volumes in highly trained male endurance athletes are very high, ranging between 150 and 200 ml per beat. (Data in B from Fox and Costill, 1972.)

heart rate is most often used as an index of circulatory function during both resting and exercising conditions. More and more coaches are teaching their athletes how to take their pulse rate and what it means with respect to work intensity, recovery from exercise, and physical training (see pp. 215 to 216).

Distribution of Blood Flow during Exercise

Along with the pumping of an increased amount of blood during exercise, there is a redistribution of the blood flow so that the working muscles receive a greater portion of the total cardiac output. This is shown in Table 8-2. Notice that 85% of the total blood flow (cardiac output) is diverted to the working skeletal muscles during maximal exercise, while only 15% is distributed to the muscles under resting conditions. Also notice that half as

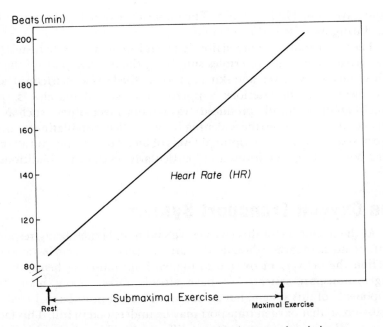

Figure 8-13 The heart rate increases during exercise, being directly related to the intensity of the work performed.

much blood is distributed to the skin, the kidney, and the liver during exercise as compared to rest. Therefore, during exercise blood is directed away from inactive tissues toward the working muscles.

Redistribution during exercise is such that of a total blood flow of 30 L per min, the amount perfusing the muscles is 25.5 L per min. If there were no redistribution, even a total blood flow of 30 L per min would provide only 4.5 L per min to the working muscles (15% of 30 L = 4.5). By extrapolation, in the absence of a redistribution of blood flow, in order for the muscle blood flow to reach values of 25 L per min during exercise, the total cardiac output

Table 8-2: Distribution of Blood Flow (Cardiac Output) During Rest and Maximal Exercise

Organ	Rest Percent	Rest L/min	Exercise Percent	Exercise L/min
Bone	5	0.3	0.5	0.15
Brain	15	0.9	4	1.2
Heart	5	0.3	4	1.2
Kidney	25	1.5	2	0.6
Liver	25	1.5	3	0.9
Muscle	15	0.9	85	25.5
Skin	5	0.3	0.5	0.15
Other	5	0.3	1	0.3
TOTAL	100	6.0	100	30

would have to be 170 L per min! The importance of redistribution of blood flow during exercise is thus obvious.

The redistribution of blood flow is dependent on two mechanisms: (1) the reflex narrowing of the arterioles supplying the inactive parts of the body, such as the kidneys, liver, and skin (a process called **vasoconstriction**); and (2) the widening of the arterioles supplying the skeletal muscles, a process brought about by locally produced "vasodilator metabolites" such as lactic acid and carbon dioxide (the widening itself is called **vasodilation**). This dual control system provides for optimal levels of blood flow to any and all organs, under both resting conditions and, particularly, exercising conditions.

The Oxygen Transport System

At the beginning of this chapter we said that, besides being responsible for the removal of carbon dioxide, the cardiorespiratory system has as a critical function the delivery of oxygen to the working muscles—hence the name **oxygen transport system**. We have already talked about many of the components of this system, but an additional factor must be included in the discussion so that oxygen transport may be understood in full. This factor is the **arterial-mixed venous oxygen difference**. The relationship of this component to stroke volume and heart rate—and the relationship of all three to the volume of transported oxygen—is expressed in the following equation:

$$\dot{V}O_2 \quad = \quad SV \quad \times \quad HR \quad \times \quad \text{a-}\bar{v}O_2\text{diff}$$

| oxygen transported | stroke volume | heart rate | arterial-mixed venous O_2 difference |

You will recall that the product of the stroke volume and heart rate equals the cardiac output. The **arterial-mixed venous oxygen difference (a-$\bar{v}O_2$)** reflects two factors: (1) how much oxygen the muscle extracts from the arterial blood—the more extracted, the less in the venous blood, with the result that the a-$\bar{v}O_2$ diff increases; and (2) the overall distribution of blood flow. An example of the latter, as just indicated, is distribution during exercise, when more blood goes to the working muscles and less to inactive tissues. Under exercise conditions, the a-$\bar{v}O_2$ diff increases, since the active muscles extract more oxygen than do the inactive tissues, thus leaving less oxygen in the venous blood.

A comparison of the oxygen transport system at rest and during exercise is presented in Table 8–3. Notice how all three components increase during exercise, each contributing to the overall increase in oxygen consumption. Notice also that the maximal stroke volume and a-$\bar{v}O_2$ difference are 30 and 10% greater, respectively, in the marathon runners than in the untrained subjects. These two factors, stroke volume and the a-$\bar{v}O_2$ difference, are entirely responsible for the 36% greater maximal oxygen consumption in the

Table 8-3: The Oxygen Transport System at Rest and During Maximal Exercise in Untrained Male Subjects and Male Marathon Runners

Condition	VO_2 ml/min		Stroke Volume L/beat*		Heart Rate beats/min		a-$\bar{v}O_2$diff ml/L
Rest	252	=	0.070	×	80	×	45.0
Maximal Exercise (untrained)	3276	=	0.120	×	195	×	140.0
Maximal Exercise (marathon runners)†	4473	=	0.156	×	185	×	155.0

*Usually expressed in ml/beat.
†Based on data from Fox and Costill (1972).

marathon runners, since the maximal heart rate of these athletes is actually lower than that of the untrained subjects.

Oxygen Transport and Endurance Performance

Since the oxygen system—aerobic metabolism—provides the major portion of the ATP required for prolonged exercise, the functional capabilities of the oxygen transport system are most important during endurance performance. There are three such capabilities that require our attention: (1) **maximal oxygen consumption**; (2) **the anaerobic threshold, that is, the percent utilization of $\dot{V}O_2$ max and lactic acid production**; and (3) **degree of efficiency**.

The Capacity of the Oxygen Transport System— Maximal Oxygen Consumption

One factor related to successful endurance performance is the maximal amount of oxygen capable of being transported to and consumed by the working muscles. As defined previously, this is the **maximal oxygen consumption ($\dot{V}O_2$ max)**. You may recall that we compared the $\dot{V}O_2$ max of participants in various sports in Figure 3–6A (p. 38), and found that the $\dot{V}O_2$ max is highest in endurance athletes. In Figure 8–14, the $\dot{V}O_2$ max of one category of endurance athletes—distance runners—is compared with the $\dot{V}O_2$ max of nonathletes. The male marathoners and female distance runners (2 to 50 miles) selected for the comparison included national and international competitors. While the $\dot{V}O_2$ max values are indeed high in these athletes, it is interesting to note that of the five champions singled out in the figure, four have only average or even below-average values for their groups. This suggests, as we will see later, that the magnitude of the $\dot{V}O_2$ max is not the only factor contributing to successful endurance performances.

One other point is evident from Figure 8–14: the relatively small change (about 10%) in $\dot{V}O_2$ max following, in this case, eight weeks of interval

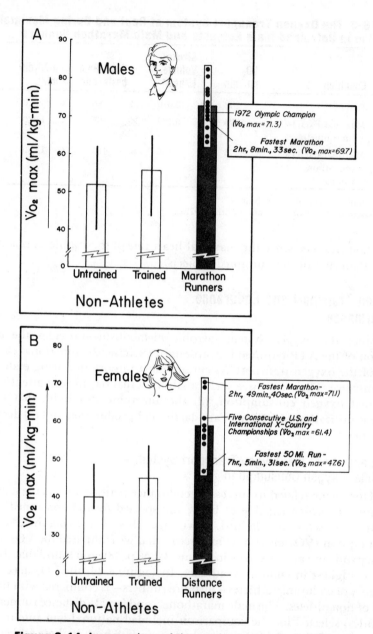

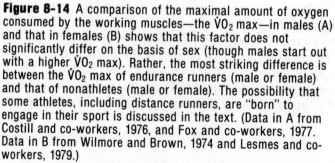

Figure 8-14 A comparison of the maximal amount of oxygen consumed by the working muscles—the $\dot{V}O_2$ max—in males (A) and that in females (B) shows that this factor does not significantly differ on the basis of sex (though males start out with a higher $\dot{V}O_2$ max). Rather, the most striking difference is between the $\dot{V}O_2$ max of endurance runners (male or female) and that of nonathletes (male or female). The possibility that some athletes, including distance runners, are "born" to engage in their sport is discussed in the text. (Data in A from Costill and co-workers, 1976, and Fox and co-workers, 1977. Data in B from Wilmore and Brown, 1974 and Lesmes and co-workers, 1979.)

training in the men and women who are not athletes. In other studies, the average increase in $\dot{V}O_2$ max following eight to 16 weeks of training varies between 5 and 15%, with individual changes as high as 20 to 25%. This means that a man who has an average $\dot{V}O_2$ max value—that is, 50 ml per kg body weight per min—may expect training to increase his $\dot{V}O_2$ max to around 60 ml/kg-min; a woman who starts out at average—i.e., 40 ml/kg-min—may expect an increase to 48 ml/kg-min. These values for trained men and women are still 18% below those for champion athletes.

The above "rough" calculations serve to point out that some factors other than training must be important in establishing the final ceiling for the oxygen transport system. It has, in fact, been determined, as shown in Figure 8-15, that the magnitude of the $\dot{V}O_2$ max has a 93% genetic component. You will recall (from p. 108) that this kind of genetic information is possible by a comparison of the variability between $\dot{V}O_2$ max values of fraternal and identical twin sets. A high genetic component is present when the scatter of points around the diagonal line is smaller for identical twins than for fraternal twins (Fig. 8-15). This prompts the question, "Are distance runners born rather than made?" Think about the question for a while; we will attempt to answer it in the next chapter.

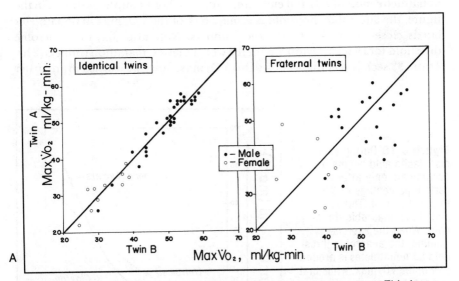

Figure 8-15 The $\dot{V}O_2$ max is genetically determined to a great extent. This is shown by the fact that the intrapair (twin A vs twin B) variability in $\dot{V}O_2$ max for fraternal twins is much greater than for identical twins, as indicated by the wide scatter of points about the diagonal line. If the $\dot{V}O_2$ max values were exactly the same for twin A and B, the points would fall on the line. (Based on data from Klissouras, 1971, and Klissouras and co-workers, 1973.)

The Anaerobic Threshold—The Percent Utilization of $\dot{V}O_2$ max and Lactic Acid Production

It is not just the magnitude of the $\dot{V}O_2$ max that is important during endurance performance; the **percentage** of the $\dot{V}O_2$ max that can be utilized without exhaustion due to lactic acid accumulation is significant as well. The percent utilization of the $\dot{V}O_2$ max is defined as the amount of oxygen consumed during exercise relative to the $\dot{V}O_2$ max. It is calculated by dividing the oxygen consumption ($\dot{V}O_2$) during exercise by the $\dot{V}O_2$ max and multiplying by 100:

$$\%\dot{V}O_2\text{max} = \dot{V}O_2/\dot{V}O_2\text{max} \times 100$$

For example, if your $\dot{V}O_2$ were 1.5 L per min while exercising and your $\dot{V}O_2$ max 3.0 L per min, then you would be utilizing $1.5/3.0 \times 100 = 50\%$ of your maximum. Someone else using the same $\dot{V}O_2$ (1.5 L per min) but with a $\dot{V}O_2$ max of 4.0 L per min would be utilizing only $1.5/4.0 \times 100 = 37.5\%$ of his or her maximum. In other words, the exercise for the latter individual, although requiring the same $\dot{V}O_2$, would be easier. Thus, $\% \dot{V}O_2$ max is useful as an index of how stressful the exercise is with respect to one's maximum capacity.

The relationship between $\%\dot{V}O_2$ max and lactic acid production during running is shown in Figure 8-16. Lactic acid begins to accumulate only after a certain $\%\dot{V}O_2$ max is reached. This "starting point" for lactic acid accumulation is called the **anaerobic threshold** and is quite different between untrained, nonathletic individuals and endurance athletes. For example, as shown in the figure, the anaerobic threshold is around 65% of the $\dot{V}O_2$ max in nonathletes but is close to 80% in the distance runners. Note also that the anaerobic threshold for Derek Clayton, one of the world's fastest marathon runners (2 hr, 8 min, 33 sec), is very high—86% of his $\dot{V}O_2$ max. Since we learned in an earlier

Figure 8-16 During exercise, lactic acid begins to accumulate only after a certain percentage of $\dot{V}O_2$ max is reached. This is called the anaerobic threshold. When the exercise is running, the anaerobic threshold for nonathletes is around 65% of the $\dot{V}O_2$ max, while that in distance runners is closer to 80% of the $\dot{V}O_2$ max. In the case of Derek Clayton, one of the world's fastest marathoners, the anaerobic threshold is 86% of the $\dot{V}O_2$ max.

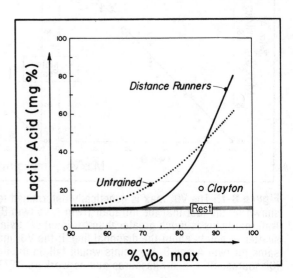

chapter that lactic acid accumulation in the blood and muscles causes temporary muscular fatigue, it is easy to understand the advantage of a high anaerobic threshold relative to endurance performance.

The relationships among the percentage of $\dot{V}O_2$ max, blood lactic acid accumulation, and competitive running distances for trained endurance athletes are shown in Figure 8-17. In studying these relationships it becomes obvious that the higher the $\dot{V}O_2$ max—and the higher the anaerobic threshold—the more successful endurance performance will be. As just mentioned, the magnitude of the $\dot{V}O_2$ max appears to be highly genetic. However, the magnitude of the anaerobic threshold is most likely a manifestation of training. More will be said about this in the next chapter.

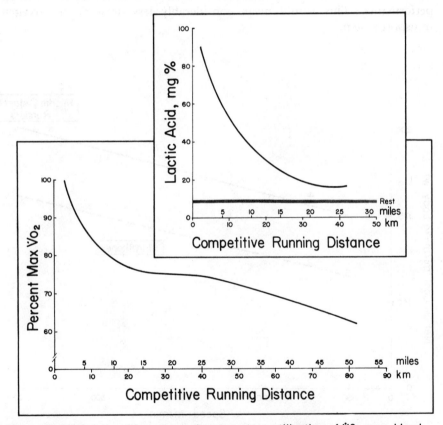

Figure 8-17 Relationships among the percentage utilization of $\dot{V}O_2$ max, blood lactic acid accumulation, and competitive running distances for trained endurance athletes. The higher one's $\dot{V}O_2$ max and the higher the percentage utilization of the $\dot{V}O_2$ max without accumulation of exhausting levels of lactic acid, the more successful endurance performance will be. (Based on data from Costill, 1970, and Costill and Fox, 1969.)

Efficiency of the Oxygen Transport System

Efficiency, or the amount of oxygen required during a given exercise level, is a further important component of endurance performance. For instance, in two runners with the same $\dot{V}O_2$ max, the one who requires less oxygen to run at the same pace will be utilizing less of his or her $\dot{V}O_2$ max, and will therefore be less fatigued. In other words, the more efficient runner will be able to run faster while experiencing no greater degree of fatigue.

In a study of the efficiency of distance runners, it was found that marathoners required less oxygen at the same speed than did middle-distance runners. The comparative degrees of efficiency are shown in Figure 8–18. It is easily seen that the marathon runners are between 5 and 10% more efficient in terms of the amount of oxygen required to run a given distance. Over a short distance, this would not be a significant factor. However, it can be calculated that between 25 and 50 L of oxygen could be saved during a 2½-hr marathon performance. This would mean considerably less stress on the oxygen transport system.

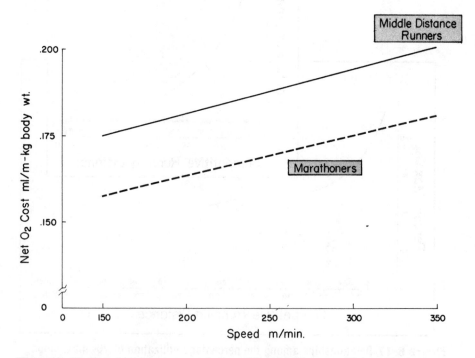

Figure 8-18 Marathon runners are between 5 and 10% more efficient than other distance runners in terms of the amount of oxygen required to run a given distance. This greater efficiency results in a savings of between 25 and 50 L of oxygen during a 2½-hour marathon performance. (Based on data from Fox and Costill, 1972.)

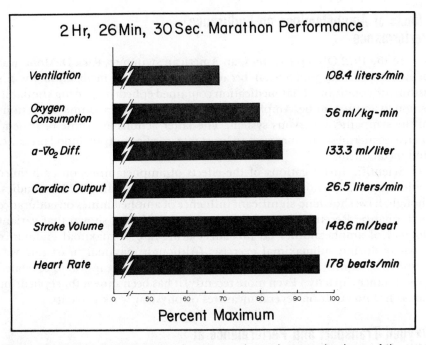

Figure 8-19 Estimated degrees of stress on the various mechanisms of the oxygen transport system during a marathon performance. As you can see, cardiac output, stroke volume, and heart rate are most heavily taxed. (Based on data from Fox and Costill, 1972.)

The importance of the oxygen transport system during endurance performance can be seen in Figure 8–19 from estimated cardiorespiratory responses during a 2-hr, 26-min, 30-sec marathon performance. Note that the circulatory responses are taxed to a much greater degree than the respiratory responses (particularly ventilation). Specifically, cardiac output, stroke volume, and heart rate are the most heavily stressed during competition. On the average, they are maintained very nearly at maximal levels throughout most of the race. In fact, it has been estimated that the heart rate and cardiac output of the winner of the 1968 Boston Marathon were maximal for at least an hour of the 2-hr, 22-min, 17-sec performance.

In summary, three physiological capacities are important for success in endurance performance:

1. A high $\dot{V}O_2$ max
2. A high anaerobic threshold
3. A high efficiency of the oxygen transport system

Effects of Amphetamines on Endurance Performance

In the 1972 Olympic Games, an American swimmer, Rick DeMont, was denied an earned gold medal because he was taking medication for his asthmatic condition. That medication contained ephedrine, a drug similar in action to amphetamine. Amphetamines are stimulants that mimic the actions of the sympathetic nervous system. The latter actions are those of general increased alertness and increases in heart rate, cardiac output, blood pressure, and metabolism.

Scientific investigations of the effects of amphetamines on endurance performance have not always produced consistent findings. Most studies, though, have shown no significant influence of amphetamines on endurance performance. Recently, in a well designed study, it was shown that variant dosages of amphetamines do not affect heart rate or maximal endurance capacity during submaximal exercise. (Although maximal heart rate was found to be significantly increased, such an effect does not appear to be related to endurance capacity.) Even more recently, it has been shown that ephedrine per se has no effect on several measures of physical work capacity.

Oxygen Transport and Performance at Altitudes above Sea Level

It has been known for some time that physical performance is reduced in areas above sea level. This is particularly evident at altitudes above 4000 to 5000 ft (1300 to 1650 m). This reduction in performance is due to **hypoxia**, a decrease in the partial pressure of oxygen in the inspired air. You will recall that the Po_2 gradients between lung and blood and between blood and tissue are vitally important with respect to the capacity of the oxygen transport system. The more severe the hypoxia—that is, the greater the altitude—the greater the decrement in performance.

Since the oxygen transport system is more and more handicapped at higher and higher altitudes, it is not surprising to find that the $\dot{V}O_2$ max declines as elevation increases. This is true for both well trained athletes and unconditioned subjects, as shown in Figure 8–20A. On the average, $\dot{V}O_2$ max for untrained individuals may be expected to decrease about 3% for every 1000 ft (305 m) above 5000 ft (1524 m). For example, at 10,000 ft (3050 m), $\dot{V}O_2$ max would be 15% below that measured at sea level.* For well trained athletes, the rate of decrease in $\dot{V}O_2$ max may not be as great; however, it starts to decrease sooner—that is, at a lower altitude. The decrease is about 2% for every 1000 ft above sea level. Thus, at 10,000 ft, the $\dot{V}O_2$ max of well trained athletes would be about 20% lower than the value measured at sea level.

From the above discussion, you may have guessed that the most difficult activities to perform at high altitudes are the endurance events. Just how

---

*The decrease in $\dot{V}O_2$ max begins at 5000 ft; for every 1000 ft of what remains—in this case 5000 ft (10,000-5000 = 5000)—the rate of decline is 3%: 3% × 5 = 15%.

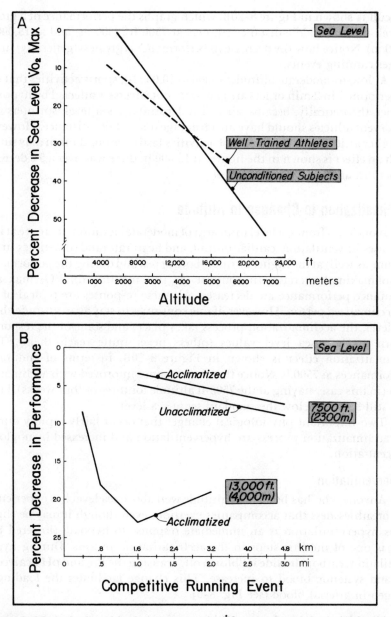

Figure 8-20 A, As the altitude increases, the $\dot{V}O_2$ max decreases in both athletes and nonathletes. B, Altitudes considerably above sea level have adverse effects on performance as well, especially in endurance events. With acclimatization, however, performance may be improved (but still will not match performance at sea level). (Data in A from Buskirk, 1969; data in B from Adams and co-workers, 1975.)

195

difficult is shown in Figure 8–20B, which graphs the performance of a group of well trained middle-distance runners at 7500 ft (2300 m) and at 13,000 ft (4000 m). Notice how the decrease in performance is greatest (generally) in the longer running events.

At low-to-moderate altitudes (5000 to 10,000 ft), sports activities that can be performed in 2 min or less are generally not adversely affected by hypoxia. In fact, theoretically, because air is less dense above sea level, sprinters and field event athletes should have an advantage due to less resistance. However, at higher altitudes, performance of activities lasting around 1 min may suffer. Such an effect is shown in the figure: at 13,000 ft, there was over a 5% decrease in performance of the 440-yd event.

Acclimatization to Changes in Altitude

If one goes from sea level to an area of moderate elevation, there are at first increases in ventilation, cardiac output, and heart rate (and sometimes stroke volume as well) at the higher altitude, both at rest and during the performance of submaximal exercise. In contrast (as just mentioned), $\dot{V}O_2$ max and endurance performance are decreased. All these responses are typical of the unacclimatized person. However, if one continues to stay at an altitude above sea level, the acclimatization process takes place, and some of the responses return to their sea level values (others never quite reach them). This acclimatization effect is shown in Figure 8–20B, in terms of endurance performances at 7500 ft. Notice that performance improved with acclimatization (in this case, staying at the 7500-ft altitude for three or four weeks), but it was still 3 to 4% below the standard set at sea level.

Two important physiological changes that occur fairly rapidly during the acclimatization process are hyperventilation and increased hemoglobin concentration.

Hyperventilation

Anyone who has been at an altitude well above sea level has experienced the breathlessness that accompanies exertion, even though it may be slight. This hyperventilation is an immediate response to hypoxia (lowered Po_2) and is one of the first steps in the acclimatization process. During hyperventilation, carbon dioxide is "blown off," causing the Po_2 and pH of alveolar air and systemic blood to increase. This change facilitates the loading of oxygen in arterial blood (see Fig. 8–6).

Increased Hemoglobin Concentration

Another very early response to hypoxia is an increase in the number of red blood cells and hence in the hemoglobin concentration. As discussed earlier, this increases the oxygen-carrying capacity of arterial blood.

Training at Moderate Altitudes

It has been suggested that a combination of training at sea level and moderate altitudes potentiates the effects of training on endurance performance. The pros and cons of training at moderate altitudes will be presented in the next chapter (p. 249).

Summary

- Pulmonary ventilation is the movement of air into and out of the lungs. The amount of air ventilated in 1 min is called the minute ventilation.

- Ventilation increases slightly before exercise begins (anticipatory rise). The increase is greatest and most rapid at the beginning of exercise, followed by a slower rise, and, in submaximal exercise, an eventual leveling off.

- In healthy individuals, physical performance is not limited by pulmonary ventilation.

- Alveolar ventilation refers to the air that enters the alveoli (terminal air sacs in the lungs), which are in contact with the blood. Air outside the alveoli (in the nose, mouth, and other respiratory passages) fills the dead space, where no gas exchange occurs.

- Chronic cigarette smoking causes increased airway resistance, which can lead to decreased endurance performance. The increased resistance can be noticeably reduced by not smoking 24 hr prior to performance.

- "Second wind" is a change from a feeling of distress early in prolonged exercise to a more agreeable feeling later in the exercise. It is associated with more comfortable breathing and other factors such as relief from muscular fatigue.

- A stitch in the side—the pain in the side that occurs in many exercises—is thought to be caused by lack of oxygen in the respiratory muscles. It is most common during running and swimming.

- Diffusion is the movement of molecules from a higher to a lower concentration. The exchange of gases at the alveolar-capillary and tissue-capillary membranes involves diffusion.

- The most important factor determining gas exchange is the partial pressure of the gases involved. The partial pressure of a gas is the pressure exerted in relation to the concentration of the gas within a volume. The partial pressure of oxygen is highest in the alveoli and lowest in the tissue. Just the opposite is true for carbon dioxide.

- The diffusion capacity of the lungs is greatest in endurance athletes.

- Oxygen and carbon dioxide are carried in the blood mostly in chemical combination with hemoglobin. Carbon dioxide is also chemically carried in the form of bicarbonate ions and carbamino compounds.

- Blood doping, the removal and subsequent reinfusion of blood and/or red blood cells, is done in an attempt to improve endurance performance by increasing the oxygen-carrying capacity of blood. Although blood doping has been shown to increase endurance performance, its effects are still controversial and not recommended, particularly for highly trained athletes. Blood doping is illegal in Olympic competition.

- The heart is a muscular pump that circulates the blood through the circulatory system. The direction of blood flow is controlled by unidirectional valves located in the heart. The myocardium (heart muscle) is a syncytium, that is, all of its fibers are interconnected. Thus the heart contracts as though it were one fiber.

- The heart has an inherent contractile rhythm that originates in the sinoatrial node (S-A node) in the right atrium and then spreads to the atrioventricular node (A-V node) and then throughout the heart muscle.

- The left and right coronary arteries are the major arteries supplying blood to the heart. They branch repeatedly throughout the entire myocardium. The major vein of the heart is called the coronary sinus.

- Cardiac output, the amount of blood pumped by the heart in 1 min, has two components: stroke volume (the amount of blood pumped per beat) and heart rate. In highly trained endurance athletes, both the cardiac output and stroke volume are very high during maximal exercise.

- During exercise, blood flow is redistributed so that the working muscles receive a greater portion of the cardiac output, with inactive tissues getting a lesser portion.

- The oxygen transport system ($\dot{V}O_2$) is made up of the stroke volume (SV), heart rate (HR), and the arterial-mixed venous oxygen difference (a-$\bar{v}O_2$ diff):

$$\dot{V}O_2 = SV \times HR \times a\text{-}\bar{v}O_2\text{diff}$$

- The capacity of the oxygen transport system—the maximal oxygen consumption ($\dot{V}O_2$ max)—is highest in endurance athletes.

- Most successful endurance athletes have a high anaerobic threshold, that is, they can utilize a high percentage of their $\dot{V}O_2$ max without lactic acid accumulating in sufficient amounts to cause exhaustion.

- Endurance runners are more efficient in terms of how much oxygen is required to run at a given speed than are other runners.

- Amphetamines, drugs that mimic the actions of the sympathetic nervous system, do not increase endurance performance.

- Endurance performance is reduced at increasing altitudes owing to the decreased partial pressure of oxygen (hypoxia).

- Acclimatization to high altitude, a process which includes such physiological responses as hyperventilation and increased hemoglobin concentration, helps overcome deficits in endurance performance, but never to the point that performance returns completely to its sea level quality.

Selected References and Readings*

Adams, W. C., et al.: Effects of equivalent sea-level and altitude training on $\dot{V}O_2$ max and running performance. *J. Appl. Physiol., 39(2)*:262–266, 1975.

Bell, R. D., et al.: Blood doping and athletic performance. *Aust. J. Sports Med., 8(2)*:133–139, 1977.

---

*For full journal titles, see Appendix A.

Buick, F. J., et al.: Effects of induced erythrocythemia on aerobic work capacity. *J. Appl. Physiol.: Respirat. Environ. Exercise Physiol.*, *48*:636–642, 1980.

Buskirk, E. R. Decrease in physical working capacity at high altitude. *In* Hegnauer, A. H. (ed.): *Biomedicine of High Terrestrial Elevations.* U.S. Army Medical Research Institute of Environmental Medicine, Natick, MA, and U.S. Army Medical Research and Development Command, Washington, D. C., 1968.

Costill, D. L., et al.: Determinants of marathon running success. *Int. Z. Angew, Physiol.*, *29*: 249–254, 1971.

Costill, D. L., W. J. Fink, and M. L. Pollock: Muscle fiber composition and enzyme activities of elite distance runners. *Med. Sci. Sports, 8(2)*:96–100, 1976.

Costill, D. L., and E. L. Fox: Energetics of marathon running. *Med. Sci. Sports, 1(2)*:81–86, 1969.

Costill, D. L.: Metabolic responses during distance running. *J. Appl. Physiol.*, *28(3)*:251–255, 1970.

Costill, D. L., H. Thomason, and E. Roberts: Fractional utilization of the aerobic capacity during distance running. *Med. Sci. Sports, 5(4)*:248–252, 1973.

Ekblom, B., G. Wilson, and P. O. Åstrand: Central circulation during exercise after venesection and reinfusion of red blood cells. *J. Appl. Physiol.*, *40*:379–383, 1976.

Ekblom, B., A. Goldbard, and B. Gullbring: Response to exercise after blood loss and reinfusion. *J. Appl. Physiol.*, *3(2)*:175–180, 1973.

Fox, E. L., et al.: Metabolic responses to interval training programs of high and low power output. *Med. Sci. Sports, 9(3)*:191–196, 1977.

Fox, E. L., and D. K. Mathews: *The Physiological Basis of Physical Education and Athletics.* 3rd ed. Philadelphia, Saunders College Publishing, 1981, pp. 183–255.

Fox, E. L., and D. L. Costill: Estimated cardiorespiratory responses during marathon running. *Arch. Environ. Health, 24*:315–324, 1972.

Gledhill, N.: Blood doping and related issues: a brief review. *Med. Sci. Sports Exercise, 14(3)*: 183–189, 1982.

Horstman, D., R. Weiskopf, and R. Jackson: Work capacity during 3-wk sojourn at 4,300 m: effects of relative polycythemia. *J. Appl. Physiol.: Respirat. Environ. Exercise Physiol.*, *49(2)*:311–318, 1980.

Klissouras, V., F. Pirnay, and J. Petit. Adaptation to maximal effort: genetics and age. *J. Appl. Physiol.*, *35(2)*:288–293, 1973.

Klissouras, V.: Heritability of adaptive variation. *J. Appl. Physiol.*, *31(3)*:338–344, 1971.

Landau, B. R.: *Essential Human Anatomy and Physiology.* Glenview, IL, Scott, Foresman and Company, 1976.

Lesmes, G. E., et al.: Metabolic responses of females to interval training programs of different frequencies. *Med. Sci. Sports*, 1979.

Magel, J., and K. Lange-Anderson: Pulmonary diffusion capacity and cardiac output in young trained Norwegian swimmers and untrained subjects. *Med. Sci. Sports, 1(3)*:131–139, 1969.

Maksud, M., et al.: Pulmonary function measurements of Olympic speed skaters from the U.S. *Med. Sci. Sports, 3(2)*:66–71, 1971.

Newman, F., B. Smalley, and M. Thompson: A comparison between body size and lung function of swimmers and normal school children. *J. Physiol.* (Lond.), *156*:9P, 1961.

Reuschlein, P., et al.: Effect of physical training on the pulmonary diffusing capacity during submaximal work. *J. Appl. Physiol., 24(2)*:152–158, 1968.

Robertson, R., et al.: Effect of red blood cell reinfusion on physical working capacity and perceived exertion at normal and reduced oxygen pressure. *Med. Sci. Sports, 10(1)*:49, 1978.

Rode, A., and R. Shephard: The influence of cigarette smoking upon the oxygen cost of breathing in near maximal exercise. *Med. Sci. Sports, 3(2)*:51–55, 1971.

Sidney, K. H., and N. M. Lefcoe: The effects of ephedrine on the physiological and psychological 'responses to submaximal and maximal exercise in man. *Med. Sci. Sports, 9(2)*:95–99, 1977.

Williams, M. H.: Blood doping and aerobic activity. *J. Phys. Educ. Rec., 51*:55–56, 1980.

Williams, M. H.: Blood doping: a review. *J. Drug Issues, 10*:331–339, 1980.

Williams, M. H.: Blood doping—does it really help athletes? *Physician and Sportsmedicine*, Jan., 1975, p. 52.

Williams, M. H.: Goodwin, R. Perkins, and J. Bocrie: Effects of blood reinjection upon endurance capacity and heart rate. *Med. Sci. Sports, 5(3)*:181–185, 1973.

Williams, M. H., and J. Thompson: Effect of variant dosages of amphetamine upon endurance. *Res. Quart., 44(4)*:417–422, 1973.

Williams, M. H., M. Lindhjem, and R. Schuster: The effect of blood infusion upon endurance capacity and ratings of perceived exertion. *Med. Sci. Sports, 10(2)*:113–118, 1978.

Williams, M. H., et al.: The effect of induced erythrocythemia upon 5-mile treadmill run time. *Med. Sci. Sports Exercise, 13(3)*:169–175, 1981.

Wilmore, J. H., and C. H. Brown: Physiological profiles of women distance runners. *Med. Sci. Sports, 6(3)*:178–181, 1974.

9

Sprint and Endurance Training: Methods and Effects

Introduction

The successful coach provides his or her athletes with a grasp of strategy, a psychological environment conducive to a model level of performance, a means of honing skills, and a proper course of training. While strategy and psychology are outside the scope of this book, and certain aspects of skill development are far too specialized for our purposes, training is in many ways the crux of our concern with sports physiology. As you will see, this chapter's focus on training relates to all other topics in this book.

Training the athlete is a matter of constructing exercise programs that develop what the individual will need for his or her specific event. The coach must, therefore, give equal consideration to increasing the athlete's skill and developing his or her energy capacities. Note that these basics of training apply to the athlete. In some respects, athletes might be considered easier to train than nonathletes, as they should know which specific energy system(s) must be developed for their particular activities and, ideally, are psychologically prepared to work hard. On the other hand, athletes might be harder to train, because their specific event requires development of a very high level of skill and an increase in the capacities of as many as two of the three energy systems.

Specificity of Training

In order for a training program to be most beneficial, it must develop the specific physiological capabilities required to perform a given sports skill or activity. As has been emphasized previously, one important physiological capability related to sports skills and to exercise in general is the supplying of energy (ATP) to the working muscles.

Metabolic Specificity

In Chapters 2 and 3, we learned that the ATP required for any exercise may be supplied by the ATP-PC or phosphagen system, the lactic acid system (anaerobic glycolysis), and/or the oxygen (aerobic) system. As shown in Table 9-1, the systems supply ATP at differing capacities and at different rates (power). Thus, for any given exercise, the predominant energy source that is used will depend on the total amount and rate of energy demanded by the exercise.

For example, in sprinting 100 m in 9.9 sec, it may be estimated that a total of only 0.43 mole of ATP is required; on a per minute basis, this is an average rate of utilization of 2.6 moles. From looking at Table 9-1, one may see that the predominant energy system in this case is the phosphagen system. To improve the performance of the sprinter, a training program that leads to greater energy output through the phosphagen stores would clearly be indicated. On the other hand, in exercises of lower power output and longer duration, in which the absolute amount of ATP rather than its rate of utilization is most important, the predominant energy system will be aerobic. A good illustration of the latter is the 42.2-km marathon race, in which a total of approximately 150 moles of ATP is required at a rate of utilization of only 1 mole or less per min. In this case, development of the aerobic capacity ($\dot{V}O_2$ max) of the athlete should be the main objective of the training program.

In many activities, all three energy systems are important suppliers of ATP, although a specific system may predominate at different times in an event. For example, in a 1500-m run, the anaerobic systems supply the majority of ATP during the sprint at both the start and the finish of the race, with the aerobic system predominating during the middle or steady-state period of the run. The involvement of both aerobic and anaerobic systems during a 1500-m race is further borne out by the fact that approximately 6.0 moles of ATP are required during the run, with an average rate of utilization of 1.7 moles per min or less—levels that can be met only by using a variety of

Table 9-1: The Capacity and Power of the Three Energy Systems (Untrained Male Subjects)*

	ATP Production	
Energy System	Capacity (total moles)	Power (moles/min)
Phosphagen stores (ATP + PC)	0.6	3.6
Anaerobic glycolysis	1.2	1.6
Aerobic (oxidative)	Theoretically unlimited	1.0

*From Fox (1977).

systems (see Table 9-1). In order to improve performance in this type of activity, a training program that increases both anaerobic and aerobic capacities must be selected.

Other Types of Specificity

Designing a training program to develop the specific energy system appropriate to an athlete's chosen sport should be just one of the coach's concerns, for other types of specificity must be taken into account as well. For example, it has been shown that a training program consisting of cycling results in an 8% increase in maximal aerobic power ($\dot{V}O_2$max) when the trainee cycles but only a 3% increase when the trainee runs on a treadmill. Similar specific training responses with respect to heart rate during submaximal cycling and running have also been reported. Swimming programs have likewise been shown to produce responses specific to swimming. These findings point to one conclusion: for maximal training benefits, the mode of exercise used during the training sessions should be consistent with that used during the performance of the skill in question.

It is important to mention here that the training effects induced by running, although still specific to the type of exercise performed, appear to be more general than those induced by cycling. Thus training programs based on running have some beneficial carry-over effects on the performance of sports skills not involving a great deal of running.

Another type of specificity is related to the muscle groups used during the training program. Researchers have examined this specificity in many ways. In one study, 15 subjects were pretested on a bicycle ergometer during submaximal exercise—once using arm work and once using leg work. Then, for five weeks, seven of the 15 subjects were trained using arm pedaling only, while the other eight subjects trained using leg pedaling only. At the conclusion of training, the subjects were again tested on the bicycle ergometer, once with arm work and once with leg work. It was found that the magnitude of post-training changes was generally greater when the exercise was performed with the trained muscle groups than when the exercise was performed with the untrained muscle groups. Specifically, when the "arm-trained" group was tested on arm work, physiological changes were more substantial than when the same group was tested on leg work. The degree of change can be readily compared. Oxygen consumption ($\dot{V}O_2$) decreased by 250 ml per min when the arm-trained group performed arm work, but the $\dot{V}O_2$ dropped by only 140 ml per min when the same group performed leg work. Levels of lactic acid in the blood of the arm-trained group decreased by 33 mg per 100 ml when arm work was tested; when leg work was tested, levels fell by only 0.8 mg per 100 ml. The heart rate dropped by 29 beats per min when arm work was tested; during leg work, the decrease was only 8 beats per min (see

Fig. 9–1). Stroke volume (SV) increased under both testing conditions, but once again values were far apart: when arm work was performed, the SV rose by 17 ml, but when leg work was carried out, the SV increased by only 1.7 ml. These results not only point out the specific nature of a large number of physiological changes induced by training but also indicate that the controlling mechanisms for such changes are to a large extent influenced by the skeletal muscles themselves. The importance of changes induced by training and physiological responses with respect to the construction of a training program is obvious.

The effects of training are specific not just to muscle groups but to the movement patterns of these muscle groups as well. In other words, neuro-muscular training appears to be motor-skill specific. Accordingly, training programs should contain, whenever feasible, exercise activities related as closely as possible to those actually performed during the execution of the sports skill in question. Motor-skill specificity may best be seen in athletes who participate in back-to-back seasonal sports; the football player who is in excellent condition for playing football can hardly run the length of the court on the first day of basketball practice.

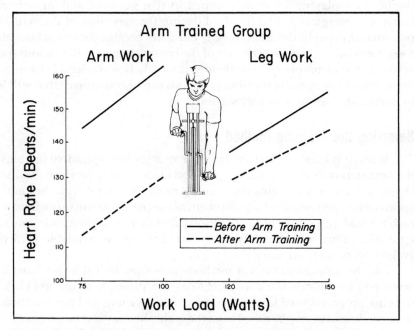

Figure 9-1 Specificity of changes in heart rate when submaximal work is performed following arm training. Note how arm training produced a greater decrease in heart rate during arm work (cycling) than during leg work (also cycling). (Based on data from Fox and co-workers, 1975.)

Construction or Selection of the Training Program

The preceding concept of specificity of physical training provides some guidelines that should be considered in constructing or selecting training programs.

Stressing the Predominant Energy System(s)

A training program should be selected that will increase the physiological capacity of the energy system(s) most used in the sport or sports activity for which the program is being designed. For example, the marathoner, who relies heavily on the aerobic system for ATP energy while running, needs a training program that leads to improvement of the aerobic system. To improve a sprinter's performance, a program that leads to improvement of the anaerobic systems should be selected.

While it is relatively easy to choose which energy system to develop in the sprinter or the marathoner, the decision is much more difficult when it comes to athletes in most other sports activities. There are, however, guidelines for estimating the emphasis that should be placed on improving the energy systems during training for various sports, and these are presented in Table 9-2. The table was developed by analysis of each sport activity with regard to the position played, the skills required in that position, and, most importantly, the energy system(s) involved during the execution of the skill. The percentages given in the table are only estimates because data from laboratory assessments of the exact interaction of the energy systems in the various sports activities are incomplete. Nevertheless, the table is very useful because with these guidelines, specific training programs can be constructed that will lead to maximum increases in performance.

Selecting the Training Method

When it is known which energy systems are to be emphasized in training, the next step is to select a training method most likely to produce the desired changes. Table 9-3 contains ten training methods, their definitions, and the approximate percentage of development of the energy systems associated with each method. (Again, it should be emphasized that these percentages are only approximations, and that laboratory data are not yet available to permit evaluation of their accuracy.)

For the most part, the ten methods presented in Table 9-3 have been developed by various track and field coaches throughout the world. Most training programs used for other sports are adaptations and combinations of these methods. As may be noted from the table, there are several programs that develop the same energy systems to approximately the same degree. One program—the interval training system—allows variations: it may be regulated so as to develop mainly the two anaerobic systems, or mainly the aerobic

Table 9-2: Various Sports and Activities and Their Predominant Energy Systems*

Sports or Sport Activity	% Emphasis per Energy System		
	ATP-PC and LA	LA-O$_2$	O$_2$
Baseball	80	20	—
Basketball	85	15	—
Fencing	90	10	—
Field hockey	60	20	20
Football	90	10	—
Golf	95	5	—
Gymnastics	90	10	—
Ice hockey			
Forwards, defense	80	20	—
Goalie	95	5	—
Lacrosse			
Goalie, defense, attack men	80	20	—
Midfielders, man-down	60	20	20
Recreational sports	—	5	95
Rowing	20	30	50
Skiing			
Slalom, jumping, downhill	80	20	—
Cross-country	—	5	95
Soccer			
Goalie, wings, strikers	80	20	—
Halfbacks, link men	60	20	20
Softball	80	20	—
Swimming and diving			
50-m freestyle, diving	98	2	—
100 m, 100 yd (all strokes)	80	15	5
200 m, 200 yd (all strokes)	30	65	5
400 m, 440 yd, 500-yd freestyle	20	55	25
1500 m, 1650 yd	10	20	70
Tennis	70	20	10
Track and field			
100 m, 100 yd; 200 m, 220 yd	98	2	—
Field events	90	10	—
400 m, 440 yd	80	15	5
800 m, 880 yd	30	65	5
1500 m, 1 mile	20	55	25
2 miles	20	40	40
3 miles, 5000 m	10	20	70
6 miles (cross-country), 10,000 m	5	15	80
Marathon	—	5	95
Volleyball	90	10	—
Wrestling	90	10	—

*Modified from Fox and Mathews (1974).

Table 9-3: Definitions of Various Training Methods and Development of the Energy Systems*

Training Method	Definition	% Development ATP-PC and LA	LA and O$_2$	O$_2$
Acceleration sprints	Gradual increases in running speed from jogging to striding to sprinting in 50- to 120-yd segments	90	5	5
Continuous fast running	Long-distance running (or swimming) at a fast pace	2	8	90
Continuous slow running	Long-distance running (or swimming) at a slow pace	2	5	93
Hollow sprints	Two sprints interrupted by "hollow" periods of jogging or walking	85	10	5
Interval sprinting	Alternate sprints of 50 yd and jogs of 60 yd for distances up to 3 miles	20	10	70
Interval training	Repeated periods of work interspersed with periods of relief	0–80	0–80	0–80
Jogging	Continuous walking or running at a slow pace over a moderate distance (e.g., 2 miles)	—	—	100
Repetition running	Similar to interval training but with longer work and relief intervals	10	50	40
Speed play (fartlek)	Alternating fast and slow running over natural terrain	20	40	40
Sprint training	Repeated sprints at maximal speed with complete recovery between repeats	90	6	4

*From Fox (1977).

system, or all three systems equally. This method of training is one of the few training systems that have been systematically and scientifically studied.

As an example of how to use Tables 9–2 and 9–3, assume that you wish to train someone to run 2 miles. From Table 9–2, you can find the degree of usage of the energy systems during a 2-mile run. Table 9–3 may then be consulted so you can determine which training methods develop the energy systems to this degree. Two programs—interval training and speed play—develop each system in the appropriate range, and another program, repetition running, approximates the development the runner will need. By looking back at Table 9–2, you can see that any one of these three programs might also be appropriate for use in training a 400-m freestyle swimmer or a rower. For the swimmer, of course, the mode of exercise would have to be swimming, just as the rower would train by rowing.

Suggested sprint and endurance training methods that are appropriate for various sports and sports activities are shown in Table 9-4. This table was constructed from the information given in Tables 9-2 and 9-3. Remember that for sports such as ice hockey, the mode of exercise for most of the training sessions should be skating rather than running. The same applies to rowing, skiing, and swimming and diving, for which the modes of exercise during training should, of course, be rowing, skiing, and swimming, respectively.

Prescription Content

It is beyond the scope of this book to describe in complete detail various training programs for athletes in all sports. What can be included here, though, are sample workouts (or prescriptions) for several different track athletes, as presented in Table 9-5. As previously mentioned, these prescriptions may be applied to other sports and activities with minimal adaptation. For example, acceleration sprints, hollow sprints, interval training, and sprint training methods may be modified for the football player along these lines: prescribe sprint distances of only 40 to 50 yd; prescribe backward and lateral running; prescribe stop-and-go sprinting (i.e., the runner sprints for 5 yd, then stops and reaches out to touch the ground, then sprints 5 more yd, reaches out and touches the ground, and so on, for a total of 40 to 50 yd). It should be noticed that these particular variations include movement patterns that are specifically involved in football skills. It is thought that such training induces changes that are quite distinct from—and more important to performance than—the training's effects on anaerobic metabolism. Essentially, the effects of training for high-power output activities (sprint training, anaerobic training) on anaerobic metabolism are small in number and degree, yet improvements in performance can be substantial. Obviously, some other changes induced by training must come into play. Presumably, changes in motor unit recruitment patterns or chemical alterations at the neuromuscular junction might be the factors that dictate performance changes in high-power output activities. Given these possibilities, repeated performance of a specific motor skill involved in a high-power activity should contribute greatly to improving performance (this effect may be related to the muscle-group specificity mentioned earlier). Any variations in prescriptions for football or other sports should take this aspect of training into account, and should also follow the principles presented in the earlier sample variation (for football).

Interval Training Prescriptions

As mentioned previously, interval training is one of the more widely studied of the popular conditioning methods. Precise definitions of terms related to the interval training system have been agreed on (see Table 9-6), and extensive guidelines for writing interval training prescriptions are available. For our purposes, the guidelines below should be sufficient when used with Tables 9-2 and 9-7:

Table 9-4: Suggested Sprint and Endurance Training Methods for Various Sports and Sports Activities

Sport or Sport Activity	Acceleration sprints	Continuous fast running	Continuous slow running	Hollow sprints	Interval sprinting	Interval training	Jogging	Speed play (fartlek)	Repetition running	Sprint training
						Suggested Training Method				
Baseball				✔		✔				✔
Basketball				✔		✔				✔
Fencing	✔			✔		✔				✔
Field Hockey						✔				
Football	✔			✔		✔				✔
Golf	✔									✔
Gymnastics	✔			✔		✔				✔
Ice Hockey*										
Forwards, defense				✔		✔				
Goalie	✔					✔				✔
Lacrosse										
Goalie, defense, attack men				✔		✔				
Midfielders, man-down						✔				
Recreational sports			✔			✔	✔			
Rowing*						✔		✔	✔	
Skiing*										
Slalom, jumping, downhill				✔		✔				
Cross-country		✔	✔							
Soccer										
Goalie, wings, strikers				✔		✔				
Halfbacks, link men						✔				
Softball				✔		✔				✔
Swimming and diving*										
50-m freestyle, diving	✔									✔
100 m, 100 yd (all strokes)				✔		✔				
200 m, 220 yd (all strokes)						✔				
400 m, 440-yd freestyle						✔		✔	✔	

*Rather than running, the mode of exercise during the training sessions should be that used in the sport.

Table 9-4: Suggested Sprint and Endurance Training Methods of Various Sports and Sports Activities (continued)

Sport or Sport Activity	Acceleration sprints	Continuous fast running	Continuous slow running	Hollow sprints	Interval sprinting	Interval training	Jogging	Repetition running	Speed play (fartlek)	Sprint training
1500 m, 1650-yd freestyle					✔	✔				
Tennis						✔				
Track and field										
100 m, 100 yd	✔									✔
200 m, 200 yd	✔			✔		✔				✔
Field events	✔			✔		✔				✔
400 m, 440 yd				✔		✔				
800 m, 880 yd						✔				
1500 m, 1 mile						✔		✔	✔	
2 miles						✔		✔	✔	
3 miles, 5000 m					✔	✔				
6 miles, 10,000 m		✔			✔	✔				
Marathon		✔	✔							
Volleyball	✔				✔	✔				✔
Wrestling	✔				✔	✔				✔

Interval Training Guidelines

Determine which energy system is to be improved (see Table 9-2).

Select the type of exercise (e.g., running, swimming, cycling) to be used during the work interval.

Using Table 9-7, write the training prescriptions according to the information appearing in the row opposite the major energy systems to be improved. The number of repetitions and sets, the work-relief ratio, and type of relief interval are all contained in the table.

The training times given in the upper part of Table 9-7 may be used for any sport. However, for running and swimming, it may be more convenient to use the training distances given in the lower part of the table.

Table 9-5: Sample Prescriptions for Various Training Methods*

Training Method	Type of Athlete	Sample Prescription
Acceleration sprints	Sprinter	Jog 50–120 yd, stride 50–120 yd, walk 50–120 yd, repeat.
Continuous fast running	Half-miler	Run ¾–1½ miles, steady, fast pace (e.g., 6-min-mile pace), repeat 1–4 times.
	6-miler	Run 8–10 miles, steady, fast pace.
Continuous slow running	Miler	Run 3–5 miles, steady, slow pace (e.g., 7½-min-mile pace).
	3-miler	Run 6–12 miles, steady, slow pace.
	6-miler	Run 12–18 miles, steady slow pace.
Hollow sprints	Sprinter	Sprint 60 yd, jog 60 yd, walk 60 yd, repeat until fatigued.
Interval sprinting	Middle-distance	Alternate 50-yd sprints with 60-yd jogs; repeat up to 3 miles.
Interval training	Sprinter	Set 1 4×220 @ 0:27 (1:21)† Set 2 8×110 @ 0:13 (0:39) Set 3 8×110 @ 0:13 (0:39)
	Miler	Set 1 1×1320 @ 3:45 (1:52) Set 2 2×1100 @ 2:58 (1:29)
Jogging	Recreational	Jog 2 miles in 14 min.
Repetition running	Miler	Run 3–4 repeats of ½ mile at a pace of 2:10 to 2:15.
Speed play (Fartlek)	Middle-distance and distance	Jog 5–10 min; run ¾–1¼ miles at fast, steady pace; walk 5 min; alternate jog-sprint (65–75 yd); sprint uphill for 175–200 yd; jog for ¾–1¼ miles.
Sprint training	Sprinter	Repeat full-speed sprints of 60–70 yd with complete recovery between repeats.

*From Fox (1977).

†Read as follows: four 220-yd runs at a pace of 27 sec with 1-min and 21-sec relief (walking) between runs.

Basic eight-week-long anaerobic and aerobic interval training programs for running are presented in Appendix D.

How many times per week should the athlete train? How intensive should the training program be and how many weeks should it last to be most effective? Coaches frequently ask these questions. Let's see what answers research provides.

Frequency and Duration of Training

For most athletes who compete in endurance activities, the frequency of training should be between four and five days per week and the duration 12 to 16 weeks or longer. However, in the case of long-distance runners and swimmers, six to seven days per week on a yearly basis may be necessary. The

Table 9-6: Definitions of Terms Related to Interval Training

Term	Definition
Work interval	That portion of the interval training program consisting of the work effort—for example, a 220-yd run performed within a prescribed time.
Relief interval	The time between work intervals in a set. The relief interval may consist of light activity such as walking (rest-relief) or mild to moderate exercise such as jogging (work-relief).
Work-relief ratio	The time ratio of the work and relief intervals. For example, a work-relief ratio of 1:2 means that the duration of the relief interval is twice that of the work interval.
Set	A group of work and relief intervals—for example, six 220-yd runs (each performed within a prescribed time) separated by designated relief intervals.
Repetition	The number of work intervals per set. Six 220-yd runs would constitute six repetitions.
Training time	The rate of work during the work interval—for example, each 220-yd run might be performed in 28 sec.
Training distance	Distance of the work interval—for example, 220 yd.
ITP prescription	The specifications for the routines to be performed in an interval training workout. For example, one set from a prescription for a running program may be written as follows: Set 1 6 $\times$ 220 @ 0:28 (1:24) where 6 = number of repetitions 220 = training distance in yards 0:28 = training time in minutes and seconds (1:24) = time of relief interval in minutes and seconds

reasons for this are twofold: (1) training volume (mileage) appears to be related to these particular types of endurance performances and therefore a greater frequency and longer duration help satisfy this requirement; and (2) as we will see later (p. 238), frequency of training is most related to changes in the anaerobic threshold and to heart rate responses during submaximal exercise. In the last chapter we discussed why these changes are extremely important to success in endurance performance.

One aspect of endurance training frequency that always needs discussing is the value of multiple daily training sessions. Are training frequencies of two and even three times per day more effective than one? Although research on this subject is slight, present evidence indicates that several daily training sessions are not necessarily more productive than a single session per day, at least in sports other than track and swimming. Two sessions per day are often necessary for endurance runners and swimmers, as just indicated, to allow for their rather large volume (mileage) of training.

For most nonendurance athletes, the training frequency should be three days per week and the duration at eight to ten weeks. The major reason for this

Table 9-7: Guidelines for Writing Interval Training Prescriptions*

Major Energy System	Training Time (min:sec)	Repetitions per Workout	Sets per Workout	Repetitions per Set	Work-Relief Ratio	Type of Relief Interval
ATP-PC	0:10	50	5	10		Rest-relief (e.g., walking, flexing)
	0:15	45	5	9		
	0:20	40	4	10	1:3	
	0:25	32	4	8		
ATP-PC-LA	0:30	25	5	5		Work-relief (e.g., light to mild exercise, jogging)
	0:40-0:50	20	4	5	1:3	
	1:00-1:10	15	3	5	1:2	
	1:20	10	2	5	1:2	
LA-O₂	1:30-2:00	8	2	4	1:2	Work-relief
	2:10-2:40	6	1	6	1:1	Rest-relief
	2:50-3:00	4	1	4	1:1	Rest-relief
O₂	3:00-4:00	4	1	4	1:1	
	4:00-5:00	3	1	3	1:½	

Major Energy System	Training Distance (yd) Run	Training Distance (yd) Swim	Repetitions per Workout	Sets per Workout	Repetitions per Set	Work-Relief Ratio	Type of Relief Interval
ATP-PC	55	15	50	5	10		Rest-relief (e.g., walking, flexing)
	110	25	24	3	8	1:3	
ATP-PC-LA	220	55	16	4	4	1:3	Work-relief (e.g., light to mild exercise, jogging)
	440	110	8	2	4	1:2	
LA-O₂	660	165	5	1	5	1:2	Work-relief
	880	220	4	2	2	1:1	Rest-relief
O₂	1100	275	3	1	3	1:½	Rest-relief
	1320	330	3	1	3	1:½	

*From Fox and Mathews (1974).

schedule is that with sprint programs, the training sessions are generally very intensive; more rest between training sessions is usually required. Remember, chronic fatigue is the enemy of effective training programs.

Once again, the exceptions to the above "rule" are the sprinters, both runners and swimmers. These athletes usually work out five or six days per week most of the year. However, the intensities of the workouts are generally alternated from day to day between "hard" workouts (intensive workouts) and "easy" workouts (less intensive workouts). Futhermore, time for skill development such as swimming mechanics, running style, relay starts, and so on, makes the workouts less intensive.

Intensity of the Training Program

How may one determine the proper intensity level of a training program? There is no ideal way of determining which training intensity is best suited to the trainee and to the demands of an effective conditioning program. However, for endurance programs, a starting point which is applicable to most athletes is to exercise at a level sufficient to raise the heart rate to 85 to 90% of the maximal level. For example, suppose a 20-year-old woman with a maximal heart rate of 200 beats per min wishes to start a training program. The intensity of the exercise should be such that her heart rate will reach between 170 and 180 beats per min (85% of 200 beats per min = 0.85 $\times$ 200 = 170; 90% of 200 = 0.9 $\times$ 200 = 180).

In order to use this method for determining training intensity, the maximal heart rate must be known. Direct determination of the maximal heart rate is difficult. However, reasonable estimates for men and women based on age may be made from the following equation:

Maximal Heart Rate = 220 − age

In the example above, the 20-year-old woman's maximal heart rate would be estimated at 220 − 20 = 200 beats per min.

For those athletes using sprint programs, the heart rate during training might be 180 beats/min or higher, as the sprints will be performed at higher intensities than the longer runs used in most endurance programs. If the sprints are only 10 to 15 sec in duration, though, it may require several repetitions for the heart rate to reach its peak.

It is a good idea to teach your athletes how and when to take their pulse rates. As shown in Figure 9-2, the pulse may be taken either by placing the hand directly over the heart (left breast) or by palpating the radial artery (at the wrist), the temporal artery (in front of the ear), or the carotid artery (in the neck). Only light pressure should be used at the carotid artery to avoid closing off the artery completely and causing a reflex slowing of the heart rate that occasionally triggers cardiac abnormalities.

At rest, the athlete should count the number of pulses he or she feels in 15 sec, and then multiply this number by four for an accurate estimate of the

Figure 9-2 Athletes should know how and when to take their pulse rates. A, The pulse may be taken by placing the hand directly over the left breast; B, by palpating the radial artery (at the wrist); C, the temporal artery (in front of the ear); or D, the carotid artery (in the neck).

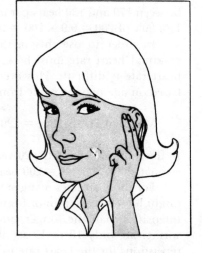

A

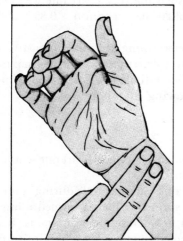

B

C

heart rate in beats per min. Although it is not possible to take the pulse accurately during exercise, the pulse count obtained in a 6- or 10-sec span immediately after exercise is a reasonable indicator of what the heart rate was during exercise (provided, of course, the 6-sec count is multiplied by ten and/or the 10-sec count is multiplied by six in order to convert the heart rate to beats per minute).

Keeping records of the athlete's resting heart rate is just as important as

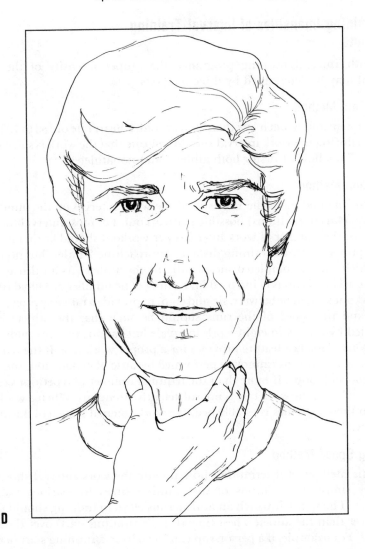

D

documenting his or her heart rate during exercise and recovery. These data provide a means of evaluating both the particular training program and the athlete's progress during the season. In the latter regard, the athlete's resting heart rate (specifically, the heart rate before he or she gets out of bed in the morning) should be expected to decrease during the season (as previously mentioned, trained athletes usually have low resting heart rates). If the heart rate does not decrease, this may be an indication of a serious problem. Of course, if the resting pulse increases suddenly from a previous low level, this too may indicate a problem (perhaps medical or emotional). In any case, the athlete with an unusual heart rate should be given special attention in order to determine the underlying cause.

Determining Intensities of Interval Training Workouts

With interval training programs, the proper intensity of the work interval may be determined by three methods.

Heart Rate Method

For men and women less than 20 years old, a heart rate of 180 to 190 beats per min during the work interval should indicate that the work is sufficiently intense. This holds true for both athletes and nonathletes.

Repetition Method

This method bases the intensity of the work interval on the number of work intervals (repetitions) possible per workout. For most interval training programs, the number of work intervals per workout should be that number which provides a total training distance approaching 2 miles (but no more) and which can be completed successfully by the athlete. As an illustration, suppose a 440-yd run is being used in training. The number of 440-yd runs in the workout should be between six and eight to provide a range approaching 2 miles, and the speed of the runs should be such that the athlete is not exhausted by the six to eight work intervals but cannot run any additional repetitions. This last feature provides for a proper work rate. If the required number of repetitions cannot be performed because of exhaustion, the work rate is too strenuous. If more than the required number of repetitions can be performed, then the work rate is not sufficiently strenuous. When a work rate between these extremes is established, the work interval is then of the proper intensity.

Running Speed Method

This method of determining how intense the work interval should be involves simple calculations of the running times for various training distances. The speed at which an athlete runs 50 yd in training should be 1.5 sec slower than the athlete's best time (from a running start) over the same distance. For example, if a person can run 50 yd from a running start in 6 sec, the training time that would guarantee the proper intensity for this distance would be $6 + 1.5 = 7.5$ sec. For training distances of 110 and 220 yd, the running times can be slower by 3 and 5 sec, respectively, than the athlete's best times (from running starts) for these distances.

For a training distance of 440 yd, the athlete's time should be 1 to 4 sec faster than one fourth of his or her time on the mile run. If an athlete runs the mile in 5 min (300 sec), this time is divided by four to yield 75 sec, from which 1 to 4 sec are subtracted. Therefore, the training time would be between $75 - 4 = 71$ sec and $75 - 1 = 74$ sec.

If the training distance is over 440 yd, each 440-yd portion of that distance should be run at an average speed 3 to 4 sec slower than the average 440-yd time in the mile run. For instance, in running 880 yd as the training distance, the 5-

min miler used in our example above would run each 440-yd length of the 880 yd in an average time of $75 + 3 = 78$ sec to $75 + 4 = 79$ sec.

This method may also be applied to swimming. However, the training distances for swimming programs will be approximately one fourth those used for running programs.

A summary of guidelines for estimating training frequency, intensity, duration, and distance for aerobic and anaerobic programs of running is presented in Table 9-8. These guidelines are appropriate for use when constructing preseason training programs for most sports except track and swimming. Guidelines for the latter sports are contained in Table 9-9. As mentioned before, two training sessions per day are often required for these sports because of the distances covered per day.

Table 9-8: Guidelines for Estimating Frequency, Intensity, Duration, and Distance of Aerobic and Anaerobic Training Programs of Running

Training Aspect	Endurance (Aerobic) Training	Sprint (Anaerobic) Training
Frequency	4-5 days/wk	3 days/wk
Intensity*	Heart rate = 85-90% of maximal heart rate	Heart rate = 180 beats/min or greater
Sessions/day	One	One
Duration	12-16 wk or longer	8-10 wk
Distance/workout	3-5 miles	1½-2 miles

*Standards of intensity besides the one used here (heart rate) are described on pages 215 to 217.

Table 9-9: Guidelines for Estimating Training Frequency and Distance in Running and Swimming Programs

Event	Training Frequency (days/wk) Run	Swim	Distance per Workout (miles) Run	Swim
50 m	—	5-6	—	4-5
100 m	5-6	5-6	4-5	4-5
200 m	5-6	6-7	4-5	5-6
400 m	5-6	6-7	7-8	7½-8½
500 yd	—	6-7	—	8-9
800 m	6	—	8-10	—
1000 yd	—	6-7	—	8½-9½
1500 m	7	—	9-10	—
1650 yd	—	6-7	—	8½-9½
1 mile	7	—	9-10	—
2 miles	7	—	10-11	—
3 miles, 5000 m	7	—	12-13	—
6 miles, 10,000 m	7	—	13	—
Marathon	7	—	13+	—

Warm-Up

It is always a good idea for the athlete to perform some preliminary exercise prior to training sessions and competitions. A warm-up makes sense for several reasons:

Reasons for Warming Up

Warming up raises the body and muscle temperatures, facilitating enzyme activity, which in turn increases the metabolism of skeletal muscle. Increases in body and muscle temperatures also promote increases in the amount of blood and oxygen reaching the skeletal muscles. Another effect of the higher temperatures is an improvement in the contraction and reflex times of the skeletal muscles.

Abrupt, strenuous exercise may be associated with inadequate blood flow to the heart. Warm-ups may lessen this danger.

Injuries associated with muscles and joints may be less likely to occur during performance if preceded by a warm-up period. This is particularly true for the high-power, sprint-like activities.

Psychologically, athletes may have a difficult time adjusting to the idea of performing without prior warm-up—so much so that their performance would almost certainly be adversely affected.*

Some of the changes just cited are shown in Figure 9-3. Notice how oxygen consumption (labelled as peak $\dot{V}O_2$ in the figure) and heart rate during maximal exercise are directly related to muscle temperature. The higher the temperature, the higher the $\dot{V}O_2$ and heart rate. Also notice that although work time was not increased at the highest muscle temperature, blood lactic acid accumulation was considerably reduced.

Warm-up procedures may be **active** or **passive**. Active procedures involve either utilizing the skill or activity that will be used during competition (so-called formal warm-up) or stretching and calisthenics (informal warm-up). Passive warm-up does not involve exercise. Instead, it involves heating the whole body or its various parts by diathermy, whirlpool baths, hot showers, and other such means. The effects of active and passive procedures have been found to be beneficial in about half of the many studies of warm-up, and few (if any) studies have shown either active or passive warm-up to be detrimental to performance (about half of the experimental work has found warm-up to have neither beneficial nor detrimental effects).

Because of the inconsistent results obtained from studies dealing with

---

*It should be noted, though, that some athletes have set records in their events without warming up prior to performing.

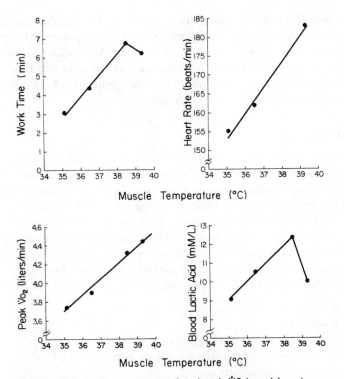

Figure 9-3 Oxygen consumption (peak $\dot{V}O_2$) and heart rate during maximal exercise are directly related to muscle temperature. The higher the temperature, the higher the $\dot{V}O_2$ and heart rate. Although work time is not increased at the highest muscle temperature, blood lactic acid is considerable reduced. (Based on data from Bergh and Ekblom, 1979.)

performance and warm-up, it is not possible to outline a definitive warm-up procedure. However, it can generally be recommended that each training session or competition should be preceded by a warm-up period lasting 15 to 30 min and consisting of stretching exercises, calisthenics, and formal activity.

Stretching Activities

Stretching should be performed before and after training or competition. During the warm-up, stretching exercises should be the first activity performed. Without being strenuous, such exercises can increase body and muscle temperature and will protect the muscle against possible tearing when more vigorous exercise is performed.

For most sports, stretching exercises should include the major muscle groups and joints of the body, such as the neck, back, hamstrings, gastrocnemius, Achilles tendon, chest, hips, groin, spine, quadriceps, shoulders, arms, ankles, abdominals, knees, and toes. Some representative stretching exercises for these various areas are shown in Appendix E. The exercises should be performed **without** bobbing or jerking, and the final stretched position should be held for 20 to 30 sec. Adequate stretching routines may require a total of 20 to 30 min to complete.

Calisthenics

Calisthenics should be performed after the stretching routines. Calisthenics are active—that is, they involve muscular contractions. Therefore, they will cause further increases in body and muscular temperatures. Calisthenic exercises should include the major muscle groups, particularly those directly involved in the sport. Athletes may unintentionally overdo calisthenics; they should be reminded that exercised muscle groups should **not** be fatigued following the calisthenic routine. The total time needed for this particular phase of the warm-up period will be only 5 to 10 min. For each body area there are calisthenics involving the appropriate muscle contractions:

Neck—bridge
Shoulders, groin—jumping jacks
Ankle, toes, gastrocnemius—toe raises, running in place
Quadriceps—half-squats
Shoulders, arms, chest—push-ups
Abdominals—bent-knee sit-ups, bent-knee leg raises

Formal Activity

The last phase of the warm-up should consist of performing the activity utilized in the sport. For example, in a warm-up for baseball, formal activities would include throwing, catching, fielding, and batting. This practice serves two purposes: (1) it ensures that physiological factors such as muscle temperature and blood flow are optimal in the muscles directly used during the sport; and (2) it provides a warm-up for hand-eye coordination and other neuromuscular mechanisms that also are directly involved in the sport.

Warm-Down

As mentioned in Chapter 5 (p. 77), it is a common practice of athletes to "warm down," that is, perform light or mild exercise immediately following competition and training sessions. As we learned earlier, there is a sound physiological basis for such a practice: levels of lactic acid in the blood decrease more rapidly during exercise-recovery than during rest-recovery (see p. 77).

Specific warm-down procedures for various sports are not available.

However, it is recommended that the warm-down be similar to the warm-up, but in reverse order. Thus, formal activity would immediately follow the training session or competition—for example, several laps of jogging would follow the mile run. Next, some calisthenics might be performed, followed by stretching exercises. The formal activity and stretching exercises should be considered the most important phases.

General warm-up and warm-down procedures are reviewed in Figure 9–4.

Year-Round Training—The Training Phases

The year-round training programs of athletes may be divided into three phases: off-season, preseason, and in-season.

Off-Season Training

Training programs during the off-season are usually nonspecific. Most often they require only that athletes keep moderately active and, perhaps of most concern, keep their body weights at or reasonably near their "playing weights."

An off-season training program might consist of some or all of the following activities:

Off-Season Training Program

A weight-training program with emphasis placed on increasing strength and power in those muscle groups most directly involved in the specific athletic event. Examples of weight-training programs that would be suited to this purpose were given in Chapter 7 (see p. 136).

A six- to ten-week training program of low intensity performed no more than twice a week. A typical program of this type is the one for running shown in Table 9–10 (an interval training program); a program for jogging, such as shown in Table 9–11), may also be adjusted to off-season needs. Either of these programs may be administered concurrently with the weight-training program. For example, if weight training is conducted on Monday, Wednesday, and Friday, the running program could be performed on Monday and Wednesday or Wednesday and Friday. It makes little difference whether the running program is performed before or after the weight-training program.

Participation in sports activities and recreational games.

Some participation in the athlete's specific sport in order to develop skill; for example, in volleyball such skills would include passing, setting up, spiking, and serving.

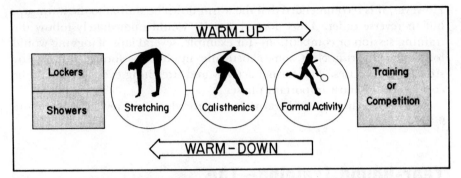

Figure 9-4 General warm up and warm-down procedures. Note that warm-down is the reverse of warm-up.

Preseason Training

During the preseason phase—that is, the eight to ten weeks prior to competition—training programs should be designed to increase to a maximum the capacities of the energy systems that are predominant when performing a specific athletic event. Examples of these programs were given earlier in Table 9-4 (see also App. D).

Another important factor to consider during this phase of training is the learning of strategies and skills specific to the sport.

Table 9-10: Example of an Off-Season Interval Training Program of Running

Week	Prescription
1	Set 1 1 × 880* @ easy
	Set 2 4 × 220 @ easy (1:3)†
2	Set 1 2 × 440 @ easy (1:2)
	Set 2 8 × 110 @ easy (1:3)
3	Set 1 2 × 440 @ easy (1:2)
	Set 2 6 × 220 @ easy (1:3)
4	Set 1 1 × 880 @ easy
	Set 2 6 × 220 @ easy (1:3)
5	Set 1 2 × 880 @ easy (1:2)
	Set 2 2 × 440 @ easy (1:2)
6	Set 1 6 × 440 @ easy (1:2)
7	Set 1 3 × 880 @ easy (1:2)
8	Set 1 2 × 880 @ easy (1:2)
	Set 2 2 × 880 @ easy (1:2)
9	Set 1 2 × 880 @ easy (1:2)
	Set 2 4 × 440 @ easy (1:2)
10	Set 1 1 × 1760 @ easy
	Set 2 1 × 1760 @ easy

*Distance in yards.

†Work-relief ratio.

Table 9-11: A Basic Jogging Schedule for Men and Women*

Steps	Time for 1 Mile (min:sec)	Total Target Time for 2 Miles (min:sec)
1. Slow walk	20:00	40:00
2. Alternate ¼ mile slow walk and ¼ mile fast walk	18:00	36:00
3. Fast walk	16:00	32:00
4. Alternate 330 yd fast walk and 110 yd slow jog	14:30	29:00
5. Alternate 220 yd fast walk and 220 yd slow jog	13:00	26:00
6. Alternate ¼ mile fast walk and ¼ mile slow jog	13:00	26:00
7. Alternate ½ mile slow jog and ¼ mile fast walk	11:30	23:00
8. Alternate ¾ mile slow jog and ¼ mile fast walk	11:30	23:00
9. Slow jog	10:00	20:00
10. Alternate ¼ mile fast jog and ¼ mile slow jog	9:30	19:00
11. Alternate ¼ mile slow jog and ¼ mile fast jog	9:00	18:00
12. Alternate ½ mile slow jog and ½ mile fast jog	9:00	18:00
13. Alternate ½ mile fast jog and ¼ mile slow jog	8:30	17:00
14. Alternate ¼ mile slow jog and ¾ mile fast jog	8:30	17:00
15. Fast jog	8:00	16:00
16. Alternate ¼ mile fast jog and ¼ mile faster jog	7:30	15:00
17. Alternate ½ mile fast jog and ½ mile faster jog	7:30	15:00
18. Faster jog	7:00	14:00

*Modified from Roby and Davis (1970).

In-Season Training

Traditionally, in-season training programs for most sports emphasize skill development. It is generally felt that drills, scrimmages, and competition will maintain the increases in energy capacities that were obtained during the preseason training program. For the majority of athletes who compete regularly, this is probably true. However, for some of the "regulars" and for most of those athletes who do not compete every week, some maintenance training might be necessary. An in-season maintenance program might include some of the following:

In-Season Training Program

One or two days of training per week, with a program similar to that used in the preseason.

Weight training with one workout per week, alternating the upper body and the lower body workouts on a weekly basis (e.g., one week, upper body, the next, lower body).

Utilizing drills not only to improve skill but also to help maintain fitness. To do this, the drills should be intense and long enough in duration to stress the muscle groups involved.

The training phases are summarized in Table 9-12.

Table 9-12: Recommended Programs for the Various Training Phases*

Training Phase		
Off-Season	Preseason	In-Season
Weight training 8 wk, 3 days per wk	Running† high intensity, 8 wk, 3 days per wk	Running† high intensity, 1 or 2 days per wk
Informal running low intensity, 8 wk, 1-2 days per wk	Weight training 2-3 days per wk	Weight training, 1 day per wk
Participation in other sports and games	Viewing films, learning strategies, some skill drills	Skill drills
		Scrimmages
Limited practice in specific sport for skill development		Regular competitive performances

*Modified from Fox and Mathews (1974).

†The training program should be specific; for example, swimmers would use a swimming program.

Effects of Sprint and Endurance Training

Most training regimens may be classified as sprint or anaerobic programs or as endurance or aerobic programs. Several examples of the two types of training were given in Table 9-3. In general, endurance training refers to exercise programs consisting of prolonged, usually continuous work bouts of relatively low intensity. Sprint training most often refers to programs of short, repeated work bouts of relatively high intensity.

In discussing the effects of sprint and endurance training, it must be remembered that skeletal muscle contains two basic fiber types or motor units that differ in their metabolic, biochemical, and neuromuscular properties. As indicated in Chapter 6, in man these fiber types are fast-twitch (FT) and slow-twitch (ST). Some training-induced changes vary according to the type of fiber.

It should be further recalled that FT and ST fibers are preferentially recruited for certain work: FT fibers for the performance of short-duration, high-power work (such as sprinting), and ST fibers for prolonged, low-intensity exercise (such as distance running). Most alterations produced within the different types of skeletal muscle fibers will therefore be specific to the design of the training program—that is, whether it consists of sprint-like or endurance-like exercise.

Changes in Skeletal Muscle Following Endurance Training

Studies of the effects of endurance training have revealed that many changes in skeletal muscle can be expected in the trainee (animal or human). Important findings are outlined below.

Changes in Myoglobin Concentration

The concentration of myoglobin in skeletal muscle has been shown to be substantially increased following prolonged exercise training in animals. As should be recalled, myoglobin is an oxygen-storing compound similar to hemoglobin. However, its main function is aiding the delivery (diffusion) of oxygen from the cell membrane to the mitochondria, where O_2 is consumed.

Changes in Oxidation of Carbohydrates and Fats

Because the aerobic capacity of skeletal muscle is greatly increased by endurance training, the ability to consume oxygen and to utilize both carbohydrates (glycogen) and fats as metabolic fuels is enhanced. This effect occurs in both FT and ST fiber types.

Two important subcellular adaptations that contribute to the increased aerobic capacity are: (1) increases in the number and size of the mitochondria in skeletal muscle; and (2) an increase in the activity or concentration of key enzymes involved in the aerobic reactions that take place in the mitochondria. With respect to increases in the number and size of mitochondria, it should be mentioned that this change appears to be less pronounced in women than in men. If there is any reason for this difference, which would appear to represent a definite biochemical limitation on the overall aerobic capacity of women, it is not evident.

Changes in Stores of Muscle Glycogen and Triglycerides

In humans who have participated in long-term physical training, stores of glycogen in skeletal muscle have been found to double; triglyceride stores have shown increases of as much as 83% in the same persons. As pointed out earlier (see p. 43), endurance performance improves when muscle glycogen levels are elevated.

Changes in Anaerobic Glycolysis (Lactic Acid System)

As might be expected, glycolytic enzymes are not normally made more active by endurance training. In fact, decreases of 20 to 25% in the activities of several key glycolytic enzymes have been found in the vastus lateralis muscle (which contains both FT and ST fibers) following endurance training.

Changes in Stores of Phosphagens

Muscular stores of ATP and PC have been shown to increase by 25 and 40%, respectively, following a training program of distance running.

Changes in Size and Number of Muscle Fibers

It was first thought that endurance training caused a conversion of FT fibers to ST fibers. However, the majority of studies have shown that this does not occur. As previously discussed, the distribution of ST and FT fibers in a muscle is probably more a function of genetics than anything else (see p. 108). It has, however, been shown that the percentage area of ST fibers (but not FT fibers) increases following endurance training, thus suggesting a selective hypertrophy (increased size).

A summary of the effects of endurance training on skeletal muscle is shown in Figure 9-5.

Changes in Skeletal Muscle Following Sprint Training

The effects of sprint training on skeletal muscle have not been extensively studied either in animals or in humans. However, judging from the specificity of results obtained following endurance training, it might be expected that sprint training would primarily result in an increased capacity for anaerobic metabolism. Although this idea appears to have some validity, the number and magnitude of the changes are not very impressive, particularly when compared to the aerobic changes produced through endurance training. Some of the changes in skeletal muscle that are induced by sprint training are outlined below.

Changes in Anaerobic Glycolysis (Lactic Acid System)

Only relatively small changes in several key glycolytic enzyme activities have been found either in animals or in humans put through sprint training. In rats, which have been the subject of most studies, the glycolytic capacity has shown little change following sprint programs. This is somewhat surprising, since the lactic acid system is used to a great extent in most sprint training programs. Apparently, most skeletal muscles possess sufficient anaerobic capacities to meet the demands of sprint work without further adaptation.

Changes in the ATP-PC System

Several key enzymes involved in the ATP-PC system in human muscle have been studied in subjects who took part in an eight-week-long sprint program consisting of repeated 5-sec-long sprints on an elevated (uphill) treadmill. As with the glycolytic enzymes, only small changes were noted following the training. However, total phosphagen stores (ATP plus PC) were found to be increased as a result of muscular hypertrophy. Anaerobic performance, as measured on a stair-climbing test, was also shown to improve following the sprint program.

Changes in Muscle Fibers

Interconversion of fiber types does not occur in persons who participate in sprint training. An increase in the diameter (hypertrophy) of both FT and

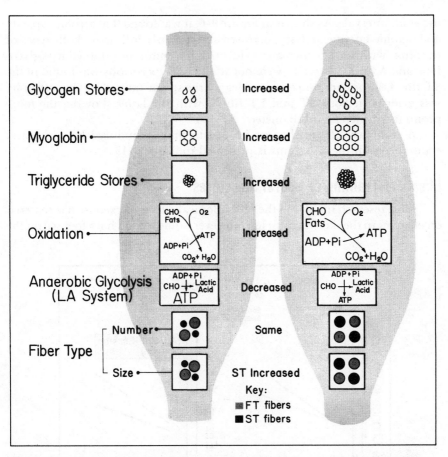

Figure 9-5 Summary of the effects of endurance training on skeletal muscle. The muscle before training is on the left and the muscle after training is on the right.

ST fibers in the vastus lateralis has, however, been linked to sprint training. In one study, the hypertrophy was more evident in the FT fibers.

Changes in the Aerobic System

Increases in some of the key aerobic enzymes have apparently been induced by sprint training. In addition, increases in maximal oxygen consumption ($\dot{V}O_2$max) have been found.

Sprint versus Endurance Training

In one especially interesting comparative study of sprint training and endurance training in humans, one leg of each subject was sprint-trained while the other was endurance-trained. The endurance training consisted of continuous bicycle exercise for 30 to 50 min; the sprint training consisted of repeated all-out efforts for 30 to 40 sec with 1½ min of relief (resting) between the work intervals. As shown in Figure 9–6, it was found that aerobic capacity and aerobic enzyme activity increased significantly following both types of training, with greater increases evident in the endurance-trained leg (glycolytic and ATP-PC enzymes were not studied). Hypertrophy was found in the ST fibers of the endurance-trained leg; in the sprint-trained leg, hypertrophy was evident in both ST and FT fibers, with the latter showing the more pronounced increase in diameter.

A summary of the changes in skeletal muscle induced by sprint and endurance training programs is presented in Table 9–13.

Effects of Training of Neural Structures

Most research involving the physiological effects of exercise has centered on changes in the skeletal muscles. However, some studies have focused on the

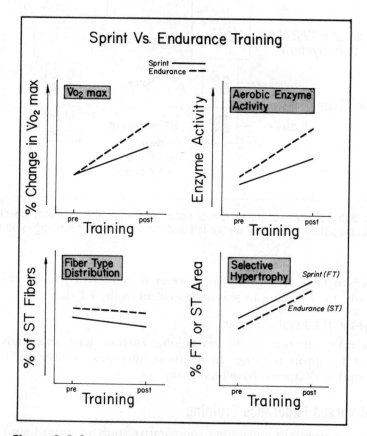

Figure 9-6 Comparative changes in maximal aerobic power ($\dot{V}O_2$ max), aerobic enzyme activity, fiber type distribution, and hypertrophy following sprint and endurance training. These comparisons were made in subjects who sprint-trained one leg and endurance-trained the other. (Based on data from Saltin and co-workers, 1976.)

Table 9-13: Summary of the Changes in Skeletal Muscle Induced by Sprint and Endurance Training Programs

Variable	Training Effect	
	Sprint Training	Endurance Training
Myoglobin concentration	?	Increased
Aerobic capacity (ability to oxidize fats and carbohydrates)	Increased or unchanged	Increased
Glycogen stores	Increased (?)	Increased
Triglyceride stores	?	Increased
Glycolytic enzyme activity	Increased (ST fibers only)	Increased, decreased, or unchanged
ATP-PC system enzyme activities	Increased	?
Phosphagen stores Concentration	Unchanged	Increased
Total stores	Increased	Increased
Fiber hypertrophy	ST and FT fibers (greater in FT)	ST fibers only
Fiber type interconversion	None	None

neuromuscular junction and motoneuron, and it has been found that these structures do show changes as a result of exercise training. These changes include cellular and subcellular adaptations in structure, modifications of transmission properties, and alterations in reflex, chemical, and biochemical responses (the latter within the motoneuron itself). Unfortunately, the significance of these neuromuscular changes remains unclear, at least insofar as they relate to specific training programs and athletic performance. However, from the fact that sprint training produces relatively small metabolic and biochemical changes but has substantial effects on performance, it can be inferred that neuromuscular alterations induced by such training are extremely important. Continued research in this area is obviously needed.

Cardiorespiratory Effects of Training Evidenced at Rest

The effects of training on the cardiovascular and respiratory systems can be broken down into those evident at rest and those evident during exercise (the latter effects are further classified in terms of submaximal and maximal exercise). The effects that are evident at rest are detailed below.

Cardiac Hypertrophy (Increased Size of the Heart)

It has been suspected for a long time that physical training results in an increase in the size of the heart (cardiac hypertrophy). However, only recently has the nature of this hypertrophy in humans (both men and women) been delineated. For example, as shown in Figure 9-7, the cardiac hypertrophy of endurance athletes (such as distance runners, swimmers, and field hockey players) consists of an increase in the size of the left ventricular cavity (pumping chamber) of the heart without an increase in the thickness of the ventricular wall. In nonendurance athletes (e.g., wrestlers and shot putters), the cardiac hypertrophy consists of just the opposite—the ventricular wall is increased in thickness while the left ventricular cavity remains normal in size.

Apparently, the type of cardiac hypertrophy found in an athlete is specific to the kind of sport in which he or she participates. This makes sense, for it is known that endurance training and performance require prolonged efforts, during which time the cardiac output is sustained at very high levels. A large ventricular volume (cavity) would, in this case, seem to be a mandatory adaptation. By the same token, athletes who participate in and train for brief, powerful activities are subjected to intermittently elevated arterial blood pressure, much like that generated during straining. Here, too, it is reasonable that a thickened ventricular wall would be required in order to repeatedly overcome such a stress.

Decreased Heart Rate (Bradycardia) and Increased Stroke Volume

Athletes, particularly endurance athletes, usually have a decreased heart rate (**bradycardia**) and an increased stroke volume while resting. Evidently, the physical training that an athlete goes through increases the pumping

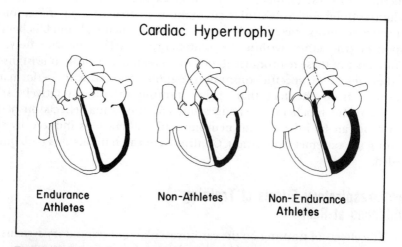

Figure 9-7 In endurance athletes (such as distance swimmers and runners), cardiac hypertrophy consists of an increase in the size of the left ventricular cavity; there is no increase in the thickness of the heart's walls. In nonendurance athletes (such as wrestlers and shot putters), cardiac hypertrophy consists of an increase in the ventricular wall's thickness; there is no increase in the size of the cavity. (Based on data from Morganroth and co-workers, 1975, and Zeldis and co-workers, 1978.)

performance (efficiency) of the heart, since, for a given cardiac output, a slower beating heart with a larger stroke volume represents more efficient energy utilization by the myocardium (see p. 183).

Increased Hemoglobin and Blood Volume

Although research in this area has not always produced consistent data, physical training is generally found to result in increased blood volume and total hemoglobin content. Most of the increase in blood volume reflects an increase in the amount of plasma rather than an actual rise in the red blood cell volume. The blood's hemoglobin concentration is, therefore, usually unchanged or slightly decreased after training.

Both total blood volume and hemoglobin are important with respect to the oxygen transport system, particularly during exercise at altitudes above sea level (see p. 194). Blood volume is also an important factor during exercise in the heat, since deep body heat is carried by the blood to peripheral areas of the body, from which heat is then dissipated to the environment (see p. 322).

Changes in Blood Pressure

Training generally does not affect the resting blood pressure of persons under 30 if their fitness level is average and their blood pressure is normal at the start of training. The resting blood pressure will be significantly reduced, however, in the middle-aged or older trainees (men or women) who start out with a below-average fitness level and higher than normal blood pressure.

Respiratory Effects

In general, most of the "lung volumes" (e.g., inspiratory and expiratory reserve volumes, residual volume, total lung volume, and vital capacity) are larger in athletes than in nonathletes of the same sex and body size. These changes may be a result of an increase in the strength of the skeletal muscles responsible for ventilation. Whatever the cause, it should be pointed out that there is little if any correlation between athletic performance and lung volumes.

With respect to pulmonary diffusion capacity, a number of studies have shown that athletes have greater capacities than do nonathletes. However, this should not be interpreted to mean that diffusion capacity is directly affected by training. On the contrary, longitudinal studies have failed to show an increase in pulmonary diffusion capacity following several weeks or months of training. In the case of athletes, the larger diffusion capacities may be related to the larger lung volumes just mentioned. The latter would provide for a greater alveolar-capillary surface area and, in turn, a greater diffusion capacity (see p. 171).

Cardiorespiratory Effects of Training Evidenced during Exercise

During exercise, major training-induced changes have been observed in: (1) the oxygen transport system; (2) the utilization of muscle glycogen; (3) the anaerobic threshold; and (4) the accumulation of lactic acid in the muscles and blood.

Changes in the Oxygen Transport System during Submaximal Exercise

When the same amount of submaximal work is performed after training as before training, the amount of oxygen consumed per minute ($\dot{V}O_2$) is in some cases unchanged and in others decreased. A decrease in $\dot{V}O_2$ is thought to be a result of an increased mechanical efficiency (skill). Although in this regard many highly skilled athletes show a much more substantial decrease in $\dot{V}O_2$ than do nonathletes, such a difference has also been observed between good and average competitive runners (see p. 192).

As pointed out in Chapter 8, the amount of oxygen transported to the working muscles is, in part, dependent upon the cardiac output, which in turn is made up of the heart rate and stroke volume. Like $\dot{V}O_2$, the cardiac output for a given amount of submaximal work has been shown to be either slightly decreased or unchanged following training. The stroke volume, however, is usually increased. As previously mentioned, such a combination of effects represents an efficient system with respect to oxygen utilization by the heart muscle (myocardium).

For a given amount of submaximal work, blood flow to the working muscles has been shown in the majority of studies to be decreased following training.* The working muscles apparently compensate for the lowered blood flow in the trained state by extracting more oxygen from the blood. An increased extraction of oxygen by skeletal muscle is probably related to the biochemical and cellular changes that are induced within the muscle itself by training. These changes were discussed earlier (see p. 227).

Changes in the Oxygen Transport System during Maximal Exercise

Under maximal exercise conditions, training increases the maximal oxygen consumption ($\dot{V}O_2$max) by 5 to 20% (on the average). This increase in $\dot{V}O_2$max is a result of two factors: (1) maximal cardiac output is higher after training; and (2) more oxygen is extracted from the blood by the skeletal muscles after training.

Since the maximal heart rate is usually **decreased** as a result of training, the increase in maximal cardiac output is due entirely to an increased stroke volume. The latter may be at least in part related to an expanded ventricular volume, referred to earlier. At any rate, one of the major differences in the oxygen transport systems of athletes and nonathletes under maximal exercise stress is the magnitude of the stroke volume.

During maximal exercise, for every kilogram of muscle that is working, the blood flow to it is the same before and after training. However, blood flow to the total working muscles has been shown to increase. This may be

---

*Some recent research suggests that the blood flow is unchanged.

interpreted to mean that the increased blood flow is distributed over a larger muscle mass, thus keeping the flow per kilogram of muscle constant.

Muscle Glycogen Utilization, Lactic Acid Accumulation, and the Anaerobic Threshold

Training enables one to use up less muscle glycogen during prolonged submaximal exercise and at the same time accumulate less lactic acid in the muscles and blood. Accumulation of less lactic acid during exercise at the same work load following training means that the anaerobic threshold has been increased (see Fig. 8-17, p. 191). It has been suggested that these effects are related either to the increase in the number and size of the muscles' mitochondria or to the increase in the muscles' ability to use free fatty acids as a fuel; perhaps both changes are involved. As mentioned previously, depletion of muscle glycogen stores and accumulation of lactic acid have both been implicated in muscular fatigue. Thus, by producing a glycogen-sparing effect during submaximal exercise—and by decreasing lactic acid accumulation during such exercise (increasing the anaerobic threshold)—training appears to help delay fatigue and increase endurance capacity.

Training also has its effects on levels of lactic acid during **maximal** exercise. It is generally found that there are higher levels of lactic acid in the muscles and blood when exhaustive work is performed after training than when such work is performed before training. Some researchers have interpreted this effect as an indication that tolerance to lactic acid is increased with training. Another possibility is that because the maximal work load is higher, the increased lactic acid production may represent a greater functional capacity to generate energy through anaerobic glycolysis.

A summary of the cardiorespiratory effects of training is given in Table 9-14.

Changes in the Oxygen Transport System: Sprint versus Endurance Training

The major differences between the effects of sprint and endurance training programs on the oxygen transport system have not been defined clearly. Based on the principle of the specificity of training, it has always been assumed that endurance training leads to greater improvement in the aerobic system, and that sprint training leads to greater improvement in the anaerobic (ATP-PC and lactic acid) systems. Yet this is not always true. For example, while some studies have shown more of an increase in the $\dot{V}O_2$max after endurance training than after sprint training (see Fig. 9-6), other studies have found the increases in $\dot{V}O_2$max to be more nearly equal in magnitude.

In these and other comparative studies, one of the conditioning methods that is tested often for its effects on the $\dot{V}O_2$max is the interval training system, since this method of training may be used with both sprint and endurance programs. For example, the effects of an interval training program consisting of repetitions of 55-, 110-, and 220-yd sprints can be compared with those of an

Table 9-14: Summary of the Major Cardiorespiratory Effects of Training

Variable	Training Effects		
	Rest	Submaximal Exercise*	Maximal Exercise
Cardiac hypertrophy	Increased	—	—
Cardiac output	Unchanged or decreased (?)	Unchanged or decreased	Increased
Heart rate	Decreased	Decreased	Decreased or unchanged
Stroke volume	Increased	Increased	Increased
Total hemoglobin and blood volume	Increased	—	—
Blood pressure			
Hypertensives	Decreased	Decreased	Decreased
Normals	Unchanged	Unchanged	Unchanged
Lung volumes	Increased	—	—
Pulmonary diffusion capacity	Increased (?)	Increased	Increased
Minute ventilation	Unchanged	Decreased	Increased
Oxygen consumption ($\dot{V}O_2$)	Unchanged	Decreased or unchanged	Increased
Oxygen extraction by muscle	Unchanged	Increased	Increased
Muscle glycogen depletion	—	Decreased	Increased
Lactic acid levels (in muscle and blood)	—	Increased	Increased
Anaerobic threshold	Unchanged	Increased	—
Blood flow to working muscles (per kg muscle tissue)	—	Decreased or unchanged (?)	Unchanged

*Same amount of work before and after training.

interval training program consisting of repetitions of 660-, 880-, 1100-, and 1320-yd runs. Such a comparison has in fact been made, and it has been found that the two programs produce much the same result: male and female trainees using the program with the shorter distances showed an average increase of 10% in $\dot{V}O_2$max, and a similar increase was measured in men and women using the longer-distance program. This information is of value to athletes in those sports that require anaerobic energy primarily **plus** some aerobic involvement, for it provides them with a means of determining the sprint interval training program that would increase both capacities.

In comparative studies of the effects of sprint and endurance conditioning on lactic acid levels, again using interval training programs, it has been found that during submaximal—but heavy—exercise, lactic acid accumulates in the blood in much smaller amounts in "endurance-trained" individuals than in "sprint-trained" individuals. Figure 9–8 shows the results of a typical study demonstrating this difference. In this study, sprint training consisted of high-intensity sprints lasting 30 sec and repeated 20 times per training session, with about 90 sec of rest-relief between sprints. Endurance training consisted of 2-min runs of lower intensity repeated seven times per workout, with about 2 min of rest-relief between runs. As you can see, the endurance trainees had a

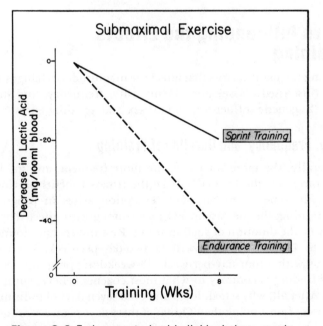

Figure 9-8 Endurance-trained individuals have much lower levels of lactic acid in the blood during submaximal exercise than do sprint-trained individuals. (Based on data from Fox, 1975, and Fox and co-workers, 1977.)

much lower level of lactic acid in the blood during demanding submaximal exercise than did the sprint trainees. These results again point out that the anaerobic threshold is increased with endurance training.

As emphasized in the last chapter, a lower level of lactic acid in the blood during submaximal exercise would prove advantageous to endurance athletes, since fatigue may be considerably reduced and thus the exercise may be continued for a longer period of time.

The effects of sprint and endurance training on the other cardiorespiratory responses, such as cardiac output, stroke volume, blood flow distribution, and respiration have not been adequately analyzed in appropriate comparative studies; this area requires more research.

Training and Changes in Body Composition

Exercise training usually leads to a reduction in body-fat content and an increase in muscle mass (lean body mass). In individuals with excessive body fat, the loss of body fat resulting from training generally exceeds the gain in muscular mass, thus total body weight decreases. As will be discussed in Chapter 11, the most important part of a training program emphasizing body composition changes (particularly loss of body fat) is the total number of calories expended during exercise.

Factors Influencing the Effects of Training

Among the many factors that affect the magnitude of changes induced by training (discussed above) are: (1) intensity, frequency, and duration of training; (2) genetic influences; and (3) sex and age differences.

Intensity, Frequency, and Duration of Training

Generally, the more intensive, the more frequent, and the longer the training program, the greater will be the fitness benefits previously mentioned, with some exceptions. One exception arises in programs using interval training: the increase in $\dot{V}O_2$max is not greatly affected by either the frequency or the duration of such training. Researchers have found gains in $\dot{V}O_2$max to be just as great with a two-day-per-week, seven-week-long program as with a four-day-per-week, 13-week-long program (see Fig. 9–9).

This finding is contrary to what most coaches believe, but it should be accepted. After all, why schedule six and even seven days of training per week for purposes of improving the $\dot{V}O_2$max if three days per week are adequate to the task? The major reason is because frequency and duration of training do affect the magnitude of the decrease in heart rate during submaximal exercise. The longer and more frequent the training, the lower the heart rate during submaximal exercise will be.

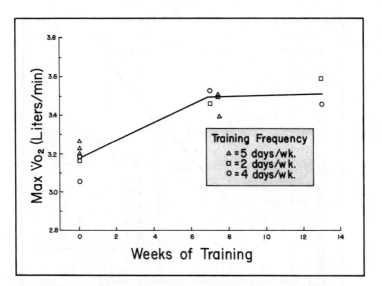

Figure 9-9 With interval training, maximal aerobic power ($\dot{V}O_2$ max) increases, but the magnitude of the increase is not greatly affected by varying the training frequency (say from two to four days per week) or by increasing the training duration (from seven to thirteen weeks). (Based on data from Fox and co-workers, 1975.)

This information is quite important when applied to endurance sports, in which the work performed is mostly submaximal. A lower heart rate under submaximal work conditions means less stress on the cardiorespiratory system. For this reason, athletes who are training for endurance sports should be advised to train more frequently and for longer periods than those training for sprint or anaerobic sports.

With interval training, the most important factor affecting gains in $\dot{V}O_2$max has been shown to be the intensity of training. The relationship between training intensity and gains in $\dot{V}O_2$max following interval training is given in Figure 9-10. Notice that the intensity of training is expressed as a relative factor—that is, each value shown is relative to each subject's initial fitness level (as measured by $\dot{V}O_2$max). (The figure also shows once again that the gains in $\dot{V}O_2$max are independent of the frequency—two, four, or five days per week—and the duration—seven weeks vs. 13 weeks—of training.)

Genetic Influences

All of us realize that our capabilities are ultimately limited by our genetic make-ups. For example, no matter how good the training program in a

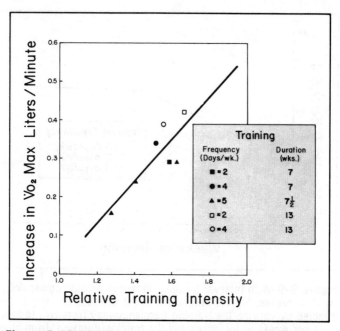

Figure 9-10 With interval training, the most important factor affecting gains in $\dot{V}O_2$ max is training intensity. Note that the gains are independent of training frequency and duration. (Based on data from Fox and co-workers, 1973, 1975.)

particular sport, only a few of us have the genetic potential to develop the capabilities required for top-flight international competition in that sport. Given this state of affairs, we must ask: how much of a person's performance is limited by heredity? Or, conversely, how much can be improved by training? The answer is still not clear. However, recent research has demonstrated that certain physiological capabilities are highly heritable. The capacity of the aerobic system ($\dot{V}O_2$max), for instance, is 93% genetically determined (see p. 189), and that of the lactic acid system is 81% genetically determined. The maximal attainable heart rate has a similar large genetic component (86%). As mentioned earlier, it also appears that the distribution of fast- and slow-twitch muscle fibers is, to a very large extent, genetically determined and cannot be altered by physical training. It just might be that if you want to become a good athlete, choose your parents wisely!

Actually, the role of the coach here is twofold: (1) to develop through training the full genetic potential of the athlete; and (2) to give each athlete a chance to participate and compete in the event or position for which he or she is best suited "genetically." The latter responsibility requires the coach to recognize the possibility that the athlete's genetic potential has in fact been fully developed through training but is inappropriate to the athlete's sport. For instance, the 6-mile runner who trains extremely hard but very seldom wins may not have the aerobic capabilities required for success in such a long run; this athlete should be encouraged to participate in shorter events, such as 2-mile runs or even 1500-m runs, where the chances of success might be greater.

Sex and Age Differences

The adaptive responses that training produces in men and women (or male and female animals) cannot be compared with any great validity because not nearly enough studies have been conducted using women as subjects. Most of the studies that **are** available indicate that there are no major differences between the training responses of women and men exposed to the same relative training stress. However, it has been pointed out that female rats develop greater degrees of cardiac hypertrophy than do male rats. In addition, the body weight of male rats does not usually follow the normal growth curve during training, whereas that of the female does. Until further comparative studies are conducted—on humans—the extent and magnitude of the differences, if any, in training responses between the sexes will remain uncertain.

Menstruation

Not too many years ago, the conclusion concerning menstruation and exercise was that neither one affected the other. Today, however, it is recognized that exercise can affect menstruation, particularly among women involved in high-intensity training and competition in sports such as long-distance running, gymnastics, swimming, and even professional ballet dancing. For example, approximately one third of female distance runners develop **amenorrhea**, an abnormal cessation of menstruation during their training and competitive seasons. This is shown in Figure 9-11. In A, the incidence of amenorrhea was 34% in a group of runners, 23% in a group of joggers, and only 4% in the nonrunning control group. In this study, runners were defined as those women who ran more than 30 miles per week and combined long, slow-distance running with speed work. Joggers, on the other hand, were defined as those women who ran slowly and easily and only 5 to 30 miles per week. The average number of menses per year for controls was 11.85, for joggers 10.32, and for runners 9.16 (Figure 9-11B).

Further evaluation of the menstrual patterns of runners is given in the inset of Figure 9-11B. Note that as many as 24% of the runners had five or fewer menses per year. Also, although not shown in the figure, the incidence of amenorrhea appears to be significantly greater in those runners and joggers with late onset of menarche (onset of menstruation), who had not experienced pregnancy, or who had taken contraceptive hormones.

The exact cause of amenorrhea in athletes is not known. However,

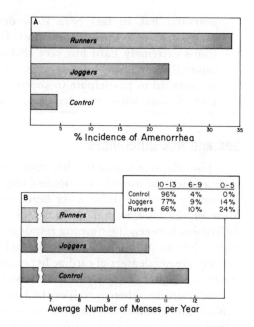

Figure 9-11 Approximately one third of female distance runners develop amenorrhea (cessation of menstruation) during their training and competitive seasons. B, The average number of menses per year is lower in runners and joggers than in controls. Further evaluation of the menstrual patterns of female runners is given in the inset. (Based on data from Dale and co-workers, 1979.)

whatever the cause, it appears to be related to the intensity of training. For example, as shown in Figure 9-12, the incidence of amenorrhea in middle-distance runners was found to be directly related to their weekly training mileage. This can be interpreted to mean that the amenorrhea is caused by the training or competition itself, or by some other factors related to chronic exercise training, such as loss of body weight, or general psychological stress. In the case of the training itself, it is important to point out that the more intense training could lead to better performance and thus more psychological stress.

Excessive weight loss through a reduction of the body fat stores has been shown to cause amenorrhea. Since fat stores of many athletes, particularly long-distance runners and gymnasts, are much lower than nonathletes' (see p. 288), this remains a possible cause of amenorrhea in these athletes. However, it should be emphasized that there is probably no single amount of body fat loss, or training for that matter, that will induce amenorrhea in every woman. Instead, each woman probably has a different threshold for amenorrhea which may be related to any of the previously mentioned factors.

Finally, the question of what happens to these kinds of menstrual disorders once exercise training and competition is stopped needs to be answered. As might be expected, the complete answer to this question is not yet available. However, based on current information, it appears that once competition and training are stopped, the menses resume a normal pattern, and the childbearing functions of the woman are normal in every respect. Presumably, this would apply to other sports as well.

Dysmenorrhea (painful menstruation) is probably neither aggravated

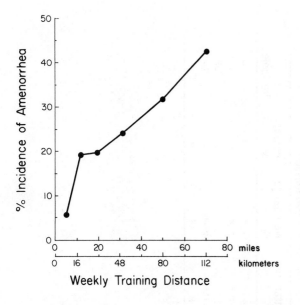

Figure 9-12 The incidence of amenorrhea in female middle-distance runners is directly related to their weekly training mileage. (Modified and redrawn from Feicht and co-workers, 1978.)

nor cured by sports participation. If anything, it may be less common in those women who are physically active than in those who are not. At any rate, dysmenorrhea, if not severe, should not hinder performance—at least from a physiological standpoint. However, it is recognized that psychological factors also play an important role.

Performance and Menstruation

In Table 9-15 is a compilation of findings obtained from a variety of athletes relative to their performances during menstruation. In general, these results show that for the majority of young athletes, physical performance itself is not materially affected by the menstrual period. However, there is considerable individual variation. Of those athletes reporting poorer performances during menstruation, a large percentage were endurance athletes (e.g., tennis players and rowers). Performances for volleyball and basketball players and swimmers and gymnasts were better than for the endurance athletes, but were still below normal. Performances by track-and-field athletes, especially sprinters, were not affected nearly so much by menstruation as were the performances by other athletes.

From a physiological standpoint, metabolic and cardiovascular responses at rest and during maximal exercise are not systematically affected during different phases of the menstrual cycle. An example of this is shown in Figure 9-13. In this study, metabolic and cardiovascular responses were determined at rest and during exercise on eight trained athletes and nine untrained women during the following three phases of the menstrual cycle: (1) seven days after ovulation (premenstrual phase); (2) three days after the

Table 9-15: Performance during Menstruation

Caliber of Performance	Reference	Sport	Performance			
			Better %	No Change %	Poorer %	Variable
Olympics	Kral and Markalous (1937)	Track and field	29	63	8	—
Olympics	Ingman (1952)	Variety	19	43	38	—
Olympics	Zaharieva (1965)	Variety	3	37	17	28
Unspecified	Erdelyi (1962)	Variety	13–15	42–48	31–38	—
Unspecified	Åstrand and co-workers (1963)	Swimming	4	48	48	—

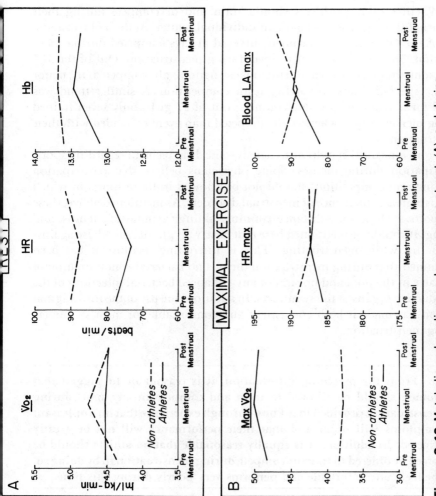

Figure 9-13 Metabolic and cardiovascular responses at rest, (A), and during maximal exercise, (B) are not systematically affected during the premenstrual phase (7 days after ovulation), the menstrual phase (3 days after the onset of bleeding), and the postmenstrual phase (13 days after the onset of bleeding) of the menstrual cycle. (Based on data from Fox and co-workers, 1977.)

onset of bleeding (menstrual phase); and (3) 13 days after the onset of bleeding (postmenstrual phase). As can be seen, none of the responses, either at rest or during exercise, was significantly affected by the different phases of the cycle. Similar results have been found by others, although some minor physiological fluctuations at rest, but not during exercise, have also been reported.

Training and Competition during Menstruation

Whether or not athletes should train and/or compete during their menstrual flow (menses) is again an individual matter. At the Tokyo games, 69% of the Olympic sportswomen surveyed always competed during menstruation. However, only 34% trained during menstruation. Out of the 31% who sometimes competed during menstruation, all competed in major meets, especially those involving team competition. A similar trend was found for a group of young swimmers: out of 27 girls, only seven trained during menstruation; whereas all competed if an event coincided with their menstruation.

From a medical standpoint, there is some disagreement regarding sports participation during menses. Some physicians believe that participation (training and competition) should not be allowed in those sports in which there is a greater incidence of menstrual disorders. As mentioned above, these are sports such as long-distance running, skiing, gymnastics, tennis, and rowing. It should be mentioned here that nearly all physicians advise against swimming while menstruating. This is interesting, because it has been determined that during menstruation there is no bacterial contamination of the water in the pool and no sign of any enhanced bacterial infections of the reproductive organs of the swimmers. In addition, the use of the intravaginal tampon has made it both convenient and comfortable for most swimmers during menstruation.

From the preceding information, it is reasonable to suggest that women should be allowed to train and compete in any sport during menstruation provided they know through experience that no unpleasant symptoms will occur and that their performance will not be greatly affected. In addition, it is equally reasonable that no athlete should be forced or ordered to train or compete during menstruation if, by doing so, she feels uncomfortable and performs very poorly during this time.

With regard to other gynecological considerations, our present state of knowledge allows us to offer the following observations:

---

1. **Complications of pregnancy and childbirth are fewer in female athletes than in nonathletes.**
2. **Following childbirth, performance returns to or even exceeds previous levels within a year or two.**

3. Pregnancy does not adversely affect athletic participation, and vice versa.
4. Serious injuries to either the breasts or the external and internal reproductive organs are very rare in female athletes, even in contact sports.

Guidelines for Female Participation in Sports

To assist those who may be involved in making decisions regarding participation in sports by girls and young women, the Committee on Pediatric Aspects of Physical Fitness, Recreation, and Sports offers the following guidelines:

Participation in Sports by Girls

There is no reason to separate prepubescent children by sex in sports, physical education, and recreational activities.

Girls can compete against girls in any sports activity if matched for size, weight, skill, and physical maturation as long as the customary safeguards for protection of health and safety in sports and competitive athletics are followed.

Girls can attain high levels of physical fitness through strenuous conditioning activities to improve their physical fitness, agility, strength, appearance, endurance, and sense of psychic well-being. These have no unfavorable influences on menstruation, future pregnancy, and childbirth.

Postpubescent girls should not participate against boys in heavy collision sports because of the grave risk of serious injury due to their lesser muscle mass per unit of body weight.

The talented female athlete may participate on a team with boys in an appropriate sport provided that the school or community offers opportunities for all girls to participate in comparable activities.

With respect to female participation in long-distance running, the American College of Sports Medicine offers the following opinion:

"It is the opinion of the American College of Sports Medicine that females should not be denied the opportunity to compete in long-distance running. There exists no conclusive scientific or medical evidence that long-distance running is contraindicated for the healthy, trained female athlete. The American College of Sports Medicine recommends that females be allowed to compete at the national and international level in the same distances in which their male counterparts compete."

The physical working capacity of both sexes declines with age. Whether this reduction is related to the aging process or to the fact that physical activity levels decrease with age is not known. However, it is known that people of all ages can and do respond to physical training programs. In addition, the responses of older people appear to be of the same **relative** magnitude as those of younger people.

Training Supplements

Over the years, coaches have developed techniques which they feel supplement regular training methods and programs. Although not all of these techniques have been adequately evaluated scientifically, they warrant mentioning.

Methods of Improving Speed

A runner can improve speed in a number of ways, but the methods that have most interested advocates of supplemental training programs are those that encourage the runner to: (1) take a longer stride; (2) lift the knees higher; (3) develop greater strength in the legs; and/or (4) increase the rate of leg movement. Among the popular methods of achieving some or all of these goals are towing (by an automobile), downhill running (or ramp running), uphill running, and treadmill sprinting.

The rationale for towing a runner by means of a tow bar and handle attached to the rear bumper of an automobile is that the car can serve as a pacing machine. It has been reported that some sprinters have reduced their average time in the 100-yd dash from 10.5 to 9.9 sec after training with towing for five weeks. Another study showed a 2.8% increase in the time required to run the last 50 m of a 70-m sprint. Readers interested in a complete towing regimen, including the proper towing speed, the number of repetitions, tow-car operation, and other training factors, will find Sandwick's program (cited in the references at the end of this chapter) to be most helpful.

Running downhill (or down a ramp) is also used in hopes of increasing speed, but this method has not been shown to be scientifically effective. In fact, many sprint coaches question the assumption that the stride length and the speed of leg movement are increased during such running. Another problematic aspect of such running is that the inclines used are often too great. The incline of the downhill terrain or of the ramp should not exceed a 5% gradient.

Running uphill, sometimes alternated with climbing steps, is a training technique intended to increase leg strength and knee lift. The actual effectiveness of this technique has not been scientifically determined, and some coaches even consider uphill running to be counter-productive. These coaches argue that both stride length and rate of leg movement are decreased during uphill running, thus offsetting any gains that might be made by increasing leg strength and knee lift. Despite its critics, uphill running is a popular training technique, particularly among track, football, and basketball coaches. It should be noted that some coaches combine uphill running with downhill running, on the assumption that trainees will develop increased knee lift and leg strength from the uphill program and a longer stride and an increased rate of leg movement from the downhill program. Obviously, research into both types of running, separately and in combination, is needed.

It has been suggested that having an athlete sprint on a motor-driven treadmill at speeds greater than those possible during actual track running will lead to a greater rate of leg movement and increased stride length. The procedure involves determining the athlete's maximum speed, which is relatively easy on the treadmill, and then slowly increasing the speed beyond the maximum with or without the athlete's knowledge. Whether the procedure produces the intended effects has not been thoroughly tested. Even if its value were proven, treadmill sprinting would still raise problems of expense (high-speed treadmills cost in excess of $5000) and expertise (the coach or handler must know how to operate the machine safely, and the runner must be skilled at performing on the treadmill at high speeds).

Treadmill Pacing

The motor-driven treadmill has also been suggested as a training supplement for cross-country runners. With this type of treadmill training, running speeds are between 9 and 11 miles per hr, much lower than those required for sprinting (20 to 25 miles per hr). Two benefits of treadmill pacing have been envisioned: (1) a sense of running pace and rhythm gained on the treadmill might be transferred to running an outdoor course; and (2) the athlete might be better trained to utilize a greater fraction of his or her maximal oxygen consumption. Although these possibilities have not been studied extensively, preliminary findings are encouraging. For example, three of four cross-country runners who participated in a three-week supplemental training program consisting of uphill and pace training and 5-mile runs on a motor-driven treadmill improved their outdoor cross-country performance times.

Training at Moderate Altitudes

As mentioned in the last chapter, it has been suggested that a combination of training at sea level and at moderate altitudes may improve endurance performance at sea level.

It would seem that training at altitudes well above sea level would enable athletes to work closer to their $\dot{V}O_2max$. Such a possibility arises because the $\dot{V}O_2max$ is progressively reduced at altitudes above 5000 ft, whereas the oxygen consumption for a given amount of work is the same. Therefore, the relative stress placed on the oxygen transport system (percent $\dot{V}O_2max$) is greater at moderate to high altitudes—an effect which should ultimately benefit the endurance athlete.

Another possible advantage of training at elevations above sea level is that endurance athletes who are not in good competitive condition may be able to train their overall functional mechanisms to their maximum at lower work loads, thus reducing the stress placed on the local musculature. In other words, high- or moderate-altitude training may stress general physiological functions to the maximum without causing undue stress on local, injured tissue.

Although these ideas appear sound, research findings on altitude training and performance have not always backed them up. Some evidence is supportive: it has been reported, for instance, that Jim Ryun, the former great middle-distance runner, hit his highest $\dot{V}O_2max$ and also established his world records for the 1-mile and 1500-m runs after he had gone through altitude training. Other evidence is incomplete: some studies that have pointed to the apparently beneficial effects of altitude training on subsequent performance at sea level have not used adequate control groups. Still other evidence (from several studies) suggests that performance at sea level may be left unaffected—or even impaired—by altitude training.

One possible disadvantage of altitude training is that the work required by athletes in especially demanding endurance programs apparently cannot be sustained at an intensity commensurate with that at sea level or at a duration corresponding to that at sea level. This limitation exists in spite of the advantages in relative stress provided by altitude training, and is particularly evident at high elevations, as is shown in Figure 9-14. The figure gives the intensity of the training workouts, at various altitudes, for six collegiate runners. Even though their coach was present at all workouts, it is quite clear that high altitude severely reduced their training efforts.

Overall, there would appear to be something of a balance between the pros and cons of altitude training for purposes of improving endurance performance at sea level. Readers who feel that the evidence favors altitude training programs should consult Table 9-16 for information on actually constructing such programs.

Summary

- The coach's responsibility in training the athlete is to construct exercise programs that will develop the energy capacities and skill needed by the individual for his or her event.

- Specificity must be considered in training; that is, training should develop the specific physiological capabilities required to perform a given sports skill or activity.

- There are several types of training specificity, among them metabolic specificity (e.g., sprint vs. endurance sports), specificity with respect to mode of exercise (e.g., cycling vs. running, running vs. swimming), and muscle group specificity (e.g., working with the arms vs. working with the legs).

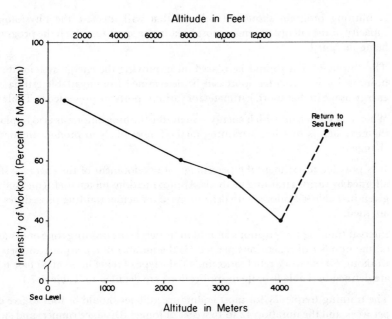

Figure 9-14 One of the problems with altitude training is the severe reduction in training intensity (not as much work can be done as at sea level). (Based on data from Kollias and Buskirk, 1974.)

Table 9-16: Guidelines for Altitude Training*

Altitude

Training should be carried out at a moderate altitude: 6500-7500 ft (2000-2400 m). Note that trainees should spend some time away from this altitude every 2 to 4 wk (see below).

Allotment of Time

1. Over the course of the entire program, the bulk of the time should be spent at the moderate altitude.
2. There should also be brief periods of time spent at other elevations. Short periods of exposure to conditions at higher altitudes should be regularly scheduled over the course of the program, as should intervals of exposure to conditions at lower altitudes (or sea level). Intermittent trips to lower altitudes ensure maintenance of muscular power, normal competitive rhythm and intensity of effort.

Emphasis of Training

The altitude training program should emphasize maintenance of muscular power yet be geared to include normal or near-normal overall amounts of work.

Scheduling of Training

Altitude training should be scheduled so that athletes who are to participate in important competition will have completed the training program about 2 wk before their scheduled events.

*Summarized from Daniels (1972).

- A training program should be selected that will increase the physiological capacity of the energy system(s) most used in the sport for which the program is being designed.

- The emphasis that should be placed on improving the energy systems during training for a particular sport can be determined from available estimates of energy usage in that sport. Estimates for various sports are presented in Table 9–2.

- When it is known on which energy systems the training emphasis is to be placed, the next step is to select a training method most likely to produce the desired change.

- It is possible to estimate the percentage of development of the energy systems afforded by various training methods. Approximations for ten useful methods are given in Table 9–3, along with definitions of the actual training procedures that are used.

- Interval training prescriptions should indicate: (1) the training time or distance; (2) the number of repetitions per set; (3) the number of repetitions and sets per workout; (4) the work-relief ratio; and (5) the type of relief interval. (These terms are defined in Table 9–6; their applications are detailed in Table 9–7.)

- The training frequency for most endurance athletes should be four to five days per week and the duration 12 to 16 weeks or longer. Distance runners and swimmers may require a training frequency of six to seven days per week the year round.

- An endurance training frequency of two or more sessions per day is not necessarily more productive (or likely to induce physiological changes) than is a frequency of one session per day.

- The training frequency for most nonendurance athletes should be three days per week and the duration eight to ten weeks. Track and swimming sprinters may require a frequency of five to six days per week, more or less on a yearly basis.

- Proper intensity levels for most endurance training programs may be determined from the heart rate of the athlete. The intensity of the exercise should be such that the heart rate reaches 85 to 90% of its maximum. If the maximal heart rate has not been measured, it may be estimated by subtracting the individual's age from 220.

- With most sprint training programs, the heart rate during training should be about 180 beats per min.

- Athletes should be taught how to count their pulse rates and why to count them.

- Proper intensity levels for interval training may be determined from the heart rate response, from the total number of repetitions performed, or from maximal running (or swimming) speeds.

- Warm-up activities raise body and muscle temperatures, an effect which promotes increased blood flow and makes more oxygen available to muscles. Warm-up may also protect against injury.

- It is recommended that a 15- to 30-min warm-up period precede each training session or competition. The warm-up should consist of stretching, calisthenics, and formal activity, in that order.

- Warm-down aids in the rapid removal of lactic acid from muscle and blood. The warm-down should be similar to the warm-up, but the order to be followed is formal activity first, then calisthenics, and then stretching.

- Off-season training programs should consist of:
  Weight training involving those muscle groups most used during the athlete's sport
  A low-intensity training program of running, swimming, or cycling, depending on the athlete's sport, scheduled for two days a week and lasting for six to ten weeks
  Participation in sports and recreational games

- Preseason training programs should be designed to increase to a maximum the capacities of the energy systems that are predominant when performing a specific athletic event.

- In-season training programs may include:
  One or two days per week of training similar to that in the preseason
  Weight training with one workout per week, alternating upper body and lower body workouts
  Drills utilized not only for skill improvement but also for fitness

- Skeletal muscle is affected in many ways by endurance training: (1) the ability to oxidize carbohydrates and fats is increased; (2) myoglobin is present in greater concentrations; (3) stores of glycogen, triglycerides, and phosphagen (ATP + PC) are increased; and (4) muscle fibers—ST fibers only—undergo hypertrophy (the fibers have a large diameter). There is also some effect on anaerobic glycolysis, but it is small (the activities of key lactic acid system enzymes are unchanged or partially decreased). There is **no** interconversion of fiber types.

- Skeletal muscle is not so extensively or intensively affected by sprint training. There is little change in the activities of glycolytic (lactic acid system) enzymes, and increases in the activities of key enzymes involved in the ATP-PC system are small. Hypertrophy does occur in both ST fibers and FT fibers, with the latter showing the more pronounced change. Again, there is no interconversion of fiber types.

- Exercise training causes adaptations in the neuromuscular junction and motoneuron.

- Cardiorespiratory effects of training that are evident at rest include: (1) cardiac hypertrophy; (2) reduction of hypertension; and (3) increases in stroke volume, total hemoglobin content, blood volume, lung volumes, and pulmonary diffusion capacity. In addition, the heart rate is **decreased**—a change toward efficiency when combined with the increased stroke volume.

- Cardiorespiratory effects of training that are evident during submaximal exercise at a fixed work load include: (1) increases in stroke volume, pulmonary diffusion capacity, and the amount of oxygen extracted by muscle; and (2) decreases in heart rate, minute ventilation, and the amount of glycogen used by muscle. In addition, levels of lactic acid are decreased in both the muscles and the blood. Cardiac output and $\dot{V}O_2$ are decreased or unchanged.

- Cardiorespiratory effects of training that are evident during maximal exercise include increases in cardiac output, stroke volume, pulmonary diffusion capacity, minute ventilation, and $\dot{V}O_2$. Moreover, a greater amount of oxygen is extracted by muscle, and usage of glycogen by muscle is increased as well. In addition, lactic acid reaches higher concentrations in both the muscles and the blood. The heart rate is, however, unchanged or decreased.

- Endurance-trained individuals have much lower levels of lactic acid in the blood when performing submaximal (but heavy) exercise than do sprint-trained individuals performing the same work (as established in studies using interval training for the sprint and endurance programs).

- Exercise training usually leads to a reduction in body fat content and an increase in muscle mass (lean body mass).

- Generally, the more intensive, the more frequent, and the longer the training program, the greater will be **some** of the fitness benefits (for example, the longer and more frequent the training, the lower the heart rate during submaximal exercise). One benefit of training, an increased $\dot{V}O_2$max, is **not** greatly affected by the frequency or duration of programs using interval training.

- With interval training, the most important factor affecting gains in $\dot{V}O_2$max has been shown to be the intensity of training.

- Certain physiological capabilities are largely determined by one's genetic make-up. Therefore, the role of the coach is to develop through training the **full** genetic potential of the athlete and give each athlete a chance to participate in the sport or event for which he or she is genetically best suited.

- There are no major differences between the training responses of women and men exposed to the same relative training stress.

- Mild exercise does not appear to have a significant effect on menstrual disorders. In fact, dysmenorrhea (painful menstruation) is less common among physically active women than among those who are sedentary.

- Heavy, intensive training has been found to induce amenorrhea (cessation of menstruation) in some athletes, particularly long-distance runners, joggers, and gymnasts. The amenorrhea is temporary and uncomplicated; it disappears upon cessation of heavy training.

- Complications of pregnancy and childbirth are fewer in athletes than in non-athletes. Pregnancy does not adversely affect athletic participation, and vice versa.

- Following childbirth, performance returns to or even exceeds previous levels within a year or two.

- Serious injuries to either the breasts or the external and internal reproductive organs are very rare in female athletes, even in contact sports.

- Although the physical working capacity declines with age, people of all ages can and do respond to physical training.

- Coaches and runners have reported increases in sprinting speed after using training supplements such as towing (by an automobile), downhill running (ramp running), uphill running, and treadmill sprinting.

- Supplemental treadmill running, from which a sense of running pace and rhythm may be gained, might help improve the performance of distance runners.

- The pros and cons of altitude training for purposes of improving endurance performance at sea level are evenly split. All advocates of altitude training should be familiar with the program guidelines presented in Table 9-16.

Selected References and Readings*

American College of Sports Medicine: Opinion statement on the participation of the female athlete in long-distance running. *Sports Med. Bull.*, *15(1)*:4-5, 1980.

Astrand, P. O., et al.: Girl swimmers. *Acta Paediat.*, Suppl. *147*, 1963.

Barnard, R., et al.: Cardiovascular responses to sudden exercise—heart rate, blood pressure and ECG. *J. Appl. Physiol.*, *34(6)*:833-837, 1973.

Bergh, U., and B. Ekblom: Physical performance and peak aerobic power at different body temperatures. *J. Appl. Physiol.: Respirat. Environ. Exercise Physiol.*, *46(5)*:885-889, 1979.

Burke, R., and V. R. Edgerton. Motor unit properties and selective involvement in movement. *In* Wilmore, J. (ed.): *Exercise and Sports Sciences Reviews.* Vol. 3. New York, Academic Press, 1975, pp. 31-81.

Clarke, H. H. (ed.): Physical activity during menstruation and pregnancy. *Physical Fitness Research Digest.* President's Council on Physical Fitness and Sports. Washington, D.C., U.S. Government Printing Office, Series 8, No. 3, July, 1978.

Clausen, J. P.: Effect of physical training on cardiovascular adjustments to exercise in man. *Physiol. Rev.*, *57*:779-815, 1977.

Costill, D. L.: *A Scientific Approach to Distance Running.* Los Altos, CA, Track and Field News, 1979.

Dale, E., D. H. Gerlach, and A. L. Wilhite: Menstrual dysfunction in distance runners. *Obstet Gynecol.*, *54(1)*:47-53, 1979.

Daniels, J. T.: Effects of altitude on athletic accomplishment. *Mod. Med.*, June 26, 1972, pp. 73-76.

Dintiman, G. B.: *Sprinting Speed.* Springfield, IL, Charles C. Thomas Publishers, 1971.

Edgerton, V. R.: Neuromuscular adaptation to power and endurance work. *Can. J. Appl. Sport Sci.*, *1*:49-58, 1976.

Ekblom, B., and L. Hermansen: Cardiac output in athletes. *J. Appl. Physiol.*, *25(5)*:619-625, 1968.

Erdelyi, G.: Gynecological survey of female athletes. *J. Sports Med.*, *2*:174-179, 1962.

Feicht, C. B., et al.: Secondary amenorrhea in athletes. *Lancet*, *2(8100)*:1145-1146, Nov., 1978.

Fox, E. L., and D. Mathews: *Interval Training: Conditioning for Sports and General Fitness.* Philadelphia, W. B. Saunders Company, 1974.

Fox, E. L., and D. Mathews: *The Physiological Basis of Physical Education and Athletics*, 3rd ed. Philadelphia, Saunders College Publishing, 1981.

Fox, E. L., D. C. McKenzie, and K. Cohen: Specificity of training: Metabolic and circulatory responses. *Med. Sci. Sports*, *7*:83, 1975.

Fox, E. L. Differences in metabolic alterations with sprint versus endurance interval training programs. *In* Howald, H. and J. Poortmans (eds.): *Metabolic Adaptation to Prolonged Physical Exercise.* Basel, Switzerland, Birkhauser Verlag, 1975, pp. 119-126.

Fox, E. L., F. L. Martin, and R. L. Bartels: Metabolic and cardiorespiratory responses to exercise during the menstrual cycle in trained and untrained subjects. *Med. Sci. Sports*, *9(1)*:70, 1977.

Fox, E. L.: Physical training: Methods and effects. *Orthop. Clin. N. Am.*, *8*:533-548, 1977.

Fox, E. L.: Physiological effects of training. *Encyclopedia of Physical Fitness.* New York, John Wiley & Sons, 1979.

Fox, E. L., et al.: Intensity and distance of interval training programs and changes in aerobic power. *Med. Sci. Sports*, *5(1)*:18-22, 1973.

---

*For full journal titles, see Appendix A.

Fox, E. L., et al.: Frequency and duration of interval training programs and changes in aerobic power. *J. Appl. Physiol., 38(3)*:481-484, 1975.

Fox, E. L., et al.: Metabolic responses to interval training programs of high and low power output. *Med. Sci. Sports, 9(3)*:191-196, 1977.

Gillespie, A. C., E. L. Fox, and A. J. Merola: Enzyme adaptations in rat skeletal muscle after two intensities of treadmill training. *Med. Sci. Sports Exercise, 14(6)*:461-466, 1982.

Gollnick, P. D., et al.: Effect of training on enzyme activity and fiber composition of human skeletal muscle. *J. Appl. Physiol., 34*:107-111, 1973.

Hickson, R., W. Heusner, and W. Van Huss: Skeletal muscle enzyme alterations after sprint and endurance training. *J. Appl. Physiol., 40*:868-872, 1976.

Holloszy, J. O., and F. W. Booth: Biochemical adaptations to endurance exercise in muscle. *Ann. Rev. Physiol., 38*:273-291, 1976.

Ingman, O.: Menstruation in Finnish top class sportswomen. *In Sports Medicine—International Symposium of the Medicine and Physiology of Sports and Athletes.* Helsinki, Finnish Association of Sports Medicine, 1952.

Kollias, J., D. L. Moody, and E. R. Buskirk: Cross-country running: Treadmill simulation and suggested effectiveness of supplemental treadmill running. *J. Sports Med., 7(3)*:148-154, 1967.

Kollias, J., and E. R. Buskirk. Exercise and altitude. *In* Johnson, W., and E. R. Buskirk (eds.): *Science and Medicine of Exercise and Sports.* 2nd ed. New York, Harper and Row, 1974, pp. 211-227.

Kral, J., and E. Markalous. The influence of menstruation on sports performance. *In* Mallwitz, A. (ed.): *Proceedings of the 2nd International Congress on Sports Medicine.* Leipzig, Thieme, 1937.

McKenzie, D. C., E. L. Fox, and K. Cohen: Specificity of metabolic and circulatory responses to arm and leg interval training. *Europ. J. Appl. Physiol., 39*:241-248, 1978.

Magel, J. R., et al.: Specificity of swim training on maximum oxygen uptake. *J. Appl. Physiol., 38*:151-155, 1974.

Morganroth, J., et al.: Comparative left ventricular dimensions in trained athletes. *Ann. Intern. Med., 82*:521-524, 1975.

Mostardi, R., R. Gandee, and T. Campbell: Multiple daily training and improvement in aerobic power. *Med. Sci. Sports, 7(1)*:82, 1975.

Pechar, G. S., et al.: Specificity of cardiorespiratory adaptation to bicycle and treadmill training. *J. Appl. Physiol., 36*:753-756, 1974.

Roberts, J., and J. Alspaugh: Specificity of training effects resulting from programs of treadmill running and bicycle ergometer riding. *Med. Sci. Sports, 4*:6-10, 1972.

Roby, F., and R. Davis: *Jogging for Fitness and Weight Control.* Philadelphia, W. B. Saunders Company, 1970.

Saltin, B., et al.: The nature of the training response; peripheral and central adaptations to one-legged exercise. *Acta Physiol. Scand., 96*:289-305, 1976.

Saltin, B.: Physiological effects of physical training. *Med. Sci. Sports, 1(1)*:50-56, 1969.

Sandwick, C. M.: Pacing machine. *Athletic Journal, 47*:36-38, 1967.

Scheuer, J., and C. M. Tipton: Cardiovascular adaptations to physical training. *Ann. Rev. Physiol., 39*:221-251, 1977.

Shaffer, T. E., and E. L. Fox: Guidelines to physical conditioning for sports. *Pediatric Basics, 18*: 10-14, 1977.

Thorstensson, A., B. Sjodin, and J. Karlsson: Enzyme activities and muscle strength after "sprint training" in man. *Acta Physiol. Scand., 94*:313-318, 1975.

Wilt, F.: Training for competitive running. *In* Falls, H. (ed.): *Exercise Physiology.* New York, Academic Press, 1968, pp. 395-414.

Zaharieva, E.: Survey of sportswomen at the Tokyo Olympics. *J. Sports Med., 5*:215-219, 1965.

Zeldis, S. M., J. Morganroth, and S. Rubler: Cardiac hypertrophy in response to dynamic conditioning in female athletes. *J. Appl. Physiol.: Respirat. Environ. Exercise Physiol., 44(6)*: 849-852, 1978.

10

Nutrition and Sports Performance

Introduction

The importance of the relationship between nutrition and exercise performance is obvious: Good nutrition is essential to proper growth and development. Too often, coaches think of good nutrition only during the season of their sport. Actually, for effective athletic performance, good nutrition is critical at all times.

In a survey of the nutritional practices of coaches in the Big Ten Conference, 78% of the coaches felt a need for more nutritional information, yet 69% of them rarely read about nutrition. In another study, it was found that the majority of coaches and trainers surveyed had up-to-date information about water replacement, but were totally uninformed about sound nutritional practices. These situations are probably typical of many coaches throughout the United States. The surveys vividly point out that scientific information aimed at the coach concerning nutrition and its effects on exercise and athletic performance is greatly needed. Our essential concern in this chapter, therefore, will be to fulfill this need.

Nutrition

In studying nutrition it is important to discuss: (1) basic nutrients; (2) food requirements; and (3) eating habits. A **nutrient** is defined as any substance which when taken into the body serves to sustain life. Our immediate interest is in food nutrients, of which there are three fundamental classes: (1) energy nutrients; (2) vitamins and minerals; and (3) water.

Energy Nutrients

Energy nutrients are those foods which when chemically broken down provide energy for synthesizing ATP. You should recall from Chapter 4 that proteins, fats, and carbohydrates are the energy nutrient foods. Of these, the primary nutrients for ATP synthesis are (1) fats stored in the adipocytes and in the muscle and, particularly (2) muscle and liver glycogen. The magnitude of the stores of these fuels within the skeletal muscles is dependent to a great extent upon our diets.

Protein is not normally used to any significant extent as an energy nutrient, although it can and does serve as such under certain unusual circumstances (e.g., during starvation). The main contribution of protein is to cellular and tissue growth and repair in the body. Proteins are complex molecules containing **amino acids**. Some, but not all, of the essential amino acids are synthesized by the body. Those that are not synthesized can only be obtained through the diet. Thus, the importance of daily dietary protein is obvious.

Protein Requirements of Athletes

The normal adult daily protein requirement is about 1 g per kg of body weight. For example, the daily protein requirement of a person weighing 75 kg (165 lb) would be 75 kg × 1g/kg = 75 g (2.6 oz). This amount of protein is easily obtained from a well balanced diet in which 10 to 15% of the calories taken in are from protein sources. If our 75-kg person has a daily caloric requirement of 3000 kcal, a well balanced diet would supply between 75 and 112 g of protein.* Contrary to what many coaches and athletes believe, the protein requirement during heavy exercise is not significantly increased in adults. Thus, amounts of protein sufficient to meet the body's ordinary

---

*10% of 3000 kcal = 300 kcal, and 15% = 450 kcal. One gram of protein contains 4 kcal. Therefore, 300/4 = 75 g, and 450/4 = 112 g of protein.

demands will also be sufficient during periods of increased physical activity—even during heavy weight training involving increases in muscle mass.

Note that since the protein requirement is estimated on a body-weight basis, it provides for greater protein intake with increases in muscle mass. For example, an active male football player who weighs 115 kg (253 lb) would have a daily protein requirement of 115 g. If his daily caloric requirement were 5000 kcal, a well balanced diet containing 10 to 15% of its calories in the form of protein would provide him with between 138 and 187 g of protein. He would easily meet his requirement.

> The consumption of excessive quantities of protein, particularly in the forms of pills and powders, during athletic training is neither required nor recommended. In fact, it may be contraindicated in many sports since a large protein diet may cause dehydration and constipation.

Some natural foods that are rich sources of fats, carbohydrates, and proteins are listed in Table 10-1.

Vitamins and Minerals

Most **vitamins** serve as essential parts of enzymes or coenzymes that are vital to the metabolism of fats and carbohydrates. Thus, although vitamins do not in themselves yield energy, they are essential to life (i.e., they are nutrients).

Vitamins are classified as **water-soluble** or **fat-soluble**. The water-soluble vitamins are vitamin C (ascorbic acid) and the B-complex vitamins. These are not stored in the body and therefore must be constantly supplied in the diet. Since they are not stored, when taken in excess (above that required), they will

Table 10-1: Natural Foods in Each of the Energy Nutrient Categories

Fat	Carbohydrate	Protein
Bacon	Baked beans	Cereal
Butter	Bread	Cheese
Margarine	Cakes	Eggs
Nuts	Cereals	Fish
Peanut Butter	Dried fruits	Lean meat
Pork	Fresh fruits	Liver
Salad Oils	Honey	Milk
	Pastries	Nuts
	Potatoes	Poultry
	Syrup	Soya beans
	Vegetables	Yeast (brewers)
		Vegetables (legumes)

be passed in the urine. The fat-soluble vitamins, A, D, E, and K, are stored in the body, principally in the liver but also in fatty tissue. While this means that these vitamins need not be supplied each day, it also means that excessive accumulations can cause toxic effects.

A deficiency of vitamins can lead to serious illness, chronic disease, and even death. However, deficiencies, particularly in the United States, are very rare. The minimum daily requirements of vitamins are small and can be easily met through a varied diet. Although most fats, carbohydrates, and protein foods contain vitamins, the richest sources are green leafy vegetables (see Table 10-2).

Table 10-2: Vitamin Sources and Principal Functions

Fat-Soluble Vitamins

Vitamins	Functions	Food Source
Vitamin A (Includes Pro-vitamin A)	Vision, resistance to infection, maintenance of healthy skin and mucous membranes	Liver, egg yolk, milk, butter, green* and yellow† vegetables, fortified margarine
Vitamin D (the "sunshine vitamin")	Facilitates absorption of calcium and phosphorus for building and maintaining bones and teeth	Cod liver oil, fish, eggs, fortified dairy products, produced in the skin following exposure to sunlight by ultraviolet radiation
Vitamin E (Tocopherol)	Prevents oxidation of essential vitamins and fatty acids (an antioxidant)	Vegetable oils, green vegetables, nuts, wheat germ, margarine, shortening, cereals
Vitamin K	Blood-clotting mechanism	Green vegetables, small amounts in cereal, fruits, meats

Water-Soluble Vitamins

B-Complex Vitamins		
Thiamine (B₁)	Carbohydrate utilization, energy metabolism, formation of niacin	Meat, whole-grain cereals, milk, wheat germ, nuts
Riboflavin (B₂)	Energy metabolism	Milk, fish, eggs, meat, green vegetables, cheese, whole-grain cereals, enriched bread
Niacin (Nicotinic acid, niacinamide, B₃)	Energy metabolism, fatty acid synthesis	Peanut butter, whole-grain cereals, greens, meat, poultry, fish, liver, nuts, enriched bread and cereals
Pyridoxine (B₆)	Protein metabolism, hemoglobin synthesis, production of energy from glycogen	Whole-grain cereals, bananas, meat, spinach, cabbage, lima beans, organ meats, fish
Folic Acid (Folacin)	Red and white-cell production, growth	Green vegetables, mushrooms, liver, whole-wheat products, nuts

Table 10-2: Vitamin Sources and Principal Functions *(continued)*

Fat-Soluble Vitamins

Vitamins	Functions	Food Source
Cyanocobalamin (B$_{12}$)	Blood-cell production, energy metabolism, central nervous system function	Liver, kidney, milk, saltwater fish, lean meat, oysters Primarily from animal food sources
Pantothenic Acid	Hemoglobin formation, fat metabolism	Whole-grain cereals, organ meats
Biotin (Vitamin H)	Carbohydrate energy metabolism, fat and protein metabolism, functional relationship with pantothenic acid may produce a growth factor	Cereal, nuts, legumes, meats, egg yolk, milk
Vitamin C (Ascorbic acid)	Formation and maintenance of teeth, bones, and capillary support tissue; wound healing; vitamin metabolism	Citrus fruits, tomatoes, strawberries, potatoes, papaya, broccoli, cabbage, peppers

*Green leafy vegetables include spinach, kale, broccoli, chard, turnip greens, mustard greens, Brussels sprouts, and lettuce.

†Yellow vegetables and fruits include carrots, squash, rutabagas, sweet potatoes, pumpkin, apricots, cantaloupes, and corn.

(Adapted from Roundtable: Nutrition in everyday practice. *Patient Care, 12(4)*:76, 1978 [Feb. 28].)

Minerals are inorganic compounds found in trace amounts in the body and are also important to proper bodily function. Calcium, phosphorus, potassium, sodium, iron, and iodine are a few of the more important required minerals. Mineral deficiencies are generally uncommon today in the United States.

Although iodine is artificially added to common table salt ("iodized" salt is the result), most minerals occur naturally in a large variety of foods. For example, milk is rich in calcium, as are other dairy products, and in potassium, as are dried fruits and wheat germ. Most animal protein foods are good sources of phosphorus, and lean meats, particularly liver, provide enough iron to meet most requirements (iron supplements are discussed below). Common table salt supplies us with sodium. Rich food sources and the functions of some important minerals are contained in Table 10-3.

Use of Vitamin and Mineral Supplements by Athletes

With respect to exercise, there does not appear to be an excessive demand for most vitamins or minerals during periods of increased physical activity. The one exception might be the requirement for **iron**, which is found in red blood cells and is responsible for the oxygen-carrying ability of the blood.

Table 10-3: Important Minerals—Their Sources, and Principal Functions

Mineral	Function	Food Source
Calcium	Required with phosphorus for the formation of teeth and bones; assists in muscle contraction, nerve conduction, blood coagulation	Milk, yogurt, cheese, egg yolk, soybeans, leafy green vegetables,* bone meal, dolomite
Phosphorus	Required for the formation of teeth and bones; also plays an important part in muscle, carbohydrate and fat metabolism	Meat, fish, poultry, eggs, cereal grains, liver, wheat germ
Iron	Necessary component of hemoglobin and as such plays an essential role in oxygen transport and cellular respiration	Liver, heart, kidney, egg yolk, dried beans, nuts, green leafy vegetables, blackstrap molasses, red meat, prune juice, wheat germ, enriched bread and cereals
Copper	Required in many enzyme systems; believed to promote iron absorption and stimulate the synthesis of iron to hemoglobin; helps form nerve-sheath material	Beef liver, nuts, dried beans, whole grains, mushrooms, avocado
Iodine	Essential for the formation of thyroid hormone which regulates body metabolism	Sea foods, marine plants, iodized salt
Zinc	Component of several enzymes which are required for vital metabolic reactions, helps maintain adequate levels of vitamin A in blood, assists in healing burns and surgical wounds	Fish, oatmeal, bran, wheat germ, yeast, liver, herring, eggs, nuts, green leafy vegetables
Magnesium	Required for many enzyme systems; cardiac and skeletal muscle depend on a proper balance of calcium and magnesium for normal function	Nuts, whole wheat, wheat germ, dried beans, dolomite, soybeans, green leafy vegetables
Sodium	Plays an important role in the regulation of the acid-base balance in the body fluids	Table salt, most foods
Potassium	Influences the contractility of smooth, skeletal, and cardiac muscle and profoundly affects the excitability of nerve tissue	Yellow† and green leafy vegetables, citrus fruits, meat, fish, watermelon
Chromium	Facilitates the action of insulin in normalizing blood sugar levels	Fats, vegetable oils, brewer's yeast, calves liver, wheat germ

Table 10-3: Important Minerals—Their Sources, and Principal Functions *(continued)*

Mineral	Function	Food Source
Manganese	Essential to enzymes involved in fat mobilization	Whole wheat flour, dry beans and peas, oatmeal
Fluorine	Formation of teeth and bones, important in maintenance of normal bone structure, protects teeth from dental caries (decay)	Drinking water, tea, seafood

*Green leafy vegetables include: spinach, kale, broccoli, chard, turnip greens, mustard greens, Brussels sprouts, and lettuce.

†Yellow fruits and vegetables include: carrots, squash, rutabagas, sweet potatoes, pumpkins, corn, apricots, cantaloupe, bananas, oranges.

Levels of iron in the blood of women have been found to be significantly decreased after heavy physical training; thus, female athletes, especially those who have heavy menstrual blood losses, may wish to consider supplementing their diets with extra iron. A note of caution is needed: overdoses of iron can be toxic. Therefore, the athlete contemplating taking iron supplements should first consult a physician.

With respect to iron deficiency and oral iron supplementation in women athletes, the following conclusion from a study conducted by Pate, Maguire, and Van Wyk (1979) is appropriate:

"We conclude that there is no basis for recommending that all women athletes routinely ingest oral iron supplements for prophylactic purposes. However, certain individual athletes (those who are iron deficient and/or anemic) may require dietary iron supplementation. We recommend that coaches, trainers, and team physicians maintain a constant awareness that a significant percentage of women are iron deficient and consequently are at increased risk of developing anemia. We suggest that tests of Hb and iron storage be included in the medical screening of women athletes and that such tests be repeated whenever an athlete experiences an unexplained drop-off in endurance performance."

Use of vitamin and mineral supplements is fairly common among athletes (as well as the general population). For example, it has been reported that 85% of the Olympic athletes use vitamin and mineral supplements. Although some of these athletes have indicated that the supplements have improved their performances, little scientific evidence is available to support their contentions. Furthermore, those authorities who recommend vitamin supplements for athletes usually do so only on theoretical grounds (the value of extra vitamins is inferred from the fact that meeting the basic vitamin requirement is essential to life).

It may be concluded that supplementing the diet with amounts of vitamins and minerals above the minimum daily requirements does not increase physical performance. Furthermore, the minimum daily requirements are easily met through a varied, normal diet.

Water

Of all the nutrients, water is probably the most essential for human life. For example, water makes up about 50 to 55% of our total body weight, 72% of our muscle weight, and 80% of our blood is water. While we can go without food for several months, we can survive only a matter of days without water. Water is important in the regulation of body temperature and it is the medium in which all the body processes occur (e.g., metabolic chemical reactions, exchange of oxygen and carbon dioxide, and so on).

The greatest sources of water intake are from drinking water and the water contained in beverages and soups. However, several food sources also contribute large quantities of water. For example, watermelon, broccoli, carrots, oranges, pineapple, potatoes, green beans, pickles, celery, and lettuce are more than 80% water.

As will be mentioned in Chapter 12, dehydration or the loss of body water is a serious problem that can lead to death. This is particularly true during exercise in hot, humid environments when large amounts of body water in the form of sweat are lost. The drinking of water under these conditions is mandatory.

Food Requirements

Food requirements are dependent upon two major factors: (1) nutritional needs; and (2) caloric needs.

Nutritional Needs

No one nutrient should supply 100% of the caloric intake. Of the total calories taken in, a certain proportion should be derived from each of the three food nutrients discussed earlier:

Protein: 10–15%
Fat: 25–30%
Carbohydrates: 55–60%

An athlete whose daily caloric requirement is 5000 kcal should thus obtain 500 to 750 kcal from proteins, 1250 to 1500 kcal from fats, and 2750 to 3000 kcal from carbohydrates. In terms of grams rather than calories, this would be 125 to 188 g of protein, 139 to 167 g of fat, and 688 to 750 g of carbohydrates.

For most individuals, athletic or otherwise, apportioning the diet along the lines given here should, under most circumstances, supply adequate amounts of the energy nutrients plus needed vitamins and minerals.

Caloric Needs

As mentioned earlier, the calories taken in as food should be approximately equal to the caloric expenditure resulting from body maintenance and physical activities. Thus, if you expend 3000 kcal daily, then you should take in 3000 kcal per day. Your body weight will, of course, remain constant. An athlete may expend 5000 or even 7000 kcal per day during heavy training and competition. Replacing these calories requires a caloric intake of the same magnitude if the body weight is to be maintained. Caloric imbalance such as required for gaining or losing weight is discussed in the next chapter.

Eating Habits

Good eating habits entail knowing how to select foods and how many meals to eat per day. It is most common to select specific foods from the following four food groups (see Fig. 10-1).

Milk and cheese
Meat and high-protein foods
Fruits and vegetables
Bread and cereals

Selection of foods from these four basic food groups will ensure a well balanced diet from a nutritional standpoint. Table 10-4 gives examples of specific foods in the food groups, their minimum daily amounts, and their main nutritional contribution. Table 10-5 provides examples of a basic five-meal diet, and a three-meal diet. Notice that the diets contain only 1200 to 1400 kcal—not nearly enough for the athlete. However, the old saying "First eat what you need and then eat what you want" is applicable here. What you need nutritionally is contained in these basic diets.

Ordinarily, three meals per day satisfy the normal caloric requirements of the nonathlete. However, since the caloric requirements of athletes are frequently doubled during periods of heavy physical activity, it is recommended that under these circumstances athletes eat five to six meals per day. An example of an eating schedule for an athlete with a 6000-kcal requirement might look like this:

	kcal %	total kcal
Breakfast	11.1	670
Snack	8.2	490
Lunch	25.2	1510
Snack	11.0	660
Dinner	27.0	1620
Snack	17.5	1050
Totals	100.0	6000

A sample 6000-kcal diet is given in Table 10-6.

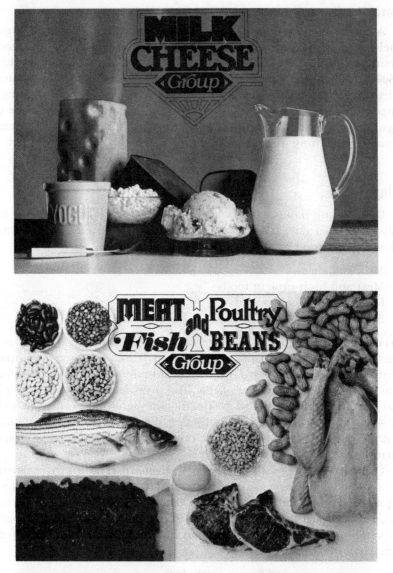

Figure 10-1 The four food groups: milk and cheese; meat and high-protein foods; fruits and vegetables; and bread and cereals. (From Food. *Home and Garden Bulletin, 228*. Prepared by the Science and Education Administration, U.S. Department of Agriculture, 1979.)

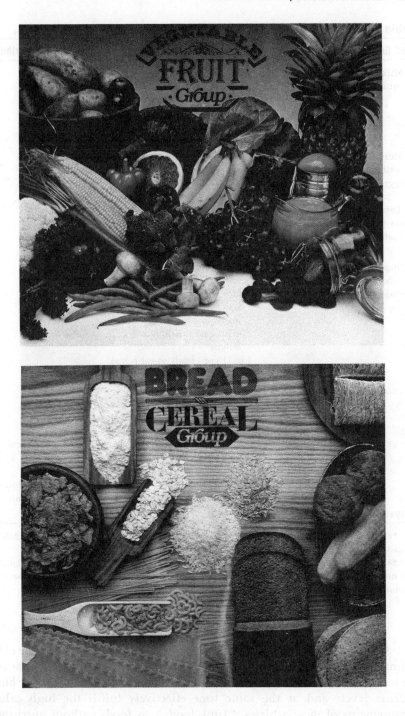

Table 10-4: Daily Food Guide for the Four Basic Food Groups*

Food Group	Daily Amounts	Main Contribution
1. Milk and cheese or equivalents†	Children under 9: 2 to 3 cups Children 9 to 12: 3 or more cups Teenagers: 4 or more cups Adults: 2 or more cups Pregnancy: 3 or more cups Lactation: 4 or more cups	Calcium Protein Riboflavin Vitamin D
2. Meat: Beef, veal, pork, lamb, poultry, fish, eggs Alternates: Dry beans, dry peas, lentils, nuts, peanut butter	2 or more servings Serving size: 2 to 3 oz lean, boneless cooked meat, poultry, fish 2 eggs 1 cup cooked dry beans, dry peas or lentils 4 tbsp peanut butter	Protein Thiamin Iron Niacin Riboflavin
3. Bread and cereals (whole-grain or enriched)	4 or more servings Serving size: 1 slice bread 1/2 to 3/4 cup cooked cereal, macaroni, spaghetti, hominy grits, kasha, rice, noodles, bulgur 1 oz (1 cup) ready-to-eat cereal 5 saltines or 2 Graham crackers	Thiamin Riboflavin Niacin Iron Protein
4. Vegetables and fruits	4 or more servings Serving size: 1/2 cup dark green or deep yellow every other day 1/2 cup or 1 medium citrus fruit (or any raw fruit or vegetable rich in ascorbic acid) Other vegetables and fruit including potato (1 medium)	Vitamin A Ascorbic acid Other vitamins and minerals
Water	6 to 8 glasses	

*From Krause, M., and Hunscher, M.: *Food, Nutrition and Diet Therapy.* 5th ed. Philadelphia, W. B. Saunders, 1972.

†Milk equivalents: 1 cup whole or skimmed milk, 1 cup buttermilk, ½ cup evaporated milk, ¼ cup non-fat milk powder, 1 oz cheddar cheese, 2 cups ice cream, 1½ cups cottage cheese. (The amount given is figured on the basis of calcium content.)

A word about snacks is appropriate here. Snacking is perhaps one of the primary causes of obesity. However, "nutritive" snacking—that is, snacking on foods of nutritional value—can aid in the maintenance of proper blood glucose levels and at the same time effectively fulfill the high caloric requirements of most athletes. "Junk foods," as foods without nutritional value are called, should be completely eliminated from the diet.

Table 10-5: Examples of Basic Diets in Three and Five Meals*

5 Meals	3 Meals
Breakfast	**Breakfast**

1/2 grapefruit
2/3 cup bran flakes
  1 cup skim or low-fat milk
    or other beverage
	1/2 cup orange juice
	  1 soft-boiled or poached
	    egg
	  1 slice whole wheat toast
	1-1/2 teasp margarine
	  1 cup skim or low-fat milk
	    or other beverage

Snack	
1 small package raisins 1/2 bologna sandwich	
Lunch	**Lunch**

1 slice pizza
1 serving of carrot sticks
1 apple
1 cup skim or low-fat milk
	1-1/2 cup Manhattan clam
	    chowder
	2 rye wafers
	1/2 cup cottage cheese
	    (uncreamed)
	1 medium bunch grapes or
	1 medium apple
	1 granola cookie

Snack	
2 oatmeal cookies	
Dinner	**Dinner**

1 baked fish with mushroom (3 oz)
1 baked potato
2 teasp margarine
1/2 cup broccoli
  1 cup tomato juice or skim or low-
    fat milk
 	
Total calories: about 1400
	1 helping of oven-barbe-
	    cued chicken (3 oz, no
	    bone)
	1/2 cup green beans
	1/2 cup cabbage and carrot
	    salad
	2/3 cup mashed potato
	1/2 cup applesauce
	  1 cup skim or low-fat milk
	    or other beverage
	
	Total calories: about 1200

*From Smith, N. J.: *Food for Sport*. Palo Alto, CA, Bull Publishing Co., 1976.

Diet and Performance

The foods the athlete eats are important because: (1) the ordinary diet can impose definite limits on performance; (2) manipulation of the diet can improve performance (specifically, manipulation involving muscle glycogen loading); and (3) the diet immediately before and during an event can be so arranged and so constituted as to help the athlete's performance.

Effects of Diet on Performance

As discussed in Chapter 4, glycogen is a preferred fuel during exercise. This is true for both short-term (sprint) exercises and long-term (endurance)

Table 10-6: Example of a High-Calorie (6000-kcal) Diet in Six Meals*

Breakfast

1/2 cup orange juice
1 cup oatmeal
1 cup low-fat milk
1 scrambled egg
1 slice whole wheat toast
1-1/2 teasp margarine
1 tbs jam

Total kilocalories: 665

Lunch

5 fish sticks with tartar sauce
1 large serving, French fries
1 bowl of green salad with avo-
   cado and French dressing
1 cup lemon sherbet
2 granola cookies
1 cup low-fat milk

Total kilocalories: 1505

Dinner

1 cup cream of mushroom soup
2 pieces oven-baked chicken
1 candied sweet potato
1 dinner roll and margarine
1 cup carrots and peas
1/2 cup coleslaw
1 piece cherry pie
1 beverage

Total kilocalories: 1615

Snack

1 peanut butter sandwich
1 banana
1 cup grape juice

Total kilocalories: 485

Snack

1 cup mixed dried fruit
1-1/2 cup malted milk

Total kilocalories: 660

Snack

1 cup cashew nuts
1 cup cocoa

Total kilocalories: 1045

Daily total kilocalories: 5975

*From Smith, N. J.: *Food for Sport.* Palo Alto, CA, Bull Publishing Co., 1976.

exercises. However, because glycogen stores are not wholly depleted during short-term exercise, the magnitude of the stores does not limit sprint performance. Figure 10-2A shows that although the muscle glycogen stores decrease during repeated bouts of sprint performance, they are not depleted even after the muscles reach exhaustion. It is the performance of endurance exercise that is profoundly affected by the magnitude of glycogen stores. Figure 10-2B shows that the muscle glycogen stores are virtually depleted after 3 hr or so of exhaustive endurance exercise. You will recall that in this case lack of glycogen is a major cause of muscular exhaustion.

Role of Muscle Glycogen in Endurance Performance

The fact that the magnitude of glycogen stores can affect performance (of endurance tasks, at least) has caused many athletes, coaches, and researchers to wonder if increased amounts of stored glycogen in the muscles would be

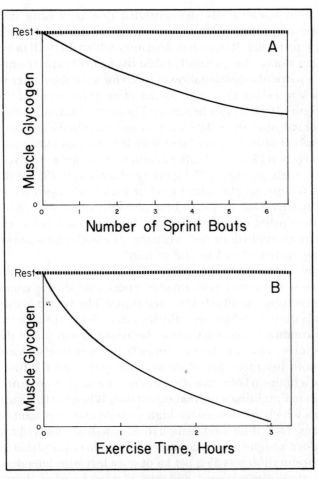

Figure 10-2 A, Muscle glycogen depletion during sprint exercise and B, endurance exercise. The glycogen stores are by no means used up following repeated sprint bouts to exhaustion. The depletion that occurs is not, therefore, a limiting factor in this kind of performance. During exhaustive endurance exercise, though, glycogen depletion is a limiting factor.

advantageous to performers. It appears from current research, which, it must be emphasized, is not complete, that increased glycogen storage is indeed helpful, at least to endurance athletes. Some researchers have suggested that more glycogen might also help performers in sprint events provided the sprinter must compete in several different sprint events in one meet and run in several races, or heats, to qualify for finals. Under these conditions, muscle glycogen could be substantially lowered. However, research as yet has not supported this idea. Methods of increasing the muscles' stores of glycogen and the effects of these methods are detailed below.

It has been scientifically demonstrated that increasing the stores of muscle glycogen by means of dietary manipulation can significantly improve endurance performance. Research to determine which diet will provide for the most glycogen storage has generally taken the form of experiments in which subjects eat a particular combination of foods for a few days, after which they perform work to exhaustion. The results of an experiment of this sort are shown in Figure 10–3. As can be seen in Figure 10–3A, not all diets increase glycogen storage: after three days on a fat and protein diet, subjects showed glycogen levels of only 6.3 g per kg of muscle (vastus lateralis); after a mixed diet, the average was 17.5 g. Only after a carbohydrate diet were glycogen levels exceptionally high, averaging 33.1 g per kg of muscle. In Figure 10–3B it can be seen that the greater the initial level of muscle glycogen the greater the endurance capacity. One subject, whose glycogen stores were only 5.8 g after the fat and protein diet, could cycle for only 1 hr and 15 min before exhaustion. However, after a carbohydrate diet, when the muscle glycogen level was 46.8 g, the work time increased to 4 hr and 45 min!

The above experiment was conducted in a laboratory. What about actual competition—is endurance performance under competitive conditions enhanced by increasing the muscle glycogen stores? The answer to this question is "yes." In a study in which ten athletes ran a 30-km (19-mile) race under competitive conditions on two separate occasions, it was found that a high-carbohydrate diet—one that increased muscle glycogen levels—was helpful to runners in both instances. Six of the runners performed the first race after maintaining a high-carbohydrate diet, whereas the other four runners ran the first race after maintaining a normal mixed diet. When the first race was over, those runners who had followed the high-carbohydrate diet went on a mixed diet for the next race (three weeks later); those who first followed a mixed diet next maintained a high-carbohydrate diet. Researchers found that the average glycogen concentration was 35 g per kg of muscle (vastus lateralis) when the high-carbohydrate diet was used, and only 17 g per kg when the normal diet was employed. In all ten runners, the best performances (shortest times) were attained when they had followed the high-carbohydrate diet (average time, mixed diet = 2 hr, 23 min; average time, carbohydrate diet = 2 hr, 15 min, 18 sec). Further analysis of the performance times showed that the enhanced muscle glycogen stores did not have a direct effect on the speed that runners could maintain at the beginning of the race. This finding is illustrated in Figure 10–4 for one of the runners. The "time loss" on the vertical axis represents the differences in minutes between the pace maintained during the race for which the mixed diet had been followed and that maintained when the high-carbohydrate diet had been followed. Notice that during both races the pace was the same during the first 12 to 16 km. However, the pace decreased considerably at about 18 km during the race for which the runner had followed a mixed diet. It was calculated that the muscle glycogen concentration at this time was equal to or less than 3 g/kg. Apparently, an optimal pace cannot be maintained with a muscle glycogen content of or below 3 g/kg.

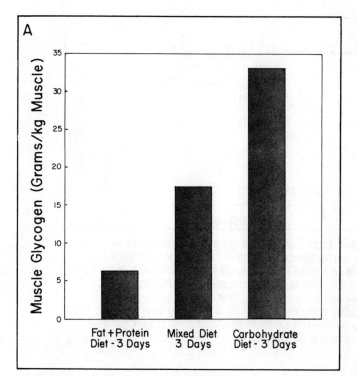

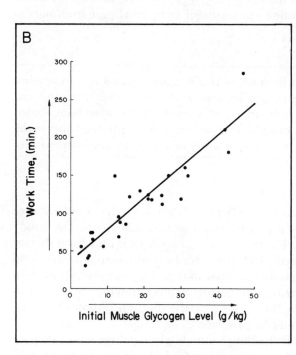

Figure 10-3 A, Effects of diet on the level of glycogen in muscle, and B, the effect of muscle glycogen level on endurance performance. The glycogen levels graphed in A are averages: 6.3 g of glycogen per kg of muscle after a high-fat, high-protein diet lasting 3 days; 17.5 g per kg after a mixed (normal) diet lasting 3 days; 33.1 g per kg after a high-carbohydrate diet lasting 3 days. The significance of the amount of glycogen present in muscle is evident in B: the greater the initial muscle glycogen level, the greater the endurance capacity. (Based on data from Bergström and co-workers, 1967.)

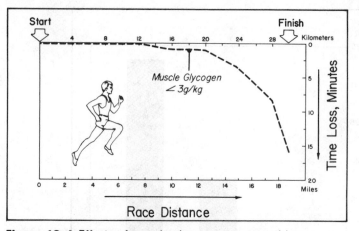

Figure 10-4 Effects of muscle glycogen on competitive endurance performance. The fall-off in the runner's pace is attributable to a drop in the muscle glycogen level to less than 3 g per kg. If the athlete is to maintain an optimal pace during competitive endurance performance, muscle glycogen levels must be sufficiently elevated (e.g., by diet) to provide more than the 3 g/kg concentration *from start to finish*. (Based on data from Karlsson and Saltin, 1971.)

Thus, a high initial level of muscle glycogen is important because it enables the athlete (in this case a runner) to maintain an optimal pace from start to finish.

In summary, it has been scientifically demonstrated that increasing the stores of muscle glycogen by means of dietary manipulation can significantly improve endurance performance. It has also been shown that such enhancement of endurance performance applies not only to the laboratory setting, but most importantly to actual athletic competition.

Muscle Glycogen Loading

Now that we know that increased stores of muscle glycogen can improve endurance performance, we must turn to procedures that are used to "load" the muscles with glycogen. The first of these procedures is the simple dietary manipulation just described. In other words, endurance athletes who consume a high-carbohydrate diet for three or four days after several days on a normal mixed diet may increase their glycogen stores from the normal 15 g to around 25 g per kg of muscle. During the period of the high-carbohydrate diet, no exhausting exercise should be performed.

A second procedure for "loading" muscle glycogen combines exercise and diet. In this procedure, the muscles that are to be loaded are first exhausted of their glycogen stores through exercise; the athlete then follows a high-carbohydrate diet for a few days. This routine has been shown to double the glycogen stores. An example of this effect is shown in Figure 10-5. Again, no exhausting exercise should be performed during the time period of the high-carbohydrate diet.

A third procedure for glycogen loading calls for exercise and two special diets. Exercise is once again used to induce glycogen depletion. The athlete then follows a diet very low in carbohyrates but high in fat and protein for three days, after which a high-carbohydrate diet is followed for an additional three days. Exhausting exercise may be performed during the period of the diet that is high in fat and protein but not during the high-carbohydrate diet. This procedure has been shown to increase the glycogen stores (in the depleted muscles) to levels approaching 50 g/kg. Examples of high- and low-carbohydrate diets, suitable for this procedure and, as needed, for the others, are given in Table 10-7.

A degree of caution should be observed whenever glycogen loading is attempted. Of the procedures described above, the third is most difficult to follow, particularly on a weekly basis. In addition, this procedure, in which exercise-induced depletion of glycogen is followed by a fat and protein diet, causes a feeling of fatigue. Therefore, for weekly competitions either of the other two procedures is suggested; the more difficult method of glycogen loading might be reserved for more important competition such as conference championships.

Whatever the procedure used, glycogen loading results in an increased muscular storage of water. A feeling of stiffness and heaviness is thus often associated with loading of the muscle. For example, increasing the glycogen

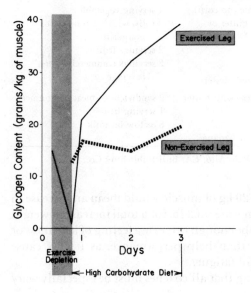

Figure 10-5 The amount of muscle glycogen stored can be increased by first depleting the muscle of its glycogen through exercise, then for three days thereafter, consuming a high carbohydrate diet. (Based on data from Bergström and Hultman, 1966.)

Table 10-7: Examples of Diets Suitable for Muscle Glycogen Loading*

	Low-Carbohydrate Diet	High-Carbohydrate Diet
	Daily Amounts	

Food Groups

Meats	20–25 oz	8 oz
Breads and cereals	4 servings	10–16 servings
Vegetables	3–4 servings	3–4 servings
Fruits	4 servings	10 servings
Fats	8–9 oz	4–6 oz
Desserts	1–2 servings (only fruits and un- sweetened gelatins)	2 servings (include ice cream, cookies, etc.)
Beverages	Unlimited (no sugar)	Unlimited (assuming proper calorie control)

	Sample Meal Plans	

Meals

Breakfast	8 oz unsweetened orange juice 4 eggs 1 slice toast 4 tsp butter or margarine 4 strips bacon	8 oz orange juice (O.K. sweetened) 1 egg 2 slices toast 2 tsp butter or margarine 1 cup cereal
Lunch	1 meat sandwich (with butter or margarine and mayonnaise) 2–3 cheese sticks 1 tossed salad with oil dressing 1 medium apple or orange	2 sandwiches—each with 1 oz meat or cheese, 1/2 tsp butter or margarine 8 oz low-fat milk 2 large bananas
Dinner	10 oz meat (not ham) 1 small baked potato, with 2–3 tsp butter or margarine and 1 tbsp sour cream 1 serving vegetable (no corn), with 1–2 tsp butter or margarine 1 tossed salad 1 small apple 1 commercial "diet" dessert	4 oz meat (not ham) 1 medium baked potato, with 1 tsp butter or margarine and 1 tbsp sour cream 1 serving vegetable 2 rolls, with 1 tsp butter or margarine 2 servings fruit 2 servings commercial "diet" beverage
Snack(s)	2 meat sandwiches (with butter or margarine) 1 cheese stick 1 medium apple or banana	2 sandwiches—meat or nonmeat 1 serving fruit 8 oz low-fat milk

*From Smith, N. J.: *Food for Sport.* Palo Alto, CA, Bull Publishing Co., 1976.

stores from 15 g/kg to 40 g/kg in 20 kg of muscle would mean an increase in glycogen of 1 lb, and an increase in water of 3 lb, for a total increase in weight of 4 lb. For some athletes, this may be enough to create a feeling of heaviness or stiffness that may hinder rather than help performance, as it may cause muscular cramping and premature fatigue.

One aspect of glycogen loading that all coaches must be especially wary of is the possibility of harmful side effects. There have been some clinical reports of myoglobinuria (myoglobin in the urine) in athletes who persistently use glycogen loading, and chest pain and electrocardiographic changes similar to those observed in patients with heart disease have been described as well. These side effects are potentially very serious (myoglobinuria may lead to acute kidney failure); if encountered, the athlete should seek medical help immediately.

A summary of the glycogen loading procedures is shown in Figure 10-6.

Role of Fat in Glycogen Sparing

One other point concerning endurance exercise and diet needs mentioning. You will recall that fat is an important fuel during the performance of endurance exercise. The effect of diet on the muscular storage and usage of fats during endurance exercise has not been extensively researched. However, a few studies of fat usage in relation to glycogen usage have been conducted recently, with interesting results. For example, in one study, seven men were analyzed during 30 min of treadmill exercise to determine the effects of increased availability of blood-borne free fatty acids (FFA) on the utilization of muscle glycogen. The free fatty acids were made available by first having the subjects consume a "fatty" meal 4½ to 5 hr before the exercise was to begin. Then, 30 min prior to exercise, heparin, an anticoagulant, was injected into a

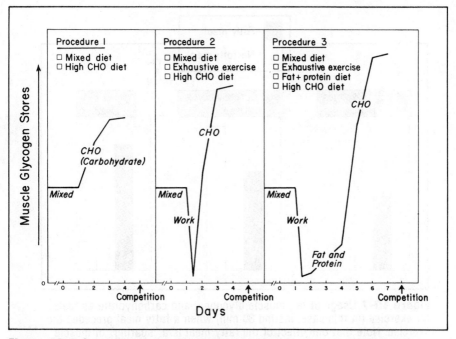

Figure 10-6 Summary of muscle glycogen loading procedures. (Modified and redrawn from Saltin and Hermansen, 1967.)

vein in the forearm to promote the breakdown of the blood triglycerides, thus elevating the free fatty acids. The results are shown in Figure 10-7. As you can see, more fat and less muscle glycogen and carbohydrate were used when a fatty meal preceded the 30-min exercise period than when no fatty meal was consumed.

The above results suggest that since muscle glycogen is "spared" when free fatty acids are available, fatigue will be delayed and endurance prolonged. Direct confirmation of this idea has been obtained, but in studies of rats only.

It is extremely important to emphasize that use of the experimental dietary regimen just described is not advised, because: (1) heparin is involved (and, in fact, must be injected); (2) large "fatty" meals prior to competition might cause considerable gastrointestinal discomfort; and (3) consumption of excessive amounts of fat has been shown to be linked to cardiovascular diseases. Therefore, dietary manipulations involving large intakes of fat must be proved safe and effective by further research before their general use is allowed.

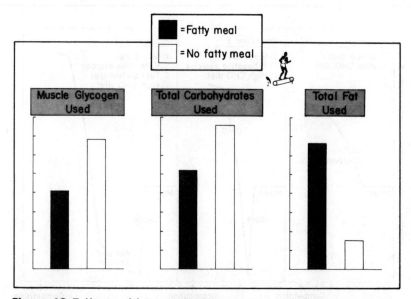

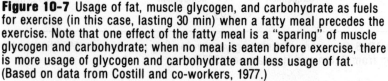

Figure 10-7 Usage of fat, muscle glycogen, and carbohydrate as fuels for exercise (in this case, lasting 30 min) when a fatty meal precedes the exercise. Note that one effect of the fatty meal is a "sparing" of muscle glycogen and carbohydrate; when no meal is eaten before exercise, there is more usage of glycogen and carbohydrate and less usage of fat. (Based on data from Costill and co-workers, 1977.)

The Pregame Meal

From what has already been stated, you should realize that there are no foods that, when taken several hours prior to physical activity, will lead to "super" performances. Proper nutrition, as emphasized throughout, is a year-round task.

There are certain foods, however, that should probably be avoided on the day of competition. For example, fats and meats are generally digested slowly. If consumed within 4 hr of an athletic event (or less), they may cause a feeling of fullness, hindering performance. Other food categories to avoid might include gas-forming foods, "greasy" foods, and highly seasoned foods.

Carbohydrates should be the major constituent of the pregame meal and should be consumed no later than 2½ hr before competition. Carbohydrates are easily digested and help maintain the blood glucose levels (the latter effect makes one "feel" better). The pregame meal can also include moderate portions of such foods as fruits, cooked vegetables, gelatin desserts, and fish (or lean meats, provided the advice given above is heeded).

Consumption of large amounts of glucose (sugar), particularly in liquid or pill form, less than an hour before exercise is not recommended. In one recent study, it was found that insulin production was stimulated by the consumption of 75 g of sugar 45 min before the start of a half-hour bout of exercise, with the result that the availability of blood-borne glucose during the exercise was actually reduced. In turn, greater dependence was placed on muscle glycogen for energy during the exercise.

Provided their sugar concentration is not excessive, liquids may be imbibed up to 30 min before physical activity without hindering performance. Water is perhaps the best liquid, but fruit and vegetable juices are suitable, as are uncarbonated fruit-flavored drinks.

An increasingly popular pregame meal with both coaches and athletes is the liquid meal. There are several liquid formulas commercially available today that can serve as excellent pregame meals (e.g., Ensure, Ensure Plus, Nutriment, Sustagen, and SustaCal). Available in a variety of flavors to suit most tastes, liquid meals are well balanced nutritionally (most contain large amounts of carbohydrate plus fat and protein). Besides being palatable and nutritious, liquid meals are easily digested and are emptied quickly from the stomach. As both "liquid" and "meals," they contribute to hydration and to energy intake. There are subjective effects as well: the athlete drinking a liquid meal will have a feeling of satiety and relief from hunger. At the very least, the occasional unpleasant sensations associated with pregame meals (nervous indigestion, diarrhea, nausea, vomiting, and abdominal cramps) are minimized when liquid meals are used.

In using the liquid pregame meal, it is important to remember that a period of adjustment will more than likely be needed, since, for most athletes, a liquid meal will be a new experience. Therefore, the coach should introduce the liquid meal early in the season, explaining to the athletes its nutritional advantages. Of course, any athlete who cannot (or will not) adjust to such a meal should not be forced to do so.

It should be emphasized that the pregame "menu" is not entirely based on strict "do's" and don't's." The athlete's diet on the day of competition should not be drastically different from that normally consumed (so long as it is remembered that nervousness and tension during intense competition may so affect the digestive system that the foods normally eaten without discomfort may now cause distress). Provided the athlete does not overeat or does not eat foods that will cause gastrointestinal discomfort, performance will not be affected by the foods consumed at the pregame meal.

Guidelines to follow in planning the pregame diet are given in Table 10-8.

Ingestion of Sugar (Glucose) during Exercise

It is fairly common to find that athletes, particularly endurance athletes, ingest glucose (usually in liquid form) during prolonged exercise. Does this practice improve performance? It is generally agreed that ingestion of some liquid glucose during prolonged physical exercise will help "spare" muscle glycogen and delay or prevent hypoglycemia (low blood sugar levels). Both the glycogen sparing effect and the deterrent effect on hypoglycemia should help reduce and/or delay fatigue. An analysis of muscle glycogen sparing following glucose ingestion during 4 hr of jogging is shown in Figure 10-8.

Table 10-8: Guidelines to Follow in Planning the PreGame Diet*

Energetics of the Diet

Energy intake should be adequate to ward off any feelings of hunger or weakness during the entire period of the competition. Although precontest food intakes make only a minor contribution to the immediate energy expenditure, they are essential for the support of an adequate level of blood sugar, and for avoiding the sensations of hunger and weakness.

Timing of the Diet

The diet plan should ensure that the stomach and upper bowel are empty at the time of competition.

Fluid Content of the Diet

Food and fluid intakes prior to and during prolonged competition should guarantee an optimal state of hydration.

Blandness of the Diet

The precompetition diet should offer foods that will minimize upset in the gastrointestinal tract.

Psychological Aspects of the Diet

The diet should include food that the athlete is familiar with, and is convinced will "make him win."

*Recommendations under each underscored heading are from Smith, N. J.: *Food for Sport.* Palo Alto, CA, Bull Publishing Co., 1976.

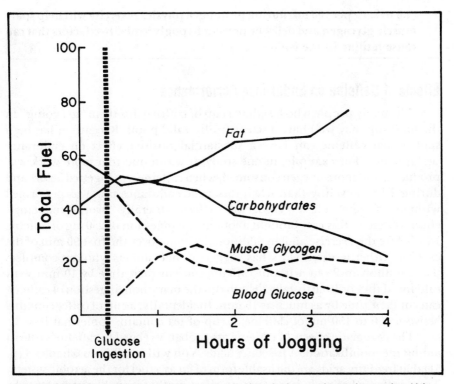

Figure 10-8 Glucose-induced glycogen sparing during prolonged exercise (4 hr of jogging). The use of muscle glycogen decreased, and that of blood glucose increased, following the ingestion of 100 g of glucose. (Based on data from Pirnay and co-workers, 1977.)

Notice how the use of muscle glycogen decreased, while that of blood glucose increased, following the ingestion of 100 g of glucose. The importance of fat as a fuel should also be noticed.

When glucose is made available to an athlete during lengthy exercise, it should be provided in low concentrations. The stomach can empty only a limited amount of glucose in a short period of time; if too much glucose is present, the rate of gastric emptying is retarded, and glucose is absorbed into the blood more slowly. Thus, ingestion of high concentrations of glucose actually delays utilization of glucose. The recommended concentration of glucose is 2.0 to 2.5 g per 100 ml of water. More will be said about liquid replacement during prolonged exercise in Chapter 12.

In summary, carbohydrates should be the major constituent of the pregame meal and should be consumed no later than 2½ hr before competition. However, consumption of large amounts of glucose or sugar, particularly in liquid or pill form, less than an hour before exercise is not recommended. Ingestion of liquid glucose in low concentrations

(2.0 to 2.5 g per 100 ml) during prolonged physical exercise will help spare muscle glycogen and delay or prevent hypoglycemia, two factors that can cause fatigue in the endurance athlete.

Effects of Caffeine on Endurance Performance

The many people who feel that a cup of coffee helps them "get going" in the morning may well have a scientifically valid point. Recently it has been shown that caffeine can have a substantial positive effect on endurance performance. For example, in one study, it was found that more work was produced, and more oxygen consumed, when caffeine was ingested before and during 2 hr of cycling than when this same endurance task was performed without caffeine. These "ergogenic" effects—literally "work-producing" effects—were in this case brought about by the ingestion of 250 mg of caffeine 1 hr before the exercise and an additional 250 mg over the first 90 min of the exercise. Other research work has suggested that runners who can complete the marathon in 2½ hr without caffeine can cut their time by 10 min with caffeine; if they ordinarily take 3½ hr to run the marathon, ingestion of caffeine can cut their time by as much as 15 min. Incidentally, a cup of coffee contains between 100 to 150 mg of caffeine; a cup of tea contains somewhat less.

The ergogenic effects of caffeine are probably related to caffeine's role in aiding the mobilization of free fatty acids. You will recall from Chapter 4 (p. 51) that free fatty acids are the usable form of fat as a fuel for the aerobic system. Thus, caffeine has a glycogen sparing effect, in that it enables more fat to be used as a fuel, with less usage of glycogen. As previously mentioned, glycogen sparing reduces muscular fatigue.

Effects of Alcohol on Sports Performance

Although it's difficult to believe, some athletes (as well as some nonathletes, for that matter) still believe that acute or short-term ingestion of small amounts of alcohol enhances athletic performance, particularly the psychological aspects of performance. Of course, nothing could be farther from the truth.

Based upon a comprehensive analysis of the available research relative to the effects of alcohol upon human physical performance, the American College of Sports Medicine draws the following conclusions:

The acute ingestion of alcohol can exert a deleterious effect upon a wide variety of psychomotor skills such as reaction time, hand-eye coordination, accuracy, balance, and complex coordination.

Acute ingestion of alcohol will not substantially influence metabolic or physiological functions essential to physical performance such as energy metabolism, maximal oxygen consumption (VO_2 max), heart rate, stroke volume, cardiac output, muscle blood flow, arteriovenous oxygen difference, or respiratory dynamics. Alcohol consumption may impair body temperature regulation during prolonged exercise in a cold environment.

Acute alcohol ingestion will not improve and may decrease strength, power, local muscular endurance, speed, and cardiovascular endurance.

Alcohol is the most abused drug in the United States and is a major contributing factor to accidents and their consequences. Also, it has been documented widely that prolonged excessive alcohol consumption can elicit pathological changes in the liver, heart, brain, and muscle, which can lead to disability and death.

Serious and continuing efforts should be made to educate athletes, coaches, health and physical educators, physicians, trainers, the sports media, and the general public regarding the effects of acute alcohol ingestion upon human physical performance and on the potential acute and chronic problems of excessive alcohol consumption.

Summary

- Good nutrition at all times is essential to effective athletic performance.

- The energy nutrient foods—proteins, carbohydrates, and fats—supply energy for ATP synthesis.

- The protein requirement of athletes, even during heavy training, is the same as that of nonathletes (1 g per kg body weight). The consumption of excessive quantities of protein, particularly in the forms of pills and powders, during athletic training is neither required nor recommended.

- Although not energy foods, vitamins and minerals are nutrients (i.e., they are essential to life). In most cases, vitamins and minerals (many of which are found in small amounts in the body) are supplied through a normal diet in sufficient quantities to ensure proper bodily function (vitamin and mineral deficiencies are uncommon).

- Consumption of vitamins and minerals in quantities above the minimum required daily dosage does not improve physical performance. The minimum daily requirements are easily met through a varied, normal diet.

- Of all the nutrients, water is the most essential for life. The greatest sources of water intake are from drinking water and the water contained in beverages and soups. Dehydration or loss of body water is a serious problem that can decrease sports performance.

- Of the total calories taken in, 10 to 15% should be derived from proteins, 25 to 30% from fats, and 55 to 60% from carbohydrates.

- While the nutritional needs of nonathletes and athletes are the same, the latter's caloric needs are usually much greater (5000 to 7000 kcal per day during heavy training).

- Foods should be selected from the four basic food groups: milk and cheese, meat and high-protein foods, fruits and vegetables, and bread and cereals.

- Because of their high caloric needs, athletes may need to eat five to six meals per day.

- It has been scientifically demonstrated that endurance performance may be significantly improved by increasing the stores of muscle glycogen.

- "Loading" the muscles with glycogen for purposes of improving endurance performance may be accomplished by means of: (1) a high-carbohydrate diet for three of four days; (2) exercise-induced glycogen depletion followed by a three-day high-carbohydrate diet; or (3) exercise-induced glycogen depletion followed first by a three-day diet high in fat and protein and then by a three-day high-carbohydrate diet.

- A feeling of stiffness and heaviness is often associated with glycogen loading because water is stored with the extra glycogen. More serious effects of persistent glycogen loading may include chest pains and myoglobinuria.

- Dietary manipulations involving large intakes of fat have not yet been proven safe and effective for use outside the laboratory.

- No known foods, when taken several hours prior to competition, will lead to "super" performances.

- Carbohydrates should be the major constituents of the pregame meal and may be consumed up to 2½ hr before competition. Liquid meals are suitable as pregame meals.

- Consumption of large amounts of glucose (sugar), particularly in liquid or pill form, less than an hour before exercise is not recommended since it promotes rather than spares muscle glycogen usage. As a result, endurance performance can be reduced.

- Since fats are digested slowly, they should be consumed no later than 3 to 4 hr prior to competition.

- It is generally agreed that ingestion of some liquid glucose during prolonged exercise will help "spare" muscle glycogen and delay or prevent hypoglycemia. The recommended concentration of glucose is 2.5 g per 100 ml of water (too much glucose retards gastric emptying).

- Caffeine increases endurance performances.

- Acute ingestion of small amounts of alcohol has a deleterious effect upon reaction time, coordination, accuracy, balance, strength, power, local muscular endurance, speed, and cardiovascular endurance.

Selected References and Readings*

American Association for Health, Physical Education, and Recreation. *Nutrition for the Athlete.* Washington, D.C.: AAHPER, 1971.

---

*For full journal titles, see Appendix A.

American College of Sports Medicine. The use of alcohol in sports. *Med. Sci. Sports Exercise,* *14(6)*:ix-xi, 1982.

Bank, W. J.: Myoglobinuria in marathon runners: Possible relationship to carbohydrate and lipid metabolism. *Ann. N.Y. Acad. Sci., 301*:942-948, 1977.

Bentivegna, A., E. J. Kelley, and A. Kalenak: Diet, fitness, and athletic performance. *Physician Sportsmed., 7(10)*:99-102, 105, 1979.

Bergström, J., and E. Hultman: Muscle glycogen synthesis after exercise: an enhancing factor localized to the muscle cells in man. *Nature, 210(5033)*:309-310, 1966.

Bergström, J., and E. Hultman: Nutrition for maximal sports performance. *J.A.M.A., 221(9)*: 999-1006, 1972.

Bergström, J., et al.: Diet, muscle glycogen and physical performance. *Acta Physiol. Scand., 71*: 140-150, 1967.

Buskirk, E. Nutrition for the athlete. *In* Ryan, A., and F. Allman (eds.): *Sports Medicine.* New York: Academic Press, 1974.

Costill, D. L. Fluids for athletic performance: Why and what you should drink during prolonged exercise. In *The New Runners Diet.* Mountain View, CA, World Publications, August, 1977.

Costill, D. L.: Performance secrets. *Runners World, 13(7)*:50-55, July, 1978.

Costill, D. L., et al.: Effects of elevated plasma FFA and insulin on muscle glycogen usage during exercise. *J. Appl. Physiol.: Respirat. Environ. Exercise Physiol., 43(4)*:695-699, 1977.

Costill, D. L., G. Dalsky, and W. Fink: Effects of caffeine ingestion on metabolism and exercise performance. *Med. Sci. Sports, 10(3)*:155-158, 1978.

Costill, D. L., and B. Saltin: Factors limiting gastric emptying during rest and exercise. *J. Appl. Physiol., 37(5)*:679-683, 1974.

Darden, E.: *Nutrition and Athletic Performance.* Pasadena, CA, The Athletic Press, 1976.

Foster, C., and D. L. Costill: Effects of preexercise feedings on endurance performance. *Med. Sci. Sports, 10(1)*:65, 1978.

Fox, E. L., and D. K. Mathews: *The Physiological Basis of Physical Education and Athletics,* 3rd ed. Philadelphia, Saunders College Publishing, 1981.

Hickson, R. C., et al.: Effects of increased plasma fatty acids on glycogen utilization and endurance. *J. Appl. Physiol.: Respirat. Environ. Exercise Physiol., 43*:829-833, 1977.

Ivy, J. L., et al.: Role of caffeine and glucose ingestion on metabolism during exercise. *Med. Sci. Sports, 10(1)*:66, 1978.

Karlsson, J., and B. Saltin: Diet, muscle glycogen and endurance performance. *J. Appl. Physiol., 31(2)*:203-206, 1971.

Krause, M., and M. Hunscher: *Food, Nutrition and Diet Therapy.* 6th ed. Philadelphia, W. B. Saunders, 1979.

Mirkin, G.: Carbohydrate loading: A dangerous practice. *J.A.M.A., 223(13)*:1511-1512, 1973.

Oscai, L., et al.: Exercise or food restriction: Effect of adipose tissue cellularity. *Am. J. Physiol., 227*:901-904, 1974.

Oscai, L., et al.: Effects of exercise and of food restriction on adipose tissue cellularity. *J. Lipid Res., 13*:588-592, 1972.

Pate, R. R., M. Maquire, and J. Van Wyk: Dietary iron supplementation in women athletes. *Physician Sportsmed., 7(9)*:81-88, 1979.

Pirnay, F., et al.: Glucose oxidation during prolonged exercise evaluated with naturally labeled [^{13}C] glucose. *J. Appl. Physiol.: Respirat. Environ. Exercise Physiol., 43(2)*:258-261, 1977.

Saltin, B., and L. Hermansen: Glycogen stores and prolonged severe exercise. *In* Blix, G. (ed.): *Nutrition and Physical Activity.* Uppsala, Sweden, Almqvist and Weksells, 1967.

Smith, N. J.: *Food for Sport.* Palo Alto, CA, Bull Publishing Co., 1976.

U.S. Department of Agriculture, Science and Education Administration, *Food, Home, and Garden Bulletin, (228)*: 1979.

Williams, M. H.: *Nutritional Aspects of Human Physical and Athletic Performance.* Springfield, IL, Charles C Thomas Publishers, 1976.

Wolf, E. M., J. C. Wirth, and T. G. Lohman: Nutritional practices of coaches in the Big Ten. *Physician Sportsmed., 7(2)*:113-114, 116-117, 119, 122-124, 1979.

11

Body Composition and Weight Control

Introduction

Basic to the understanding of obesity and nutrition are the principles of body-weight control. These principles apply to the nonathlete as well as to the athlete, but for different reasons. The nonathlete must always be concerned with the problem of obesity, whereas the athlete is more concerned with gaining muscle mass or fat-free weight. In either case, the "do's and don'ts" of body-weight control must be learned and thoroughly understood by the physical educator and coach. The purpose of this chapter is to help you do just that.

Body Composition

For our purposes, the body may be regarded as being composed basically of two fractions: (1) **body fat**; and (2) **fat-free weight (lean body mass)**.

Body Fat

The amount of body fat (adipose tissue) that is stored is determined by two factors: (1) the number of fat-storing cells, or **adipocytes**; and (2) the size, or capacity, of the adipocytes. It has been shown that the number of fat cells cannot be effectively decreased by exercise or dietary restrictions once adulthood is reached; during weight reduction involving fat loss in adults, it is the size but not the number of adipocytes that decreases. However, exercise and diet programs introduced during early childhood lead to a reduction in both the number and size of fat cells during the adult years. This is true even though the exercise and diet programs may not be continued into adulthood. This emphasizes how important the formulation of good nutritional habits and of good exercise habits are early in life as well as throughout life.

Body Fat of Athletes

In nonathletic college-aged men, body fat accounts for approximately 15% of the total body weight; the corresponding figure for women is approximately 26%. Among athletes, regardless of sports preference, the body fat is generally lower, with the percentages again differing on the basis of sex. For example, male marathon runners are extremely lean, with body fat ranging between 1 and 9% of total body weight and averaging at under 5%. Female long-distance runners are also exceptionally lean, but the lowest individual values are about 6% fat. The percent body fat among various men and women athletes is given in Figure 11-1. A more complete list of body fats among athletes is presented in Table 11-1. In studying both the figure and the table, keep in mind that since athletes are low in body fat, their muscle mass is generally greater than that of their nonathletic counterparts.

Fat cells and adipose tissue per se are not biochemically active in generating ATP energy (at least not in the same sense that muscle cells actively generate ATP energy). Thus, excess fat contributes weight but not the metabolic wherewithal for its movement. In physical activities that demand weight-bearing skills (e.g., walking, running, and gymnastics), excess fat tissue is, accordingly, a hindrance. In this respect, those most "handicapped" by fat are women, because their fat-to-muscle ratio is greater than that of men (even those of the same total body weight). However, in swimming, women have the advantage over men. In this case, the woman's greater fat content leads to less body drag in the water and thus to less energy expenditure per unit of distance swum.

Fat-Free Weight (Lean Body Mass)

When the weight of body fat is subtracted from the total body weight, the remaining weight is referred to as **fat-free weight**, or **lean body mass**. The fat-free weight (FFW) reflects mainly the skeletal muscle mass but also includes the weight of other tissues and organs such as bone and skin. The muscle mass makes up about 40 to 50% of the fat-free weight. The less body fat, the more fat-free weight. The average fat-free weight of college-aged men is about 85% of their total body weight, and that of college-aged women about 75% of their total body weight.

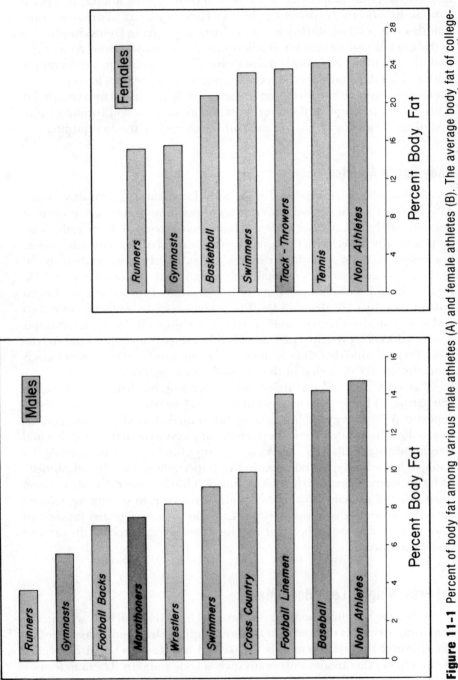

Figure 11-1 Percent of body fat among various male athletes (A) and female athletes (B). The average body fat of college-age nonathletes is approximately 15% for men and 26% for women. Among athletes, regardless of sports preference, the body fat is generally lower for both sexes. (Based on data from Boileau and Lohman, 1977.)

Fat-Free Weight of Athletes

The absolute and relative fat-free weights of men and women athletes are shown in Figure 11-2. Relative FFW refers to the percentage of total body weight that is lean body mass. The 85% FFW of the average college-aged man just mentioned is expressed *relative* to his total body weight. Absolute FFW, on the other hand, refers to the actual weight of the lean body mass and is calculated by the following formula:

actual FFW = (total body weight × relative FFW)/100

For example, if our average college man has a total body weight of 160 lb (72.6 kg), then his absolute FFW would be 160 lb × 85%/100 = **136 lb** or 72.6 kg × 85 %/100 = **61.7 kg**.

Fat-free weight is usually considered to be positively related to athletic performance, because a large FFW component means a large muscle mass and thus greater force potential. Large muscular forces are important in contact sports (particularly football) and in the track-and-field throwing events. Note in the figure that the male athletes with the largest absolute FFW are in fact the football players (both linemen and backs), and that the women with the largest FFW are the throwers. Of course, in certain activities, a large fat-free weight component may have a negative influence on performance. Activities involving sustained movement of the body mass would not be benefited by a large absolute FFW because, like fat, it adds body weight. Thus, runners, wrestlers, and gymnasts have rather small absolute FFW components. It is important to point out, however, that these athletes have a large relative FFW component. This means that they have low total body weights, with very little fat.

One other point is obvious from Figure 11-2—women athletes have much lower FFW components than do their male counterparts. For example, female gymnasts have about 44 kg of FFW, whereas male gymnasts have about 63 kg. As previously mentioned, in most sports this is a definite disadvantage for women.

In summary, then, athletes of both sexes generally have less body fat than do nonathletes. In sports that demand weight-bearing activities, the less fat the better, for excess fat is a hindrance.

Athletes generally have a greater fat-free weight (FFW) than do nonathletes. Male athletes have a greater FFW than do female athletes. The smaller FFW of the latter is a disadvantage in most sports.

Assessment of Body Composition

There are few techniques that allow one to readily assess body composition in humans in a precise way. One widely used method is shown in Figure 11-3. It involves underwater weighing and measurement of lung residual volume, an approach that provides for a considerable degree of accuracy but obviously not for ease of measurement. What actually is measured with

Table 11-1: Body Composition Values in Male and Female Athletes*

Athletic Group or Sport	Sex	Age (yr)	Height (cm)	Weight (kg)	Relative Fat %
Baseball	male	20.8	182.7	83.3	14.2
	male	—	—	—	11.8
	male	27.4	183.1	88.0	12.6
Basketball	female	19.1	169.1	62.6	20.8
	female	19.4	167.0	63.9	26.9
Centers	male	27.7	214.0	109.2	7.1
Forwards	male	25.3	200.6	96.9	9.0
Guards	male	25.2	188.0	83.6	10.6
Canoeing	male	23.7	182.0	79.6	12.4
Football	male	20.3	184.9	96.4	13.8
	male	—	—	—	13.9
Defensive backs	male	17–23	178.3	77.3	11.5
	male	24.5	182.5	84.8	9.6
Offensive backs	male	17–23	179.7	79.8	12.4
	male	24.7	183.8	90.7	9.4
Linebackers	male	17–23	180.1	87.2	13.4
	male	24.2	188.6	102.2	14.0
Offensive linemen	male	17–23	186.0	99.2	19.1
	male	24.7	193.0	112.6	15.6
Defensive linemen	male	17–23	186.6	97.8	18.5
	male	25.7	192.4	117.1	18.2
Quarterbacks, kickers	male	24.1	185.0	90.1	14.4
Gymnastics	male	20.3	178.5	69.2	4.6
	female	19.4	163.0	57.9	23.8
	female	20.0	158.5	51.5	15.5
	female	14.0	—	—	17.0
	female	23.0	—	—	11.0
	female	23.0	—	—	9.6
Ice hockey	male	26.3	180.3	86.7	15.1
	male	22.5	179.0	77.3	13.0
Jockeys	male	30.9	158.2	50.3	14.1
Orienteering	male	31.2	—	72.2	16.3
	female	29.0	—	58.1	18.7
Pentathalon	female	21.5	175.4	65.4	11.0
Racketball	male	25.0	181.7	80.3	8.1
Lightweight	male	21.0	186.0	71.0	8.5
	female	23.0	173.0	68.0	14.0
Skiing	male	25.9	176.6	74.8	7.4
Alpine	male	21.2	176.0	70.1	14.1
	male	21.8	177.8	75.5	10.2
	female	19.5	165.1	58.8	20.6
Cross-country	male	21.2	176.0	66.6	12.5
	male	25.6	174.0	69.3	10.2
	male	22.7	176.2	73.2	7.9
	female	24.3	163.0	59.1	21.8
	female	20.2	163.4	55.9	15.7
Nordic combination	male	22.9	176.0	70.4	11.2
	male	21.7	181.7	70.4	8.9
Ski jumping	male	22.2	174.0	69.9	14.3
Soccer	male	26.0	176.0	75.5	9.6

Table 11-1: Body Composition Values in Male and Female Athletes *(continued)*

Athletic Group or Sport	Sex	Age (yr)	Height (cm)	Weight (kg)	Relative Fat %
Speed skating	male	21.0	181.0	76.5	11.4
Swimming	male	21.8	182.3	79.1	8.5
	male	20.6	182.9	78.9	5.0
	female	19.4	168.0	63.8	26.3
Sprint	female	—	165.1	57.1	14.6
Middle distance	female	—	166.6	66.8	24.1
Distance	female	—	166.3	60.9	17.1
Tennis	male	—	—	—	15.2
	male	42.0	179.6	77.1	16.3
	female	39.0	163.3	55.7	20.3
Track and field	male	21.3	180.6	71.6	3.7
	male	—	—	—	8.8
Runners	male	22.5	177.4	64.5	6.3
Distance	male	26.1	175.7	64.2	7.5
	male	26.2	177.0	66.2	8.4
	male	40–49	180.7	71.6	11.2
	male	55.3	174.5	63.4	18.0
	male	50–59	174.7	67.2	10.9
	male	60–69	175.7	67.1	11.3
	male	70–75	175.6	66.8	13.6
	male	47.2	176.5	70.7	13.2
	female	19.9	161.3	52.9	19.2
	female	32.4	169.4	57.2	15.2
Middle distance	male	24.6	179.0	72.3	12.4
Sprint	female	20.1	164.9	56.7	19.3
	male	46.5	177.0	74.1	16.5
Discus	male	28.3	186.1	104.7	16.4
	male	26.4	190.8	110.5	16.3
	female	21.1	168.1	71.0	25.0
Jumpers and hurdlers	female	20.3	165.9	59.0	20.7
Shot-put	male	27.0	188.2	112.5	16.5
	male	22.0	191.6	126.2	19.6
	female	21.5	167.6	78.1	28.0
Volleyball	female	19.4	166.0	59.8	25.3
	female	19.9	172.2	64.1	21.3
Weight lifting	male	24.9	166.4	77.2	9.8
Power	male	26.3	176.1	92.0	15.6
Olympic	male	25.3	177.1	88.2	12.2
Body builders	male	29.0	172.4	83.1	8.4
	male	27.6	178.8	88.1	8.3
Wrestling	male	26.0	177.8	81.8	9.8
	male	27.0	176.0	75.7	10.7
	male	22.0	—	—	5.0
	male	23.0	—	79.3	14.3
	male	19.6	174.6	74.8	8.8
	male	15–18	172.3	66.3	6.9
	male	20.6	174.8	67.3	4.0

*Adapted from J.H. Wilmore, et al., Body physique and composition of the female distance runner. *Ann. NY Acad. Sci.* 301:764–776, 1977.

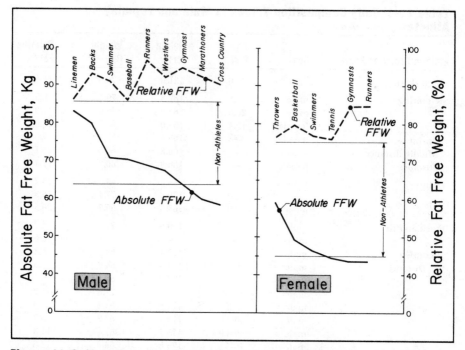

Figure 11-2 Absolute and relative fat-free weights (FFW) of male and female athletes. Fat-free weight is usually considered to be positively related to athletic performance. (Based on data from Boileau and Lohman, 1977.)

underwater weighing is body density. **Density (D)** is defined as mass (M) per unit volume (V) or:

$$D = M/V$$

Because the body is 70% water, its density is very close to that of water, that is, 1 g per cm^3 of volume ($1g/cm^3$). However, the density of pure fat tissue is only 0.9 g/cm^3 whereas the density of fat-free tissue is 1.10 g/cm^3. Therefore, by knowing the density of the body, the percentage of body fat can be calculated.

Body fat and composition may also be reasonably estimated from measurements of subcutaneous fat as reflected by skinfold thicknesses. Such measurements, which are relatively uncomplicated, have been adopted by physicians, trainers, coaches, and physical educators as a means of assessing the body composition of various persons, including athletes. For example, as shown in Table 11-2, skinfold measurements at the triceps, scapula, and abdomen may be used to classify men and women athletes with respect to acceptable values of body fat. The skinfold measurements are taken with an instrument called a **skinfold caliper.*** The caliper should be used to measure

---

*Lange Skinfold Caliper, Cambridge Scientific Industries, Cambridge, MD; Harpenden Caliper (No. 3496), Quinton Instruments, 2121 Terry Avenue, Seattle, WA 98121.

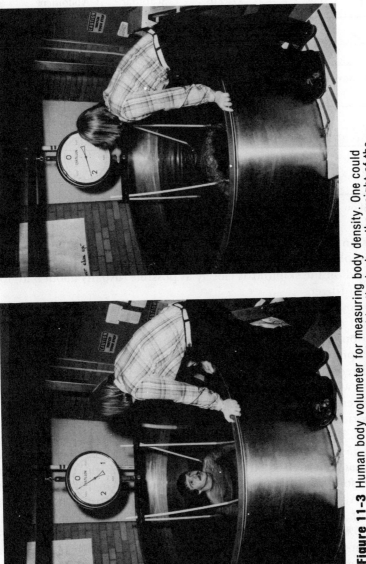

Figure 11-3 Human body volumeter for measuring body density. One could measure either weight of the water displaced by the body or the weight of the body when completely submerged. (Photographs by Tom Malloy. Courtesy of the Department of Photography, The Ohio State University, Columbus, OH.)

Table 11-2: Classification of Body Fat from Skinfold Thicknesses for Male and Female Athletes

		Male Athletes*			
Classifi-cation	Body Fat	Skinfold Thickness (mm)			
		Triceps	Scapular	Abdomen	Sum
Lean	<7%	<7	<8	<10	<25
Acceptable	7-15%	7-13	8-15	10-20	25-48
Overfat	>15%	>13	>15	>20	>48

*From Buskirk (1974).

		Female Athletes†			
Classifi-cation	Body Fat	Skinfold Thickness (mm)			
		Triceps	Scapular	Abdomen	Sum
Lean	<12%	<9	<7	<7	<23
Acceptable	12-25%	9-17	7-14	7-15	23-46
Overfat	>25%	>17	>14	>15	>46

†Based on data from Hall (1977).

folds of skin only—no muscle tissue should be included. As shown in Figure 11-4, skinfold is held firmly between thumb and index finger. The caliper is then placed on the skinfold as closely as possible (usually about ½ in) to the thumb and finger.

The body fat and skinfold measures presented in Table 11-2 should not be thought of as absolute values but rather as rough estimates of the body composition status of the athlete. They are meant to provide information with respect to preparing the athlete for competition. For example, suppose you wish to determine whether two linemen for a high school football team will have any "weight problem" if each weighs 100 kg (220 lb) at the start of the season. By establishing from skinfold measurements where the linemen fit in the categories given in Table 11-2, you will be able to identify any potential difficulties. If, for example, skinfold measurements of lineman A add up to less than 25 mm whereas those of lineman B total more than 48 mm, it is obvious that, although equal in weight, the athletes are not equally prepared for the season (one is "lean" and the other "overfat" in Table 11-2's terms). Lineman A, at 220 lb, has less than 7% fat, or less than 15 lb of fat (7% of 220 = 15.4). Lineman B, also at 220 lb, has more than 15% fat, or more than 33 lb of fat (15% of 220 = 33.0). This means that lineman A has at least 220−15 = 205 lb of fat-free weight and lineman B has at most 220−33 = 187 lb of fat-free weight. You may conclude from this information that lineman B has a "weight problem," in that he should lose about 18 lb of fat and gain about 18 lb of fat-free weight. Lineman A has no weight problem and should concentrate on maintaining or gaining fat-free weight.

Let's apply Table 11-2 to another sport. Suppose you are the coach of a high school wrestler who wants to drop from his present 167 lb class to the

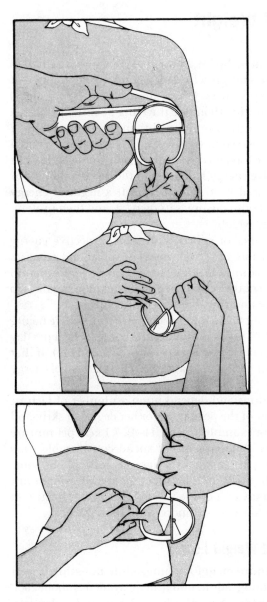

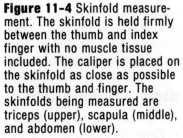

Figure 11-4 Skinfold measurement. The skinfold is held firmly between the thumb and index finger with no muscle tissue included. The caliper is placed on the skinfold as close as possible to the thumb and finger. The skinfolds being measured are triceps (upper), scapula (middle), and abdomen (lower).

next lower class (155 lb). You assess his skinfolds and find from Table 11-2 that he is in the "lean" category—he has less than 7% fat. At his midweek weight of 170 lb, this means that he has less than $170 \times .07 = 12$ lb of fat. Since, for health reasons, it is recommended that wrestlers not go below 5% body fat (see p. 307), he should have about $155 \times .05 = 8$ lb of fat at the 155-lb weight class. Therefore, he has only 4 lb of "excess" fat to lose—not enough to make the drop from 170 to 155 safely.

Energy Balance and Weight Control

The quantity of food required by an individual above that which is necessary for body maintenance and growth depends upon the amount of physical activity that he or she experiences. Just as an automobile traveling 60 miles each day requires more gasoline than one traveling 30 miles per day, a person walking 20 miles a day requires more food than a person walking 2 miles each day. For body weight to remain constant, food intake must equal energy needs. If, in fact, too much food is consumed, we will gain weight or be in what is referred to as a **positive energy balance**. On the other hand, if our energy needs exceed that produced by the food we eat, a **negative energy balance** occurs. In this case, the body consumes its own fat, and then protein, with a concomitant loss in body weight.

Table 11-3 contains a number of sports with their respective energy requirements in kcal* per day. Table 11-4 contains a few sports and exercises in terms of total kcal expended per minute. Of what value is this information to us? By knowing the energy cost of the activity, we can better plan our diets to maintain proper energy balance and thus body weight control.

For example, a man weighing 68 kg and participating in bicycle racing would expend 5450 kcal (plus 10% utilized in digestion) or 5995 kcal per day (Table 11-3). A person playing golf uses 5 kcal per min (Table 11-4). If that person were to play for 3 hr, he or she would have expended 900 kcal of energy (5 kcal per min times 180 min).

These data are approximations and depend upon a number of factors, including the physical condition of the person, his or her degree of skill, and the degree of effort employed. For example, (Table 11-4), 7.1 kcal per min are expended while playing tennis. A novice might spend considerable time walking after balls, while the expert engages in vigorous rallies. The same would be true for golf. Terrain, skill, and body weight are also important considerations related to the energy cost of the activity. Usually, it costs you more in the rough than on the fairway—in more ways than one!

Negative Energy Balance and Weight Loss

The average daily caloric requirement for young, adult, nonathletic men is about 3000 kcal, and that for young, adult, nonathletic women is about 2000 kcal. If the daily caloric expenditure through physical activity for the man were also 3000 kcal, then his body weight would remain constant. However, if he were to climb for an hour each day without changing his caloric intake, he would be expending between 642 and 792 kcal more than he takes in; his body weight would decrease. The magnitude of the decrease may be calculated in terms of how long it would take 1 lb of pure fat, which contains about 3500

---

*To convert from kcal to liters of oxygen consumed, divide kcal by 5.

kcal, to be lost. In this case, it would take 4½ to 5½ days for the pound of fat to be lost ($3500/642 = 5½$ and $3500/792 = 4½$).

As mentioned in the last chapter, for highly active men and women athletes, the daily caloric requirements might be as high as 5000 to 6000 kcal and 3500 to 4500 kcal, respectively. Although these might appear to be excessively high, remember that athlete's daily energy expenditures are also high (e.g., running a 26.2-mile marathon requires about 2500 to 2800 kcal).

Positive Energy Balance and Weight Gain

If our average man from the preceding example were consuming 3500 kcal and expending only 3000 kcal, then he would be in positive energy balance as previously mentioned and would gain body weight. The question to answer is whether he would gain fat weight or fat-free weight. If he were not engaged in an exercise program, the weight gain would be mainly in the form of stored fat. In this case, it would require an excess caloric intake of 3500 kcal to gain 1 lb of fat. With a + 500 kcal balance per day, this would take seven days.

On the other hand, if an exercise program is undertaken at the same time during positive energy balance, the weight gain would be mainly in the form of lean (muscle) weight or fat-free weight. In this case, it requires about 2500 kcal of excess intake to gain 1 lb of lean or fat-free weight. Assuming the same + 500 kcal balance per days as before, this would take five days.

Figure 11-5 may help in summarizing the relationship of food consumption and energy expenditure (energy balance) to body weight control.

Guidelines for Losing Body Fat in Athletes

While male athletes who have an estimated body fat of less than 7% and female athletes of less than 12% (Table 11-2) should not be concerned about losing fat (except under medical advisement), many nonathletes and other athletes will find it necessary to shed body fat. For athletes, this is especially true at the beginning of the season. At the same time, these "overfat" athletes may want to gain, or at least maintain, their fat-free weight. The following guidelines should be helpful in achieving these goals:

Guidelines for Losing Body Fat

Remember, it requires an excess expenditure of 3500 kcal in order to lose 1 lb of pure fat.

It is recommended that the caloric deficit not exceed 2000 to 2500 kcal/day or 4 lb of fat per week. An ideal loss is 2 lb per week. An attempt to estimate daily or weekly caloric intake and expenditure should be made. This is not easy, but it can be done with the help of the athlete's parents and perhaps the home economics teacher.

Table 11-3: Median Energy Consumption and Corresponding Daily Food Requirements (in kilocalories)

Selected Disciplines 1	Expenditure of Energy/kg of Body Weight/ Day (kcal) 2	Average Body Weight (kg) 3	Normative Daily Net Needs Based On Computed Energy Requirements (Column 2 × Column 3) (kcal) 4	Nutritional, Physiological, Optimal Daily Gross Requirements with 10% Added for Consumption (kcal) 5
Group A				
Cross-country skiing	82.14	67.5	5550	6105*
Crew racing	69.21	80.0	5550	6105
Canoe racing	72.72	75.0	5450	5995
Swimming	69.87	76.0	5300	5830*
Bicycle racing	80.39	68.0	5450	5995
Marathon racing	79.07	68.0	5400	5940
Average values (men)			5450	5995*

Rounded-off norm: 6000 kcal

Also belonging to sports of Group A are skiing, Norwegian combination, middle-distance racing, walking, ice racing, modern pentathlon, equine sports, military, and touring (Alpine climbing).

Group B				
Soccer	72.28	74.0	5350	5885
Handball	68.06	75.0	5100	5610
Basketball	67.93	75.0	5100	5610
Field hockey	69.18	75.0	5200	5720
Ice hockey	71.87	68.0	4900	5390
Average values (men)			5130	5643

Rounded-off norm: 5600 kcal

Also belonging to Group B are rugby, water polo, volleyball, tennis, polo, and bicycle polo.

Group C				
Canoe slalom	67.16	68.0	4550	5005
Shooting	62.71	72.5	4550	5005
Table tennis	59.96	74.0	4450	4895
Bowling	62.69	75.0	4700	5170
Sailing	63.77	74.0	4700	5170
Average values (men)			4590	5049

Rounded-off norm: 5000 kcal

Also belonging to Group C are circuit cycle racing (1000–4000 m), fencing, ice sailing, and gliding.

The caloric deficit should represent both an increased expenditure and a reduced caloric intake. A caloric deficit that is solely the result of diet restriction will cause fat-free weight loss.

For most active athletes, the lower limit of a restricted diet is a 2000-kcal intake per day. Caloric reductions below this level should be medically supervised. An example of a 2000-kcal diet is presented in Table 11-5. Note that all of the essential nutrients are provided in amounts adequate for most athletes.

Table 11-3: Median Energy Consumption and Corresponding Daily Food Requirements (in kilocalories) *(continued)*

Group D				
Sprinting	61.77	69.0	4250	4675
Running: short to middle distances	65.62	65.0	4250	4675
Pole vault	57.83	73.0	4200	4620
Diving	69.24	61.0	4200	4620
Boxing (middle and welter weight: to 63.5 kg)	67.25	63.0	4250	4675
Average values (men)			4230	4653

Rounded-off norm: 4600 kcal

Also belonging to Group D are hurdle races, broad- and high-jump, hop-skip-and-jump, ballet, swimming, figure skating, figure roller skating, and skiing, ski jump, bob sled, and tobogganing.

Selected Disciplines 1	Expenditure of Energy/kg of Body Weight/ Day (kcal) 2	Average Body Weight (kg) 3	Normative Daily Net Needs Based on Computed Energy Requirements (Column 2 × Column 3) (kcal) 4	Nutritional, Physiological, Optimal Daily Gross Requirements, with 10% Added for Consumption (kcal) 5
Group E				
Group I				
Judo (lightweight)	79.92	62.5	4550	5005
Weight lifting (light-weight)	69.15	67.5	4650	5115
Javelin	56.95	76.0	4350	4785
Gymnastics with apparatus	67.14	65.0	4350	4785
Steeplechase	63.96	68.0	4350	4785
Ski: Alpine competition	71.29	67.5	4800	5280
Average values (men)			4508	4959
		Rounded-off norm: 5000 kcal		
Group II				
Hammerthrow	62.46	102.0	6350	6985
Shot put and discus	62.47	102.0	6350	6985
		Rounded-off norm: 7000 kcal		

Also belonging to Group E/I are wrestling, automobile rallies, motor racing, gymnastics, acrobatics, parachute jumping, equine sports shows, decathlon, and bicycle gymnastics.

*Deviations of a few percent from the median values are, in the field of biology, to be taken as basically insignificant.

From Encyclopedia of Sport Sciences and Medicine (1971) pp. 1128–1129.

Table 11-4: Approximate Energy Cost (in Kilocalories) of Various Physical Activities*

Sport or Activity	Kilocalories Expended Per Minute (kcal/min) of Activity
Climbing	10.7–13.2
Cycling 5.5 mph	4.5
9.4 mph	7.0
13.1 mph	11.1
Dancing	3.3–7.7
Football	8.9
Golf	5.0
Gymnastics	
Balancing	2.5
Abdominal exercises	3.0
Trunk bending	3.5
Arm swinging, hopping	6.5
Rowing 51 str/min	4.1
87 str/min	7.0
97 str/min	11.2
Running	
Short distance	13.3–16.6
Cross-country	10.6
Tennis	7.1
Skating (fast)	11.5
Skiing, moderate speed	10.8–15.9
Uphill, maximum speed	18.6
Squash	10.2
Swimming	
Breaststroke	11.0
Backstroke	11.5
Crawl (55 yd/min)	14.0
Wrestling	14.2

*From The American Association for Health, Physical Education, and Recreation. *Nutrition for the Athlete.* Washington, D.C. AAHPER, 1971.

ACSM Guidelines for Proper and Improper Weight-Loss Programs

Millions of individuals are involved in weight-loss programs, not just athletes. Therefore, guidelines for proper weight-loss programs for everyone are very much needed. This is even more apparent when one stops to think about how many "fad diets" are available today (most of which are undesirable) and how widespread are the misconceptions concerning weight-loss programs.

Based on the existing evidence concerning the effects of weight loss on health status, physiologic processes and body composition parameters, the American College of Sports Medicine (ACSM) makes the following statements and recommendations for weight-loss programs.

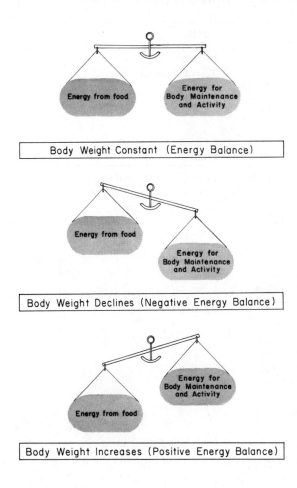

Figure 11-5 Relationship of food consumption, energy expenditure, and body weight.

Prolonged fasting and diet programs that severely restrict caloric intake are scientifically undesirable and can be medically dangerous.

Fasting and diet programs that severely restrict caloric intake result in the loss of large amounts of water, electrolytes, minerals, glycogen stores, and other fat-free tissue (including proteins within fat-free tissues), with minimal amounts of fat loss.

Mild calorie restriction (500–1000 kcal less than the usual daily intake) results in a smaller loss of water, electrolytes, minerals, and other fat-free tissue, and is less likely to cause malnutrition.

Dynamic exercise of large muscles helps to maintain fat-free tissue, including muscle mass and bone density, and results in losses of body weight. Weight loss resulting from an increase in energy expenditure is primarily in the form of fat weight.

Table 11-5: Example of a Low-Calorie (2000-kcal) Diet in Five Meals*

Breakfast	Snack
1/2 cup orange juice 1 soft-boiled egg 1 slice whole wheat toast 2 teasp margarine 1 glass skim milk or other beverage Total kilocalories: 345	1 banana Total kilocalories: 100

Lunch	Snack
1 hamburger (3 oz) on a roll with relish 1/2 sliced tomato 1 glass skim milk 1 medium apple Total kilocalories: 510	1 carton fruit-flavored yogurt 1 cup grape juice Total kilocalories: 385

Dinner	
1 serving of baked chicken marengo (1/2 breast) 3/4 cup rice 5–6 Brussel sprouts 1 bowl of green salad with French dressing 1 small piece gingerbread 1 cup skim milk or other beverage Total kilocalories: 660	

Daily total kilocalories: 2000

*From Smith, N. J.: *Food for Sport*. Palo Alto, CA, Bull Publishing Co., 1976.

A nutritionally sound diet resulting in mild calorie restriction coupled with an endurance exercise program along with behavioral modification of existing eating habits is recommended for weight reduction. The rate of sustained weight loss should not exceed 1 kg (2 lb) per week. To maintain proper weight control and optimal body fat levels, a lifetime commitment to proper eating habits and regular physical activity is required.

Guidelines for Gaining Fat-Free Weight in Athletes

For most people, gaining weight is easy. Unfortunately, the gain is mostly in body fat, which can lead to health problems. Ideally, increases in weight should reflect gains in fat-free weight. Such gains are often desired by athletes, since fat-free weight is generally positively correlated with athletic performance. However, for many athletes, gaining or at least maintaining fat-free weight during the long, difficult season is a real problem. One way of handling this problem is to follow the guidelines for gaining fat-free weight presented below. While reviewing these guidelines, keep in mind that **no athlete should be encouraged to participate in weight-gaining programs if his or her family has a history of heart disease.**

Guidelines for Gaining Fat-Free Weight

As previously mentioned, in order to gain weight, caloric intake must be greater than caloric expenditure. In order to gain 1 lb of fat-free weight (muscle), an excess intake of about 2500 kcal is required. An excess of this size should not be taken in in one day.

It is recommended that the daily caloric intake not exceed expenditure by more than 1000 to 1500 kcal. On the basis of five diet days per week, this would mean a gain of 2 to 3 lb per week.

An estimate of how many calories are being taken in and how many are being expended daily or weekly should be made (just as in the weight-loss program).

Note that calories needed to maintain weight must be added to excess intake for an accurate picture of the diet of an athlete on a weight-gain plan. In this regard, an intake of 6000 kcal a day is a realistic diet for young male athletes, since their average daily caloric expenditure may be about 5000 kcal. An example of a 6000-kcal diet is given in Table 11-6. Note the quality of the food—low levels of large-bulk foods (such as cereals, grains, beverages, and salads), low amounts of animal fats, and an abundance of low-bulk carbohydrates.

To ensure that the excess calories will be laid down primarily as muscle, a vigorous training program, particularly of weight training, should be undertaken during the high caloric diet period. The skinfold measures mentioned earlier can be used to determine whether any excess fat is being added.

Examples of programs of weight gain and weight reduction are given in Table 11-7.

Weight Reduction in Wrestling

Athletes in any sport may follow the guidelines just presented and successfully lose body fat. Wrestlers, however, often go in for weight reduction that involves far more than food restriction, using methods that commonly include fluid restriction and dehydration (e.g., inducing excessive sweating). In a recent review of the literature, The American College of Sports Medicine

Table 11-6: Example of a High-Calorie (6000-kcal) Diet in Six Meals*

Breakfast

1/2 cup orange juice
1 cup oatmeal
1 cup low-fat milk
1 scrambled egg
1 slice whole wheat toast
1-1/2 teasp margarine
1 tbs jam

Total kilocalories: 665

Lunch

5 fish sticks with tartar
    sauce
1 large serving, French
    fries
1 bowl of green salad with
    avocado and French
    dressing
1 cup lemon sherbet
2 granola cookies
1 cup low-fat milk

Total kilocalories: 1505

Dinner

1 cup cream of mushroom
    soup
2 pieces oven-baked
    chicken
1 candied sweet potato
1 dinner roll and
    margarine
1 cup carrots and peas
1/2 cup coleslaw
1 piece cherry pie
1 beverage

Total kilocalories: 1615

Snack

1 peanut butter sandwich
1 banana
1 cup grape juice

Total kilocalories: 485

Snack

1 cup mixed dried fruit
1-1/2 cup malted milk

Total kilocalories: 660

Snack

1 cup cashew nuts
1 cup cocoa

Total kilocalories: 1045

Daily total kilocalories: 5975

*From Smith, N. J.: *Food for Sport*. Palo Alto, CA, Bull Publish-Co., 1976.

concluded that the simple and combined effects of these practices are generally associated with: (1) a reduction in muscular strength; (2) a decrease in work performance times (the athlete cannot work as long); (3) lower plasma and blood volumes; (4) a reduction in cardiac functioning during submaximal work conditions; (5) a lower oxygen consumption, especially when food restriction is a critical part of the weight-reduction plan; (6) an impairment of thermoregulatory processes; (7) a decrease in renal blood flow and in the

Table 11-7: Examples of Fat-Free Weight (FFW) Gain and Fat Reduction Programs

Athlete	Present Body Composition	Daily Caloric Intake	Means of Achieving Goal		Goal (after 3 months)
			Daily Caloric Expenditure	Difference between Intake & Expenditure	
Football player	Total body weight: 200 lb Fat: 10% FFW: 180 lb	6000 kcal; see Table 9-3	4940 kcal, including calories spent in training*	6000 − 4940 = 1060 kcal excess	Total body weight: 225 lb Fat: 8% FFW: 207 lb
Field hockey player	Total body weight: 127 lb Fat: 25% FFW: 95 lb	2000 kcal; see Table 9-4	3000 kcal, including calories spent in training†	3000 − 2000 = 1000 kcal deficit (500 from restricted diet, 500 from exercise)	Total body weight: 112 lb Fat: 15% FFW: 95 lb

*Training for the football player interested in gaining fat-free weight might include repeated 40-yd sprints (two days per week) and weight-resistance training (three days per week).

†Training for the field hockey player interested in losing body fat might include jogging 3 miles per day, calisthenics, and weight-resistance training (two days per week).

volume of fluid being filtered by the kidney; (8) a depletion of liver glycogen stores; and (9) an increase in the amount of electrolytes being lost from the body. Some studies have shown that weight losses caused by dehydration of 3% or more result in diminished athletic performance. Prolonged semistarvation diets, unbalanced diets, and excessive sweating combined with dehydration may cause severe harm to the athlete.

The Committee of Medical Aspects of Sports of the American Medical Association has posed several questions raised by the wrestling community:

1. What are the hazards of indiscriminate and excessive weight reduction?
2. How much weight can a wrestler lose safely?
3. What are defensible means of losing weight?
4. What weigh-in plan would best serve the purpose intended?

The committee also states that the amount of weight that a wrestler can safely lose should be related to his **effective weight level** (the weight level which yields his best performance) rather than the minimal weight. It is difficult to define scientifically the limits of safe weight control. Argument is in favor of a good preparticipation medical examination. Such a plan involves the weight history which allows the physician a more valid judgment regarding how much weight a boy can safely lose.

The committee is quick to emphasize that there is no alternative to:

1. A balanced diet at a sustaining caloric level.
2. Adequate fluid intake.
3. High energy output for attaining and maintaining an effective competitive weight.

Finally, the committee suggests the weight of the wrestling candidates can best be assessed through a natural approach:

1. Educate youth who are interested in athletics regarding the importance of periodic medical examinations and the advantages of a general, year-round conditioning program for cardiovascular-pulmonary endurance, muscular fitness, and nutritional readiness.
2. Building on this orientation, assist any aspiring wrestler in an intensive conditioning program related to the demands of wrestling for at least four weeks, preferably six, without emphasis on weight level.
3. At the end of this period and without altering his daily training routine, take his weight in a prebreakfast, postmicturition state.
4. Consider this weight his minimal effective weight for competition as well as certification purposes.
5. Educate the boy and his parents in the concept of defensible weight control to avert fluctuation from his effective weight level.

The Iowa Studies

Tipton and colleagues at the University of Iowa have performed extensive studies concerning the effect of weight loss in high-school wrestlers. Their studies show:

1. A large number of young athletes lose an excessive amount of weight in a relatively short period of time. This holds true for all classes below 175 lb. The lightest lose the highest percentage (circa 10%) of body weight during a 17-day period [Fig. 11-6].
2. The majority of weight loss occurs immediately preceding the date of certification.
3. Weight-losing methods were suggested by either coach or teammate.
4. Of the 835 boys measured, the average percentage of fat is 8%, whereas the state finalists (N = 224) had a 4 to 6% body-fat content.

Dr. Tipton is particularly concerned with the lack of professional supervision dealing with the method or amount of weight which an athlete should lose. He recommends a body weight containing 7% fat (not less than 5% without medical supervision) and one which does not exceed 7% loss of the initial weight. Ideally, one would predict minimal weight at the beginning of the school year; then under professional guidance, a proper and gradual weight reduction could take place.

Predicting Minimal Weight Values for Wrestlers

Research by Dr. Tipton and co-workers resulted in an equation which allows prediction of minimal weight values. Several anthropometric mea-

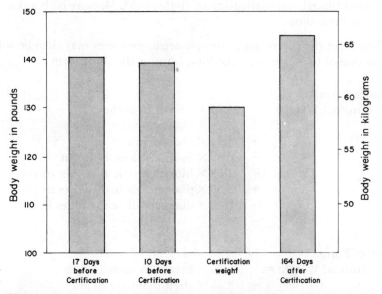

Figure 11-6 During a 17-day period, 6.8 lb or 4.9% of the body weight was lost, most of which occurred during the last 10 days. An average increase of 13.6 lb above the certification weight occurred at the end of the season. (From Tipton and Tcheng, 1970.)

surements are obtained six to eight weeks before the start of the wrestling season. The minimal weights are computed; the results are then used as a screening device along with the physician's judgment concerning the proper minimal weight for the particular boy.

Anthropometric Measurements (Fig. 11-7)

The following anthropometric measurements are necessary for predicting minimal weights in wrestlers:

1. **Chest Diameter.** Subject stands with both hands on the crests of the ilium. Calipers are placed in the axillary region with ends placed on the second or third rib. At the end of the expiration, the measurement is obtained.
2. **Chest Depth.** Subject stands with right hand behind head. One end of the caliper is placed on the tip of the xiphoid process while the other end is placed over the vertebrae of the twelfth rib. Measurement is taken at the end of the expiration.
3. **Bi-iliac Diameter.** Distance between most lateral projections of the crests of the ilium is measured.
4. **Bitrochanteric Diameter.** Distance between the most lateral projections of the greater trochanters is measured.
5. **Wrist Diameter.** Distance between the styloid processes of the radius and ulna is measured. Measure both wrists and use their sum.
6. **Ankle Diameter.** The foot is placed on a stool or chair with caliper ends placed over malleoli at an angle of 45°. Measure both ankles and use their sum.

Data from the preceding anthropometric measures may then be substituted in one of two formulas, the long form or the short form.

Long Form:
Minimal Weight =   1.84 × height in inches
                 +   3.28 × chest diameter in cm
                 +   3.31 × chest depth in cm
                 +   0.82 × bi-iliac diameter in cm
                 +   1.69 × bitrochanteric diameter in cm
                 +   3.56 × diameter of both wrists in cm
                 +   2.15 × diameter of both ankles in cm
                 −   281.72

Short Form:
Minimal Weight =   2.05 × height in inches
                 +   3.65 × chest diameter in cm
                 +   3.51 × chest depth in cm
                 +   1.96 × bitrochanteric diameter in cm
                 +   8.02 × left ankle diameter in cm
                 −   282.18

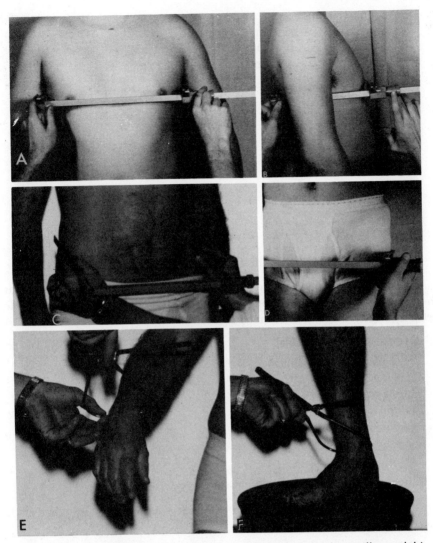

Figure 11-7 Measurements required for predicting minimal wrestling weight for high school men. A, Chest diameter; B, chest depth; C, bi-iliac diameter; D, bitrochanteric diameter; E, wrist diameter; and F, ankle diameter. (A, B, D, courtesy of Churchill, 1971.)

As an example of how to use the equations, an Ohio State Big Ten finalist was measured at the beginning of the wrestling season with the following results:

Wt = 150 lb
Ht = 71 in
Chest diameter = 25.4 cm
Chest depth = 18.5 cm

Bitrochanteric diameter = 32.3 cm
Bi-iliac diameter = 25.7 cm
Wrist diameter (sum of both wrists) = 11.4 cm
Ankle diameter (sum of both ankles) = 14.2 cm

Minimal Weight (Long Form)

$(1.84) \times (71 \text{ in})$	= 130.64
$(3.28) \times (25.4)$	= 83.31
$(3.31) \times (18.5)$	= 61.24
$(.82) \times (25.7)$	= 21.07
$(1.69) \times (32.3)$	= 54.59
$(3.56) \times (11.4)$	= 40.58
$(2.15) \times (14.2)$	= 30.53
	421.96
	− 281.72

Minimal weight = 140.24 lb

The boy's predicted minimal weight equals 140.24 lb. Weighing 150 lb at the beginning of the season, this wrestler could lose a maximum of 10 lb. He actually wrestled at a body weight of 142 lb.

Minimal Weight (Short Form)

$(2.05) \times (71 \text{ in})$	= 145.55
$(3.65) \times (25.4)$	= 92.71
$(3.51) \times (18.5)$	= 64.94
$(1.96) \times (32.3)$	= 63.31
$(8.02) \times (7.1)$	= 56.94
	423.45
	− 282.18

Minimal weight = 141.27 lb

You can see that the short form produces results almost identical with those of the long form.

ACSM Guidelines for Weight Loss in Wrestlers

The American College of Sports Medicine (ACSM) suggests that the potential health hazard created by the procedures that are used by wrestlers to "make weight" can be eliminated if state and national organizations will:

Guidelines for Weight Loss in Wrestlers

"Assess the body composition of each wrestler several weeks in advance of the competitive season. Individuals with a fat content less than

5% of their certified body weight should receive medical clearance before being allowed to compete.

"Emphasize the fact that the daily caloric requirements of wrestlers should be obtained from a balanced diet and determined on the basis of age, body surface area, growth, and physical activity levels. The minimal caloric needs of wrestlers in high schools and colleges will range from 1200 to 2400 kcal/day; therefore, it is the responsibility of coaches, school officials, physicians, and parents to discourage wrestlers from securing less than their minimal needs without prior medical approval.

"Discourage the practice of fluid deprivation and dehydration. This can be accomplished by:

Educating the coaches and wrestlers . . . [so that they are aware of] the physiological consequences and medical complications that can occur as a result of these practices.

Prohibiting the single or combined use of rubber suits, steam rooms, hot boxes, saunas, laxatives, and diuretics to 'make weight.'

Scheduling weigh-ins just prior to competition.

Scheduling more official weigh-ins between team matches.

"Permit more participants per team to compete in those weight classes (119–145 lb) which have the highest percentages of wrestlers certified for competition.

"Standardize regulations concerning the eligibility rules at championship tournaments so that individuals can participate only in those weight classes in which they had the highest frequencies of matches throughout the season.

"Encourage local and county organizations to systematically collect data on the hydration state of wrestlers and its relationship to growth and development."

Summary

- Good nutrition at all times is essential to effective athletic performance.

- The body is composed basically of body fat and fat-free weight (lean body mass).

- The amount of body fat that humans and animals store is determined by the size and number of fat cells. The number of fat cells is determined during the growing years, and in humans is fixed by the time adulthood is reached.

- Athletes generally have less body fat than do nonathletes. In sports that demand weight-bearing activities, the less fat the better, because excess fat is a hindrance.

- Female athletes have a greater fat-to-muscle ratio than do male athletes and are thus more subject to the effects of body fat—which in most sports (except swimming) is a drawback.

- Fat-free weight (FFW) reflects mainly skeletal muscle mass but also includes the weight of tissues and organs such as bone and skin. The less body fat, the more fat-free weight.

- Athletes generally have a greater muscle mass and thus a greater FFW than do nonathletes. Men athletes have a greater FFW than do women athletes. The smaller FFW of the latter is a disadvantage in most sports or sports activities.

- Fat-free weight is usually considered to be positively related to athletic performance.

- Body composition is most accurately assessed by underwater weighing but may be reasonably estimated from measurements of subcutaneous fat as reflected by skinfold thicknesses. Evaluating the body composition of athletes aids in their preparation for competition.

- Energy balance means consuming the same amount of energy through food intake as is being expended through physical activity.

- Positive energy balance means that more energy is consumed than is expended. As a result, body weight is gained.

- Negative energy balance means that less energy is consumed than expended, and body weight will be lost.

- Energy intake can be reasonably estimated by knowing the caloric content of the food eaten whereas energy expended can be estimated by knowing the energy requirement of various activities.

- In order to lose 1 lb of fat, an excess expenditure of 3500 kcal is required.

- To maintain proper weight control and optimal levels of fat, a lifetime commitment to proper eating habits and to regular physical activity is required.

- In order to gain 1 lb of FFW (muscle mass), an excess intake of about 2500 kcal is required.

- Weight-reduction methods that include fluid restriction and dehydration (both popular in wrestling) are a potential health hazard.

- Minimal weights for wrestlers can be safely predicted from anthropometric measurements.

- Wrestlers wishing to lose weight should follow the guidelines set forth by the American College of Sports Medicine.

Selected References and Readings*

American Association for Health, Physical Education, and Recreation. *Nutrition for the Athlete.* Washington, D.C.: AAHPER, 1971.

American College of Sports Medicine. *Encyclopedia of Sport Sciences and Medicine.* New York, Macmillan Co., 1971.

---

*For full journal titles, see Appendix A.

American College of Sports Medicine. Proper and improper weight loss programs. *Med. Sci. Sports Exercise, 15(1)*:ix–xiii, 1983.

American College of Sports Medicine. Weight loss in wrestlers. *Med. Sci. Sports Exercise, 8(2)*: xi–xiii, 1976.

Boileau, R. A., and T. G. Lohman: The measurement of human physique and its effects on physical performance. *Orthop. Clin. N. Am., 8(3)*:563–581, 1977.

Buskirk, E. Nutrition for the athlete. *In* Ryan, A., and F. Allman (eds.): *Sports Medicine.* New York: Academic Press, 1974.

Churchill, E., et al.: Anthropometry of U.S. Army Aviators—1970. *Technical Report 72-52-CE.* Natick, MA, U.S. Army Natick Laboratories, Dec., 1971.

Fox, E. L., and D. K. Mathews: *The Physiological Basis of Physical Education and Athletics.* 3rd ed. Philadelphia, Saunders College Publishing, 1981.

Hall, L. K.: Anthropometric Estimations of Body Density of Women Athletes in Selected Athletic Activities. Doctoral Dissertation, The Ohio State University, 1977.

Hirsch, J.: Adipose cellularity in relation to human obesity. *Advances Internal Med., 17*:289–300, 1971.

Malina, R. M., et al.: Fatness and fat patterning among athletes at the Montreal Olympic Games, 1976. *Med. Sci. Sports Exercise, 14(6)*:445–452, 1982.

Oscai, L., et al.: Exercise or food restriction: Effect on adipose tissue cellularity. *Am. J. Physiol., 227*:901–904, 1974.

Oscai, L., et al.: Effects of exercise and of food restriction on adipose tissue cellularity. *J. Lipid Res., 13*:588–592, 1972.

Smith, N. J. *Food for Sport.* Palo Alto, CA, Bull Publishing Co., 1976.

Tcheng, T. -K., and C. M. Tipton: Iowa wrestling study: anthropometric measurements and the prediction of a "minimal" body weight for high school wrestlers. *Med. Sci. Sports Exercise, 5(1)*:1–10, 1973.

Tipton, C. M., and T. -K. Tcheng: Iowa wrestling study. *J.A.M.A., 214(7)*:1269–1274, 1970.

Widerman, P. M., and R. D. Hagan: Body weight loss in a wrestler preparing for competition: a case report. *Med. Sci. Sports Exercise, 14(6)*:413–418, 1982.

Wilmore, J. H.: Body composition in sport and exercise: directions for future research. *Med. Sci. Sports Exercise, 15(1)*:21–31, 1983.

12

Dehydration, Heat Problems, and Prevention of Heat Illness

Introduction

Performing in the heat involves problems that can be more serious than the immediate discomfort that the athlete and coach alike may feel. For instance, sweating will cool the body in the heat but can result in the loss of too much water, or dehydration. Even if water is provided in abundance, certain activities are almost inevitably risky in the heat—football and distance running in particular. Recognizing when activities must be limited or halted

314

is a critical responsibility of the coach (and the athlete). If the coach and player are not aware that a hot and/or humid environment can cause heat illness, the consequences can be life-threatening. Given the seriousness of heat illness, this chapter is devoted entirely to the handling of this problem and its many components (environmental factors, bodily adjustments, clothing, etc.).

Dehydration (Water Loss)

During heavy physical activity, particularly on hot and/or humid days, large quantities of water and some salt are lost by the body through sweating. Dehydration and heat illness may result if they are not replaced within a 24-hr period. Although replacement of lost water is by far the more serious requirement, the uninformed person is concerned more with the taking of salt tablets (to replace salt) than with the drinking of water. This is a very poor health practice.

It is not unusual for athletes to lose 5 to 15 lb of water (1 lb equals 1 pint of water) during physical activity over a period of 1½ to 2 hr. The wide range in how much can be lost is attributable to variations in environmental temperature, relative humidity, the duration of the exercise, the athletes' clothing, and the intensity of the activity. For example, in a not overly demanding practice session, football players may lose an average of 5 lb of water (5 pints). On a hot, humid day, some players may lose as much as 20 lb of water—equivalent to 2.5 gallons. For a player weighing 200 lb, this would represent a loss of 10% of the body weight! In this case, health may be seriously jeopardized, for a water loss of just 3% of the total body weight may significantly diminish exercise performance and provoke heat illness.

Effects of Dehydration on Sports Performance

As pointed out in the last chapter, the physiological effects of dehydration are: (1) a reduction in muscular strength; (2) a decrease in work performance times (the athlete cannot work as long); (3) lower plasma and blood volumes; (4) a reduction in cardiac functioning during submaximal work conditions; (5) a lower oxygen consumption, especially when food restriction is also involved; (6) an impairment of thermoregulatory processes; (7) a decrease in renal blood flow and in the volume of fluid being filtered by the kidney; (8) a depletion of liver glycogen stores; and (9) an increase in the amount of electrolytes being lost from the body. Remember, some studies have shown that weight losses caused by dehydration of 3% or more result in diminished athletic performance. Furthermore, prolonged semi-starvation diets, unbalanced diets, and excessive sweating combined with dehydration may cause severe harm to the athlete.

Water Loss Versus Fat Loss

Water has no caloric value; therefore drinking water in large amounts **does not** result in obesity. Nor does loss of water play any role in the loss of body fat. Thus, deliberately causing excessive water loss through sweating for purposes of losing weight is uncalled for. Such a practice is in fact very hazardous; persons who garb themselves in sweatsuits, rubber jackets, and other similar clothing on hot days run the risk of serious heat illness and other health problems. They may think they are "melting off" pounds, but this has nothing to do with real weight loss. Real weight loss is the loss of body fat, and **body fat does not melt.** As previously indicated, it is increased physical activity that aids in the loss of body fat—a loss that takes place over a considerable period of time. Remember, the single most important aspect of loss of body fat is this: **caloric intake (calories due to food) must be less than caloric output (energy spent during activity).**

The Body-Weight Chart

The thirst mechanism—that is, the natural desire to drink water—is not always adequate to the task of replacing a sufficient amount of fluid, particularly during day-to-day exposure to high environmental heat and/or humidity. Therefore, continued measurements of daily body weight (which mainly reflect water loss) should be taken. The body weight should be recorded before and after practice or training so that possible excessive water loss may be detected. A 3% weight (water) deficit is cause for concern if it is not made up in a 24- to 48-hr period. Figure 12–1 contains an example of a chart that may be used for measuring weight as needed (instructions for using the chart are included in the figure).

As an example of how to use the body-weight chart, suppose that a football player weighed 215 lb prior to the morning practice. After practice he weighed 200 lb, a loss of water equaling 7% of his body weight. During weigh-in prior to the afternoon practice, he weighed 210 lb. Since this is within 3% of his original morning weight, he should be able to safely participate in the afternoon practice session. However, if he were not within the 3%-limit, his afternoon practice should be postponed or at least limited.

Environmental Heat Problems in Athletics

Heat problems in athletics are not uncommon; there is a possibility of heat illness occurring in football and several other sports, such as long-distance running, tennis, and as pointed out in the last chapter, wrestling.

Football

Prior to 1972, about five deaths per year occurred among young men playing or practicing football under conditions of high environmental

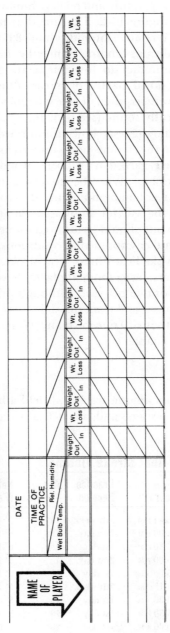

WEIGHT CHART

For Prevention of Heat Illness in Football Players

NAME OF
SCHOOL _____

YEAR _____

"Weight chart adapted from chart prepared by Joint Advisory Committee on Sports Medicine, Ohio State Medical Association and the Ohio High School Athletic Association, 17 South High Street, Columbus, Ohio 43215."

USE OF PSYCHROMETER TO RECORD TEMPERATURE AND HUMIDITY ON THE FOOTBALL FIELD

The wet bulb reading is an accurate method of determining environmental conditions which would predispose football players to problems with heat. The dry bulb and wet bulb temperatures are measured by using a sling psychrometer. This is an instrument used for measuring relative humidity in the atmosphere. Its operation depends upon the comparative readings of two similar thermometers, with the bulb of one being kept wet so that it is cooled as a result of evaporation. It always shows a temperature equal to or lower than that of the dry bulb thermometer. The difference between the thermometer readings constitutes a measure of the dryness or wetness of the surrounding air. The relative humidity is calculated from the difference between the dry and wet bulb readings.

TECHNIQUE

At the beginning and one hour into each practice, a coach or trainer should sling the psychrometer for 1½ minutes after dipping wick in distilled water. The wet bulb readings should be taken and recorded. Also record relative humidity.

PROCEDURES TO BE FOLLOWED

BEFORE PRACTICE

1. Assign a trainer or manager to regularly maintain this chart.

2. Post chart on Locker Room wall near shower.

3. Place scales near the chart.

4. Weigh each player before practice in T shirt and shorts.

5. Record weight in "out" section under day's practice. (If there are 2-a-day practices use 2 spaces.)

DURING PRACTICE

6. Measure wet bulb temperature and relative humidity by means of a sling psychrometer and record at beginning of practice and one hour later.

7. Record wet bulb temperature and relative humidity on chart.

8. Inform coach of condition which should be observed on the field. (See Wet Bulb Chart)

AFTER PRACTICE

9. Weigh each player after practice and record in "in" space.

10. Record weight loss for each practice session for each player.

11. Inform coach of all players with any significant weight loss.
    120 # -150 # — 4 #   180 # -210 # — 6 #
    150 # -180 # — 5 #   over 210 # — 7 #

12. Have water, salt tablets or replacement solutions available.

Figure 12-1 Example of a weight chart including instructions for its use. (Modified from Murphy, 1979.)

temperature and/or humidity. Information about nine of these deaths is assembled in Table 12-1. All players were interior linemen, and seven of the nine were stricken during the first two days of practice. All were clothed in full football equipment. The temperature and relative humidity at the time of the fatalities are indicated in Figure 12-2. The line drawn from 100% relative humidity and 60°F to 40% relative humidity and 89°F indicates that the deaths occurred under conditions ranging from either high temperature (dry bulb) and low relative humidity to low temperature and high relative humidity. It should also be noted that five of the casualties were not permitted water during practice but were required to take salt tablets, a practice which is far from being physiologically sound (see p. 320).

This shocking statistic suggests how uninformed some coaches apparently were with regard to the circumstances underlying heat illness. In one instance, a 15-year-old athlete, garbed in a rubber suit and, over this, a football uniform, was ordered to run laps. When he attempted this, he collapsed and died of heat stroke. The player had been instructed to run laps as a means of losing weight. This is not the way for an overweight athlete to lose weight (fat). More to the point, no one should be allowed (or be advised) to exercise excessively under hot, humid environmental conditions, and/or in a rubber suit, because this may provoke heat illness, heat stroke, and death.

During the past few years, fewer football players have died of heat stroke; fatalities now number one or two per year. Although this decrease in deaths indicates that coaches, trainers, and team physicians are now more aware of heat problems, a single death is still one too many. Heat stroke is preventable, as we will see later in this chapter.

Other Sports

Heat illness also occurs among track-and-field athletes, long-distance runners, tennis players, wrestlers, and, in fact, anyone performing heavy

Table 12-1: Description of Heat Stroke Victims

Position	Date	Hour	Practice Session	Age (Years)	Height (Feet, Inches)	Weight (Pounds)
Guard-tackle (1)*	9/25/61	2-4 P.M.	5th week	17	5′ 11″	190
Tackle (2)	8/21/59	4:00 P.M.	2nd day	16	6′ 1″	185
Tackle (3)	8/29/60	3:30 P.M.	1st day	15	6′ 1″	180
Guard (4)	8/27/62	5:00 P.M.	2nd day	15	5′ 10″	165
Tackle (5)	8/22/62	10:00 A.M.	1st day	15	6′ 1-1/2″	244
Tackle (6)	10/8/62	4:15 P.M.	7th week	15	5′ 10″	190
Guard (7)	8/20/59	10:00 A.M.	1st day	15	5′ 8″	180
Guard (8)	9/1/62	5:50 P.M.	1st day	19	5′ 11″	190
Center (9)	9/2/62	10:00 A.M.	1st day	20	6′ 0″	200

*The numbers in parenthesis correspond to the circled numbers in Figure 12-2.

From Fox, E. L., et al.: Effects of football equipment on thermal balance and energy cost during exercise. *Res. Quart.*, 37:332-339, 1966.

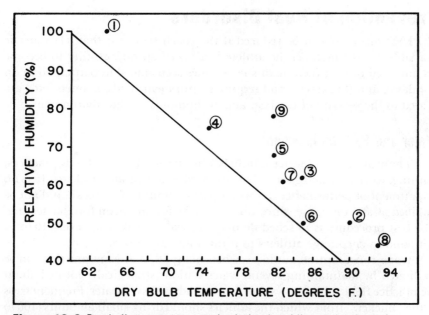

Figure 12-2 Dry bulb temperature and relative humidity at the time of heat stroke fatality. Note football casualty number one occurred at a temperature of 64° F and relative humidity of 100%. Although the temperature was low,heat could not be lost through evaporation because the atmosphere was saturated with water vapor. (Fox, E. L., et al.: Effects of football equipment on thermal balance and energy cost during exercise. *Res. Quart., 37*:332–339, 1966.)

exercise in the heat. Some athletes have recognized that the heat can in some cases pose very real dangers. When the weather for the marathon race in the 1956 Olympic Games turned out to be hot (85°F) and humid, Emil Zatopek, the former great Czechoslovakian runner, was reported to have said, "Today we die!" It is not surprising that a French Algerian, who was heat-acclimatized, won that particular marathon race.

Unfortunately, not all athletes are sufficiently wary of the effects of heat. It has been reported, for instance, that a college wrestler left alone in a "sweat box" nearly died (he was rescued by a janitor, who found him unconscious). Apparently, the wrestler was trying to lose weight in order to qualify for an upcoming away match. Unless he were a certain weight by the next morning, he would not make the trip. So, on his own, he went to the "sweat box." The fact that tragic consequences were avoided is scant argument against the conclusion that there is no place for such a device—in any sport. It must be hoped that more and more high school and college organizations will adopt in full the recommendations for safe and effective weight control set forth by the American College of Sports Medicine (these are presented on p. 310).

Prevention of Heat Disorders

Heat disorders can be reduced if the coach sees to it that: (1) water is available at all times; (2) the athlete is allowed an opportunity to become acclimatized to heat (i.e., he or she becomes accustomed to participation on hot days); and (3) exercise and required equipment (pads, helmets, etc.) are geared to the severity of the heat and/or humidity of the environment.

Water and Salt Replacement

The availability of water should be unrestricted during athletic practices, training, workouts, and games. The so-called superhydrated athlete suffers no impairment of performance. However, large amounts of water should not be imbibed at any one time, since this can make for an uncomfortable feeling. The best procedure is to schedule frequent water breaks (e.g., every 10 to 15 min) and to encourage athletes to drink water as needed.

Water consumption outdoors, where many athletic teams practice, can be facilitated by maintaining several water stations strategically located about the practice field. This allows the players ready access to water. Frequent trips to the "bucket," from which the athletes should drink small amounts (100 to 200 ml, or 3 to 6 oz), are ideal. This procedure is more physiologically sound than having a break every hour or so, during which the athlete might gulp copious amounts of water. It also allows for more efficient use of practice time. Ice-water buckets, pressure gardenspray containers, and thermos-type jugs can all be located for the athletes' convenience and can be adequately maintained.

A person normally consumes anywhere between 3 and 10 g of salt each day. This is more than adequate when we consider that the daily requirement for sodium is only 200 mg or 0.2 g! As was mentioned previously, some salt is lost through sweating, and when excessive, supplemental salt might be required.

There are basically two ways to supplement with salt: through the food you eat (diet), and by taking salt tablets. Probably the safest and best way is through the diet. In other words, during prolonged, excessive sweating, you should make an effort to salt your food a little more than you normally do. If this is done consistently, the salt lost in the sweat should be adequately replaced. Taking salt tablets is usually not necessary with most sports activities. Too often salt tablets are taken in excess and without drinking sufficient water. Such a practice can actually **promote** rather than prevent the possibility of serious heat injury. Provided extra salt (from the "shaker") is supplied during meals, salt tablets are not recommended for most athletes.

What the Athlete Should Drink

During competition and training in hot and/or humid weather, coaches and athletes should follow the "drinking" guidelines outlined in Table 12-2. Many liquids may be taken in to replace lost water and satisfy thirst, but what

Table 12-2: Guidelines for the Drinking Athlete*

Content of Drink

The drink should be
  hypotonic (few solid particles per unit of water)
  low in sugar content (less than 2.5 g per 100 ml of water)
  cold (roughly 45–55°F, or 8–13°C)
  palatable (it will be consumed in volumes ranging from 100
    to 400 ml, or 3 to 10 oz)

Amount to be Ingested before Competition

Drink 400–600 ml (13.5 to 20 oz) of water or the above drink 30
min before the start of competition.

Amount to be Ingested during Competition

During the competition, 100 to 200 ml (3 to 6.5 oz) of the above
drink should be taken at 10- to 15-min intervals throughout the
activity.

Postcompetition Diet

Following the competition, modest salting of foods and the
ingestion of drinks with essential minerals can adequately replace the electrolytes (sodium and potassium) lost in sweat.

Detection of Dehydration

The athlete should keep a record of his or her early morning
body weight (taken immediately after rising, after urination,
and before breakfast) to detect symptoms of a condition of
chronic dehydration.

Value of Drink(s)

Drinks are of significant value in races lasting more than 50 or
60 min.

*Text appearing beneath each underscored heading is from
Costill, D. L.: Fluids for athletic performance: Why and what you
should drink during prolonged exercise. In *The New Runners
Diet*. Mountain View, CA, World Publications, August, 1977.

is needed most is a drink that will provide for hydration without "lying in the stomach" for too long. A cold drink that is hypotonic and has a concentration of sugar below that which retards gastric emptying (see p. 281) is ideal. Contrary to popular belief, cold (45 to 55°F) drinks do not cause stomach cramps. Such cramps are probably related to the volume taken in rather than to temperature. Note that fluid replacement is of significant value mainly in activities lasting more than 50 to 60 min.

Acclimatization to Heat

The problems posed by heat obviously are compounded when an athlete must follow a heavy schedule of all-out training; in fact, it is during the first few days of such activity that most heat stroke deaths occur. There is, therefore, a need for an increase in the athlete's resistance to heat illness. Acclimatization to the heat will provide such an increase, and will also improve physical performance during exercise in hot weather. As shown in Table 12-3, acclimatization improves the circulatory and sweating responses that dissipate heat, thus minimizing increases in skin and body temperatures.

A four- to eight-day program of progressively longer periods of exercise performed in the heat should induce acclimatization. Workouts must occur in the heat for the athlete to become fully acclimatized. The program should begin one week prior to the start of regular practice, with the team's first "acclimatizing" workout consisting of a few minutes of exercise performed in light clothing (shorts). On each succeeding day, 10 to 20 min should be added to the workout. Some states have legislated a mandatory week of such workouts prior to the regular practice schedule for many sports. Such action on the part of these state athletic associations is to be commended, for not only does acclimatization take place but the athletes gain valuable conditioning as well.

In those states where such programs are not in existence, coaches (especially football coaches) should be strongly urged to construct an acclimatizing plan, one that could perhaps be administered by the team captains. For football, the Big Ten Conference has designed a three-day-long acclimatization program in which no equipment is permitted (i.e., no pads, helmets, etc.). It is hoped that all state athletic associations will eventually

Table 12-3: Changes Produced by Heat Acclimatization

System Affected	Change Due to Acclimatization
Circulation	
Heart rate	Decreased
Skin blood flow	Decreased
Muscle blood flow	Increased
Blood volume	Increased (sometimes)
Blood pressure	Adequately maintained
Evaporative Cooling (Sweating)	
Sweat production	Increased
Evaporation of sweat	Increased
Salt lost in sweat	Decreased
Central Nervous System	
Level of consciousness	Made more resistant to dizziness, nausea, discomfort, and syncope (fainting)
Heat-Regulating Systems	
Skin temperature and core (rectal) temperature	Both decreased, but there is no change in overall metabolism

consider requiring a week of heat acclimatization prior to the usual first week of practice for all outdoor sports. During the first few days of acclimatization, no equipment should be permitted; at no time during the week, or thereafter, should "sweat gear" be allowed. Of course, adequate water should always be available; withholding water retards the acclimatization process.

An example of an acclimatization schedule designed for football (and adaptable to other sports) is given in Table 12-4. Within a five-day period that begins with light exercise performed in shorts, acclimatization is induced by gradually increasing the intensity of exercise, the amount of equipment that is worn, and the length of practice time. In the latter regard, going from an initial hour-long session to a 2-hr session in the course of the five days is recommended, with variation and relief possibly provided by 5- to 10-min breaks for every 20 min of practice.

Clothing

Regardless of how well heat-acclimatized or hydrated athletes are, they may still suffer heat illness if they wear clothing and/or protective equipment that prevents evaporative cooling. Without sufficient exposure of the body surface area, sweat cannot evaporate from the skin, and heat will not dissipate (the body will not be cooled). Dissipation of heat is particularly hindered in football players, for the padding of the football uniform covers 50% of the body. If the environmental conditions are severe or the work load heavy, the football uniform has the potential of seriously limiting the heat loss provided by evaporative cooling.

The magnitude of the heat loss limit imposed by the football uniform is shown in Figure 12-3. In this study, nine men ran on a treadmill for 30 min at 9.6 km/hr (6 mph) under three conditions: (1) in shorts only; (2) in a football uniform; and (3) in shorts plus a backpack weighing the same as the uniform (13 lb). The temperature of the room for all runs was only 23.9° C (78° F), with a relative humidity of 35%—in other words, a normally comfortable situation. As shown in Figure 12-3A, the increase in rectal temperature while wearing the uniform was 1.5 times greater (average, 39.0° C) than when only shorts were worn.

The weight of the uniform alone, as shown by the increase in rectal temperature while carrying the pack, was as important a factor as was the

Table 12-4: Sample Heat Acclimatizations Schedule for Football and Other Sports

Requirement	Day 1	Day 2	Day 3	Day 4	Day 5
Time (minutes)	60	80	100	119	120
Uniform	Shorts	Shorts	Pants	Pants and helmet	Full
Workout	Calisthenics and jogging	Calisthenics and sprints	Drills and sprints	Drills and sprints	Full practice

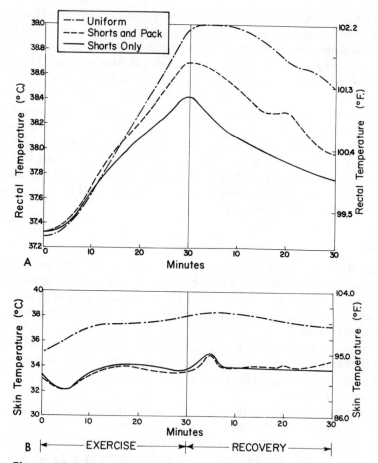

Figure 12-3 The effects of football uniform on rectal and skin temperatures during 30 min of running at 6 mi per hour. A, the uniform retards heat loss, causing rectal temperature to climb during exercise and remain elevated during recovery. B, Skin temperatures while wearing the uniform also rise considerably owing to reduction in evaporative cooling. Environmental conditions were 78°F and 35% relative humidity. (Adapted from Mathews, Fox, and Tanzi, 1969.)

heat-loss barrier imposed by the clothing and protective pads of the uniform. The heat-loss barrier of the uniform showed its effect by the excessively high skin temperatures of those areas covered by both pads and clothing, compared with conditions obtained by shorts and shorts plus pack (Fig. 12-3B). In other words, the uniform prevented the evaporation of sweat, greatly impairing body cooling. Concomitant with this was a twofold greater loss of body water because of profuse sweating and a significantly higher heart rate of circulatory strain—both of which reduce tolerance to heat.

Perhaps even more startling was the slow return of rectal temperature during recovery in the uniform, as compared with the other conditions. This is an extremely important point to remember. For example, a 16-year-old boy reported to his first football practice on a hot day and was required to wear a complete uniform. After a period of time, he felt ill. The coach placed him in the shade but did not remove his uniform; practice was then resumed and the boy was left unattended. About 2 hr later the boy was found unconscious. He was then taken to the hospital, where he died of heat stroke.

Obviously the coach must ensure that the uniform can be tolerated. The jersey, for instance, should be short-sleeved and made of light-weight netted material. Any taping over exposed skin must be conservative. The players themselves can help increase the extent of the body surface from which sweat can evaporate: during rest periods, each athlete should take off his helmet, raise the jersey to expose the skin of the abdominal area, roll down his socks, and so on.

Athletes and coaches in other sports should act on the principle underlying all the measures cited above: the less body covering, the more evaporative cooling that takes place. No player or coach should choose clothing that is intended to cut off evaporative cooling. Wearing such clothing, particularly a rubberized suit, raises the body temperature and increases the tendency toward heat illness, along with causing excessive stress on the cardiovascular system. There is absolutely no place for rubberized suits in athletics.

Assessment of Environmental Heat Stress

Perhaps the simplest measurement of environmental heat stress is the **wet-bulb temperature (WBT)**. The WBT is obtained by first wetting a wick wrapped around the bulb of a thermometer and then determining the effects of evaporation of moisture in the wick on the thermometer's temperature reading. The thermometer used in this assessment is called a wet-bulb thermometer. Together with a regular (dry-bulb) thermometer, it is contained in a device called a sling psychrometer, which is used to produce evaporation. Actual measurement of the WBT involves dipping the wick of the wet-bulb thermometer into water, after which the psychrometer housing the thermometer (see Fig. 12-4) is spun by its handle for 1½ min (a process known as "slinging"). As the water in the wick evaporates, the bulb of the thermometer is cooled, just as your skin is cooled when sweat evaporates. The amount of evaporation depends upon wind currents and, more importantly, the amount of water vapor in the air. Therefore, a high wet-bulb temperature would reflect considerable moisture in the air (little evaporation possible), whereas a low wet-bulb temperature would reflect little moisture (a high rate of evaporation possible). The wet-bulb temperature never exceeds the dry-bulb temperature; when they are equal, the air is completely saturated with water vapor (relative humidity = 100%), and no evaporation is possible.

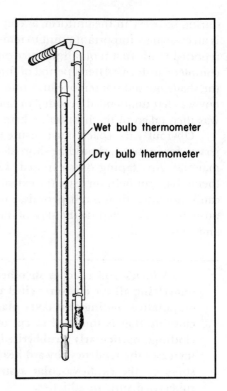

Figure 12-4 The sling psychrometer for assessment of environmental heat stress. The psychrometer contains a dry bulb thermometer and a wet bulb thermometer; with these, the temperature and the relative humidity of air may be measured.

Wet bulb thermometer
Dry bulb thermometer

The WBT Index

The following wet-bulb temperatures have been suggested by Murphy and Ashe (1965) as guides to the degree of environmental stress on persons wearing heavy, protective clothing such as a football uniform:

Wet-bulb Temperature	Precautions
less than 60° F	No precaution necessary.
61 to 66° F	Alert observation of all squad members, particularly those who lose considerable weight.
67 to 72° F	Insist water be given on field.
73 to 77° F	Alter practice schedule to provide rest periods every 30 min, in addition to above precautions.
78°F or higher	Practice postponed or conducted in shorts.

The Wet-bulb Globe Temperature

The **wet-bulb globe temperature (WBGT)** consists of: (1) ordinary air temperature (measured with a dry-bulb thermometer); (2) temperature as affected by wind and humidity (measured with a wet-bulb thermometer); and

(3) temperature as affected by radiant heat from the sun (measured with a black-globe thermometer). Figure 12–5 shows the combination of thermometers used to take the WBGT. The assembly shown is inexpensive; the black-globe thermometer, for instance, consists of an ordinary thermometer, the bulb of which is placed inside a copper toilet float painted black.

The assembled device is placed in the open, away from trees, buildings, or other objects that cast shadows or influence air movement. Readings should not be made for at least 30 min after the unit is in place. To compute the WBGT, the following formula is used:

$$WBGT (°F) = (0.7 \times wb) + (0.2 \times bg) + (0.1 \times db)$$
$$\text{where wb} = \text{wet-bulb temperature}$$
$$\text{bg} = \text{black-globe temperature (radiant energy)}$$
$$\text{db} = \text{dry-bulb temperature}$$

If, for example, the wet-bulb temperature is 75°F, the black-globe temperature is 110°F, and the dry-bulb temperature is 85°F, then:

$$WBGT = (75 \times .7) + (110 \times .2) + (85 \times .1) = 83° \text{ F}$$

A wet-bulb-globe temperature of 83°F is quite high. It falls in the upper range of the WBGT Index, which, like the WBT Index, is designed to identify conditions of heat stress. (Specifically, the WBGT Index was developed by the armed forces for use in determining stress on unconditioned trainees

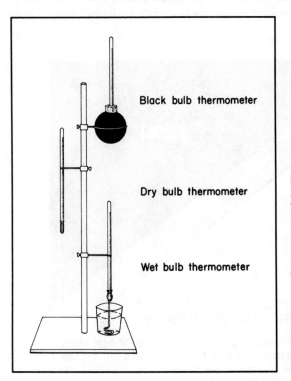

Black bulb thermometer

Dry bulb thermometer

Wet bulb thermometer

Figure 12-5 An example of an instrument incorporating the three thermometers that yield the measurements needed to calculate the wet bulb globe temperature (WBGT). The black bulb or globe thermometer measures solar radiation (radiant heat); the dry bulb thermometer measures air temperature; and the wet bulb thermometer measures humidity (expressed as the wet bulb temperature).

participating in physical activity while wearing army fatigues; the standards derived by the armed forces are widely applicable to many aspects of sports.) The portion of the WBGT Index listing the temperatures at which heat stress is the strongest threat is presented below, along with precautions to take at such temperatures. These precautions apply to tennis, track and field, soccer, field hockey, training workouts, and those activities in which heavy protective clothing is not a problem.

WBGT	Precautions
80 to 85° F	Caution; frequent water breaks; alert to heat illness symptoms.
85 to 88° F	Activity for nonconditioned and unacclimatized personnel suspended. Very limited activity for those conditioned and used to working in heat (acclimatized). Frequent water breaks.
Greater than 88° F	Activity for all personnel suspended.

The Football Weather Guide

The football weather guide shown in Figure 12-6 was constructed from the weather data gathered at the time of the heat stroke fatalities shown in Figure 12-2. Note that any combination of environmental conditions in Zone

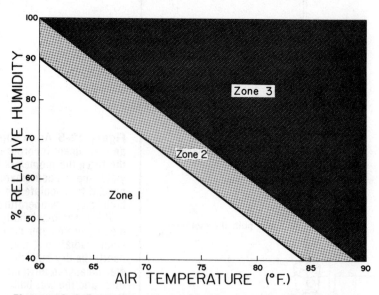

Figure 12-6 Football weather guide for prevention of heat illness. The combination of relative humidity and air temperature in Zone 1 can be considered safe; in Zone 2, use caution; and in Zone 3, use extreme caution when working in a football uniform.

1 would be considered safe. Under conditions obtained in Zone 2, all players should be carefully observed for symptoms of heat illness, for example, nausea, profuse sweating, lack of good color, headache, and lack of coordination. When conditions meet those of Zone 3, practice should be postponed, or only moderately light workouts in shorts should be permitted. Unacclimatized players should be closely observed for the symptoms previously mentioned. Note that all the heat stroke fatalities plus the marine survivors referred to earlier occurred in this zone. It should be mentioned that the marines were wearing the usual fatigue uniforms and were engaged in heavy exercise.

Guidelines for Distance Running

The need to assess environmental conditions—and to take appropriate measures when conditions are severe—is perhaps most pressing in distance running. Recognizing the necessity of preventing heat illness during distance running, the American College of Sports Medicine has issued the following position statement:

Guidelines for Distance Running

"Distance races (16 km, or 10 miles) should not be conducted when the wet-bulb globe temperature exceeds 82.4° F (28.0° C).

"During periods of the year when the daylight dry-bulb temperature often exceeds 80° F (27° C), distance races should be conducted before 9 A.M. or after 4 P.M.

"It is the responsibility of the race sponsors to provide fluids which contain small amounts of sugar (less than 2.5 g of glucose per 100 ml of water) and electrolytes (less than 10 milliequivalents or 230 mg of sodium and 5 milliequivalents or 195 mg of potassium per liter of solution).

"Runners should be encouraged to frequently ingest fluids during competition and to consume 400 to 500 ml (13 to 17 oz) of fluid 10 to 15 min before competition.

"Rules prohibiting the administration of fluids during the first 6.2 miles (10 km) of a marathon race should be amended to permit fluid ingestion at frequent intervals along the race course. In light of the high sweat rates and body temperatures during distance running in the heat, race sponsors should provide 'water stations' at 2- to 2½-mile (3- to 4-km) intervals for all races of 10 miles (16 km) or more.

"Runners should be instructed in how to recognize the early warning symptoms that precede heat injury. Recognition of symptoms, cessation of running, and proper treatment can prevent heat injury. Early warning symptoms include the following: piloerection [the hair stands on end] on chest and arms; chilling; throbbing pressure in the head; unsteadiness; nausea; and dry skin.

"Race sponsors should make prior arrangements with medical personnel for the care of cases of heat injury. Responsible and informed personnel should supervise each 'feeding station.' Organizational personnel should reserve the right to stop runners who exhibit clear signs of heat stroke or heat exhaustion."

What to Do When Heat Illness Is Present

All coaches and athletes should be familiar with the symptoms of heat illness, either on an overall basis or on the basis of type of illness, as in Table 12-5. Heat cramps, heat exhaustion, and heat stroke are all emergencies. The first two may not appear to be life-threatening, but remember that they may progress to heat stroke, the most dangerous heat illness. The danger lies in failure of the sweating mechanism: the affected person's skin is, in fact, dry to the touch and, of course, warm. Body temperature rises rapidly in the heat stroke victim; when the temperature exceeds 105°F, irreversible changes may occur. Heat stroke should be recognized from earlier signs than these (signs suggestive more of impaired functioning of the central nervous system than of a breakdown in the sweating mechanism): headache, confusion, staggering gait, and subsequent unconsciousness. Whatever the specific signs, if they indicate heat illness (heat stroke or otherwise), immediate treatment is called for:

Emergency Treatment for Heat Stroke

Remove all the victim's clothing at once.

Provide immediate cooling by whatever means are available (e.g., garden hose, containers of ice water, or cold shower).

Summon an emergency vehicle and notify the hospital of a possible heat casualty.

While en route to the hospital, use sponges or towels to apply ice water continuously and generously to the victim.

Ideally, there will never be a need to carry out these steps. However, if a problem should exist, a prearranged and printed plan for prompt emergency

Table 12-5: Heat Illnesses and Their Symptoms

Heat Illness	Symptoms
Heat cramps	Muscle spasms (cramps); heavy sweating; fatigue; normal body temperature.
Heat exhaustion	Extreme weakness; exhaustion; headache; dizziness; nausea; profuse sweating; cool skin; normal body temperature; rapid pulse; sometimes unconsciousness.
Heat stroke	No sweating; hot, dry skin; headache; nausea; confusion; staggering gait; extremely high body temperature; collapse; unconsciousness; sometimes death.

care and medical assistance, regardless of the illness or injury, should be available. This includes immediate access to a phone. In addition, assistants who are familiar with emergency procedures that have been well thought out and rehearsed should be present.

A Guide to Fluid Replacement

The convenience of having a guide to fluid replacement available at one's fingertips is obvious. Such a guide is shown in Figure 12-7. This ten-point

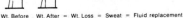

1 ACCLIMATIZATION — GETTING YOUR MEN IN CONDITION

Get your athlete in condition by getting him used to working in heat. Start with light exercise in gym shorts and gradually increase workout time and clothing to full uniform over a 5 day period. Workout sessions starting with 1 hour and working up to 2 hours in 5 days is recommended. Consider 10 minute breaks every 20 minutes of workout.

Day	1	2	3	4	5
Time in Minutes	60	80	100	110	120
Gear	Shorts	Shorts	Pants	Pants & Helmet	Full Gear
Workout	Calisthenics & Jogging	Calis. & Sprints	Sprints & Drills	Sprints & Drills	Practice

2 WEIGHT CHARTS — KEY TO GOOD TRAINING PRACTICE

The weight charts are prepared to help you in your work. Set up a procedure of lining up your men for weigh-in and weigh-out before and after practice or workout. The difference in weight is the athlete's loss of sweat. Replacement of fluid loss is important. Replacement is necessary for performance. At least 80% replacement must be achieved before next practice session.

Wt. Before — Wt. After = Wt. Loss = Sweat = Fluid replacement needed.

3 WEIGHT LOSS CHECK — FOCUS ON REHYDRATION NEED

The weight loss check is a convenient, reliable way of keeping tabs on the athlete's rehydration needs. If an athlete is given adequate access to fluids (Gatorade thirst quencher, water) by providing water breaks and encouraged to drink, he may be able to diminish his dehydration and replenish his fluid requirements. Such athletes will not show large losses in weight. If an athlete's weight loss is high, then his rehydration needs are great and should be satisfied. It is better to drink frequently, replace the fluid needed gradually, and maintain maximum rehydration throughout practice workout and game performance.

4 WATER REPLACEMENT — MAJOR INGREDIENT OF SWEAT

What goes out as sweat must be put back in the form of a fluid replacement. Since sweating helps to keep our body temperature from becoming excessive, it is in line to least, to minimize body temperature rise. Rehydrating the body of fluid lost is one of the best ways of insuring a continued cycle of performance. Rehydration must be encouraged — fluid replacement made available to make up for the fluid lost in sweat.

5 SALT REPLACEMENT — THE OTHER INGREDIENTS OF SWEAT

Along with water, when one sweats one loses electrolytes and body salts, primarily sodium chloride. In rehydrating the athlete with the water lost, we must replenish the lost salts as well. Gatorade has been formulated to supply those body salts in their proper ratios with respect to water and rehydration. If you drink water, however, make certain you use the proper ratio of water to salt tablets in order to keep the concentrations in balance. It is easier to stick to Gatorade and have the properly prepared, physiologically sound fluid replacement for your needs. No salt tablets should be used if one is drinking Gatorade.

6 WORK-HEAT RELATIONSHIP — ELEMENTARY BUT BASIC FACTS

Work produces heat and increases body temperature. If we were not able to lose the heat produced, our body temperature could go from 98.6°F (normal body temperature) to as high as 114°F (fatal to humans) in one hour. Fortunately, our body has a built-in temperature regulator and control. Our body sweats, loses water and salts and cools the skin while evaporation is taking place. Under normal conditions this cycle and regulation is adequate. In periods of heavy work and/or heavy uniform and insulation, the regulation system needs a helping hand to be able to maintain reasonable temperature control. The properly hydrated athlete in top shape is able to perform to his capacity. Remember that even a 3% weight loss is sufficient to show up significant performance loss. The percent weight loss can easily be calculated.

$$\frac{\text{Wt. loss of athlete}}{\text{Wt. before workout}} \times 100 = \text{Percent wt. loss.}$$

If you want the athlete's best performance, keep a sharp lookout on his heat-work relationship. Give him fluid replacement to help keep that temperature in control. Rehydrate him continually.

7 WEATHER EFFECTS — THE OVERLOOKED FACTOR

Hot and humid days can materially contribute to taking the zing out of your athlete's performance. On such days, the dehydration of the athlete is greater. His chances of heat illness are greater and your needs for rehydration are more acute. Use of the wet bulb thermometer is a means of quickly determining what the conditions on the field during practice or a game. The sling psychrometer (about $15.00) may be purchased at any industrial supply company and assigned to a student manager, trainer or assistant coach. Careful observations of the wet bulb temperature and following the recommendations on the chart, can minimize dehydration. Frequent drinking breaks, fluid drinking encouragement, as well as allowing the body to dissipate heat, will be needed. The higher the temperature, the greater the humidity of the day, the greater is the degree of dehydration. Rehydrate your athletes — do it with Gatorade. It works.

8 DANGER SYMPTOMS — KEEP A SHARP LOOKOUT

They say an ounce of prevention is worth a pound of cure. A coach or trainer who is on the lookout for the danger signs will not only catch a situation before it becomes dangerous, but will also recognize that something must be corrected if it is producing such dangerous conditions. He then takes steps to correct the situation. Watch out for Muscle Cramps, Heat Exhaustion, Heat Stroke, Heat Fatigue and Sloppy Coordination. They all spell danger.

9 PROPER DRESS — EVERY LITTLE BIT HELPS

Particularly in football, the athlete is forced to wear heavy clothing which retards heat dissipation and acts as an insulator. Whenever and wherever it is possible, the body should be given a chance to throw off heat and become cooler. Clothing which can breathe and ventilate rather than insulate, can be helpful. Loosening the garments when not in action will help to cool. Keep using every means to bring your athlete close to normal body condition.

10 EMERGENCY MEASURES

If you practice good performance habits you will cut down on dangerous incidents. When an emergency occurs, however, be prepared to handle it with professional efficiency. Have a telephone handy. Give quick, effective treatment on the spot by cooling the body, removing clothing and applying cold applications such as a sponge, towel or bath in cold water or ice. Transport to a hospital immediately while applying the cold applications. Give the doctor the background information so that he can quickly anticipate what must be done. Even with all this, you must orient and teach all your personnel to carry out such a program when the necessity arises.

Figure 12-7 The 10-Point Fluid Replacement Guide. (Courtesy of Stokely-Van Camp, Inc., P.O. Box 1113, Indianapolis, IN, 46206.)

fluid replacement guide, including emergency measures, is reproduced through the courtesy of Stokely-Van Camp, Inc. The chart itself, which is large and is printed in color, may be obtained free of charge by writing Stokely-Van Camp, Inc., PO Box 113, Indianapolis, IN 46206. It would appear wise to post such a chart in the locker or training facility for all participants, coaches, trainers, and athletes to study.

Summary

- During exercise in hot, humid weather, large quantities of water and some salt are lost by the body through sweating. Heat illness may result if lost water is not replaced within 24 hr.

- Wearing a rubber sweatsuit on a hot day will neither melt body fat nor cause fat to be lost in any other way. Only water (sweat) will be lost—at considerable risk to one's health.

- A water loss of just 3% of the total body weight may significantly diminish exercise performance and provoke heat illness.

- Deliberately causing excessive water loss through increased sweating for purposes of losing weight is a very hazardous practice. It does nothing but provoke serious heat illness and other health problems.

- Recording the body weight before and after practice enables one to detect possible excessive water loss.

- Heat problems in athletics are not uncommon, with the possibility of heat illness occurring in football, distance running, tennis, and wrestling.

- The football uniform has the potential of seriously limiting heat loss through evaporative cooling (sweating).

- The availability of water should be unrestricted during athletic practices and games. Water breaks should be scheduled every 10 to 15 min, with the drinking of small amounts (3 to 6 oz) encouraged.

- The safest and best way to supplement the salt lost through excessive sweating is through the diet. The taking of salt tablets is usually not necessary with most sports activities.

- Participants in activities lasting more than 50 to 60 min should imbibe a cold, low-sugar drink 30 min before—and every 10 to 15 min during—the activities.

- Heat acclimatization improves the circulatory and sweating responses that serve to dissipate heat, thus minimizing increases in skin and body temperatures.

- Acclimatization may be induced by means of a four- to eight-day conditioning program in which the work load becomes progressively greater and exercises are performed in the heat.

- Regardless of how well heat-acclimatized or hydrated athletes are, they may still suffer heat illness if their clothing and/or protective equipment prevents evaporative cooling.

- There is absolutely no place for rubberized sweatsuits in athletics.

- Environmental heat loads may be effectively assessed by consulting the football weather guide or by finding the wet-bulb temperature or the wet-bulb-globe temperature. The WBT Index or the WBGT Index may then be consulted as a guide to permissible activities in the heat.

- Heat injuries during distance running may be considerably reduced by following the guidelines set forth by the American College of Sports Medicine.

- Every coach and athlete should be able to recognize the symptoms of heat illness (heat stroke, heat exhaustion, and heat cramps). Whenever heat illness is suspected, emergency treatment should begin immediately.

Selected References and Readings*

American College of Sports Medicine. Position statement on prevention of heat injuries during distance running. *Med. Sci. Sports, 7(1)*:vii-ix, 1975.

Bass, D. E., et al.: Mechanisms of acclimatization to heat in man. *Medicine, 34*: 323, 1955.

Blyth, C. S., and J. J. Burt: Effect of water balance on ability to perform at high ambient temperatures. *Res. Quart., 32*:301-307, 1961.

Buskirk, E., and D. Bass. Climate and exercise. *In* Johnson, W., and E. Buskirk (eds.): *Science and Medicine of Exercise and Sports*. 2nd ed. New York, Harper and Row Publishers, 1974, pp. 190-205.

Buskirk, E. R., P. F. Iampietro, and D. E. Bass: Work performance and dehydration: Effects of pysical condition and heat acclimatization. *J. Appl. Physiol., 12*:189-194, 1958.

Costill, D. L. Fluids for athletic performance: Why and what should you drink during prolonged exercise. In *The New Runners Diet*. Mountain View, CA, World Publications, August, 1977.

Craig, E. N., and E. G. Cummings: Dehydration and muscular work. *J. Appl. Physiol., 21*:670-674, 1966.

Fox, E. L., and D. K. Mathews: *Interval Training: Conditioning for Sports and General Fitness*. Philadelphia, W. B. Saunders, 1974.

Fox, E. L., and D. K. Mathews: *The Physiological Basis of Physical Education and Athletics*. 3rd ed. Philadelphia, Saunders College Publishing, 1981.

Fox, E. L., et al.: Effects of football equipment on thermal balance and energy cost during exercise. *Res. Quart., 37*:332-339, 1966.

Gisolfi, C. V.: Work-heat tolerance derived from interval training. *J. Appl. Physiol., 35*:349-354, 1973.

Lind, A. R., and D. E. Bass: Optimal exposure time for development of acclimatization to heat. *Fed. Proc., 22*:704, 1963.

Mathews, D. K., E. L. Fox, and D. E. Tanzi: Physiological responses during exercise and recovery in a football uniform. *J. Appl. Physiol., 26*:611-615, 1969.

Minard, D., H. S. Belding, and J. R. Kingston: Prevention of heat casualties. *J.A.M.A., 165*:1813-1818, 1957.

Murphy, R. Heat injury. *In* Strauss, R. H. (ed.): *Sports Medicine and Physiology*. Philadelphia, W. B. Saunders, 1979, Chapter 21.

Murphy, R. J.: The problem of environmental heat in athletics. *Ohio State Med. J., 59*, No. 8, 1963.

Murphy, R. J., and W. F. Ashe: Prevention of heat illness in football players. *J.A.M.A., 194*:650-654, 1965.

---

*For full journal titles, see Appendix A.

Pitts, G. C., R. E. Johnson, and F. C. Consolazio: Work in the heat as affected by intake of water, salt, and glucose. Am. J. Physiol., 142:253–259, 1944.

Saltin, B.: Aerobic and anaerobic work capacity after dehydration. *J. Appl. Physiol., 19*:1114–1118, 1964.

Saltin, B.: Circulatory response to submaximal and maximal exercise after thermal dehydration. *J. Appl. Physiol., 19*:1125–1132, 1964.

Turner, H. S.: Environmental heat exposure and athletic competition. *J. Am. Coll. Health Assoc., 23(3)*:211–214, 1975.

13

Frequently Asked Questions Concerning Sports Performance and Physiology

Introduction

The main purpose of this chapter is to present answers to frequently asked questions relating to athletic performance and physiology. The answers, although abbreviated, contain pertinent information that may be directly applied by the coach and physical educator. For more detailed explanations, references to pages in text are provided at the end of each answer.

The questions have been classified according to subject as well as

335

possible. Generally, the subject areas follow the outline of the book. However, since many questions and answers include several different subjects, there is some overlapping. Therefore, if the desired question and answer cannot be found under one subject area, look for it under a related subject heading.

Questions Related to Human Energy Production

Question: How is energy defined?

Answer: Energy is the capacity to perform work. Work is the product of a force acting through a distance. Kinetic energy is associated with motion, such as a swinging bat or club. Potential energy is energy by virtue of position, such as in a bent bow. Chemical energy is potential energy, such as in the foods we eat. (For further discussion, see p. 10.)

Question: What is a calorie or kilocalorie?

Answer: These are units of measure of energy. A calorie is the amount of heat energy required to raise the temperature of 1 g of water 1° Celsius (°C). The kilocalorie (kcal) is equal to 1000 calories. (For further discussion, see p. 10.)

Question: What is ATP?

Answer: Adenosine triphosphate (ATP) is the immediately usable form of chemical energy for muscular activity; it is stored in all muscle cells. The energy needed to synthesize ATP comes from energy released during the breakdown of foods and other chemicals in the body. The coupling of energy release and energy usage—a system called coupled reactions—is the fundamental principle involved in the metabolic production of ATP. (For further discussion, see pp. (11–13.)

Question: What is meant by aerobic and anaerobic metabolism?

Answer: The term metabolism refers to the various series of chemical reactions that take place within the body in making ATP. Aerobic means in the presence of oxygen, whereas anaerobic refers to without oxygen. Therefore, aerobic metabolism refers to a series of chemical reactions whereby ATP is synthesized that requires the presence of oxygen. Anaerobic metabolism means just the opposite—a series of chemical reactions that does not require the presence of oxygen. (For further discussion, see pp. 13–14.)

Question: Which sports activities primarily depend on aerobic metabolism for their source of ATP energy?

Answer: The oxygen or aerobic system utilizes both glycogen and fats as fuels for ATP resynthesis. By chemical reactions that take place in the mitochondria of the cells, the aerobic system yields large amounts of ATP but no fatiguing by-products. Therefore, the aerobic system is used predominantly during endurance tasks or low-power-output activities. (For further discussion, see pp. 16–22, 26–37.)

Question: Which sports activities primarily depend on anaerobic metabolism for their source of ATP energy?

Answer: First, there are two anaerobic systems. One, called the ATP-PC or Phosphagen system, resynthesizes ATP from energy released when phosphocreatine (PC) is broken down. It is a very rapid but limited source of ATP that is used predominantly during the performance of high-power, short-duration activities. Sprinting 100 m is a good example. The other anaerobic system is called the lactic acid system or anaerobic glycolysis. It resynthesizes ATP from energy released during the breakdown of glycogen (sugar) to lactic acid. Accumulation of the latter in the blood and muscles causes temporary muscular fatigue. This system, then, is used predominantly during activities that require between 1 and 3 min to perform. Running 800 m would be a good example. (For further discussion, see pp. 14–16, 26–37.)

Question: Which foods serve as the major fuel during exercise?

Answer: The primary food fuels for exercise are carbohydrate and fat. Overall, carbohydrate (glycogen and glucose) is probably the more important fuel. However, during prolonged endurance performances lasting several hours or more, fat is also important. It has been observed that muscular fatigue coincides with muscle glycogen depletion; thus, maintaining adequate muscle glycogen stores at all times is essential. (For further discussion, see pp. 40–55.)

Questions Related to Recovery from Exercise

Question: What is the oxygen debt and how does it relate to recovery from exercise?

Answer: Oxygen debt is defined as the amount of oxygen consumed during recovery from exercise above that which would have ordinarily been consumed at rest in the same time period. The concept of oxygen debt means the oxygen consumed above the resting level during recovery is primarily used to provide ATP energy for restoring the body to its pre-exercise condition. This means replenishing the depleted energy stores and removing any lactic acid accumulated during exercise. Actually, there are two components to the oxygen debt, a very rapid portion called the alactacid oxygen debt component and a much slower portion termed the lactacid oxygen debt component. (For further discussion, see pp. 59–60, 63–64, 79–80.)

Question: How much time is needed between performances for adequate recovery?

Answer: This depends on the kind of performance in question. Usually, for activities that are high in intensity but short in duration (e.g., sprinting), a recovery period of perhaps 1 hr or less will be satisfactory for a repeat performance. However, with prolonged endurance performances—for example, the marathon—several days of recovery may be required. Important factors in complete recovery are: (1) the replenishment of stores of phosphagen, oxymyoglobin, and muscle glycogen; and (2) the removal of lactic acid from the blood and muscles. Restoration of phosphagen and oxymyoglobin is rapid, but glycogen is slow to be replaced (see question and answer following). Removal of lactic acid is accomplished within 1 to 3 hr. (For further discussion, see pp. 60–68, 75–80.)

Question: How long does it take to replenish the stores of muscle glycogen?

Answer: That depends on what kind of exercise caused the depletion in the first place. For example, replenishment of muscle glycogen in an athlete recovering from prolonged, continuous exercise is complete within 46 hr, provided the athlete follows a high-carbohydrate diet during the recovery period. About 60% of the stores are replenished in the first 10 hr of recovery.

Replenishment of glycogen stores following short-term, high-intensity, intermittent exercise is complete within 24 hr (carbohydrate intake can be normal during recovery). In this case, about 45% of the stores are replenished in the first 5 hr of recovery. Also, independent of food intake, some glycogen replenishment takes place within 30 min of recovery from intermittent exercise. (For further discussion, see pp. 68–75.)

Question: What is "staleness?"

Answer: No one knows for sure, but is is probably related to or caused by chronic fatigue. In some sports, particularly distance running, chronic fatigue may result when stores of muscle glycogen are lowered over the course of several days of intensive endurance training. (Such a training schedule has been shown to drastically reduce the glycogen stores in the working musculature even when normal amounts of carbohydrates are consumed in the diet.)

Possible causes of staleness besides chronic fatigue may be related to psychological factors such as boredom, depression, and lack of interest. (For further discussion, see pp. 69–70.)

Question: What does a "warm-down" do physiologically?

Answer: Perhaps the single most important physiological effect of a warm-down is the rapid removal of lactic acid from the muscles and blood (without warm-down, lactic acid removal may take twice as long). Rapid removal of lactic acid may help reduce subsequent soreness and stiffness. (For further discussion, see pp. 75–77.)

Questions Related to Muscle Function and Weight Training

Question: What causes muscular soreness, and how may it be minimized?

Answer: Although muscular soreness can have many origins, one of the major causes appears to be damage to the connective tissue of the muscle. Such damage would account for the pronounced soreness that follows eccentric contractions, for these place the greatest tension on connective tissue. (Isokinetic contractions cause the least amount of soreness, apparently because the control of tension through a range of movement minimizes damage to connective tissue.) No sure-fire method of overcoming soreness is available, but adequate stretching appears to help not only the prevention of soreness but also the relief of it when present. Thus, adequate warm-up (along with gradually increasing the intensity of the exercises) should minimize muscular soreness. (For further discussion, see pp. 96–99.)

Question: What is the significance of the two basic kinds of motor units or muscle fibers with respect to sports performance?

Answer: First, it must be remembered that the two basic motor units or fiber types, fast-twitch (FT) and slow-twitch (ST), cannot be interconverted to any extent through any type of physical training program. So, we are more or less "stuck" genetically with a given fiber type distribution in our muscles. However, both FT and ST fibers can be increased in size and metabolic potential through proper training methods. For example, since FT fibers are preferentially used during short-term, high-intensity exercise and ST fibers during longer, less intense exercises, it follows that in order to improve a given fiber type, a specific kind of exercise must be used. In other words, to increase the size and metabolic potential of FT fibers, high-intensity exercises must be used; to increase the size and metabolic potential of ST fibers, exercises of lower intensity and longer duration must be used. In any athletic program, the exercises used during training must simulate as closely as possible those used in the sport for which the athlete is training. (For further discussion, see pp. 99–101, 108.)

Question: Do athletes whose sport requires high speeds of motion (e.g., sprinters, high-jumpers, shot-putters) have higher than normal percentages of FT units in the muscles involved in the motion?

Answer: Yes. It has been found that athletes who participate in and train for sprint-like activities have higher-than-normal percentages of FT fibers in their muscles. By the same token, athletes who participate in and train for endurance-like activities have higher-than-normal percentages of ST fibers in their muscles.

It should be mentioned, however, that the variability of fiber-type distribution in these athletes is quite large. For example, it is possible to have two athletes, one a marathoner, the other a sprinter, who have the same fiber-type distribution in their gastrocnemius muscles. (For further discussion, see pp. 103–104, 108–109.)

Question: Isn't fiber-type distribution mainly a function of genetics, and, if so, as a coach, what can I do about it?

Answer: It is true that fiber-type distribution is mainly a function of genetics. As a coach, you can do nothing about this. However, all coaches should seek to: (1) develop through training the full genetic potential of the athlete; and (2) give each athlete a chance to participate and compete in events or activities for which he or she is "genetically" best suited. If you as a coach are convinced that the athlete has in fact reached his or her full genetic potential through training, but the potential is not up to that required for success in a particular event, you should encourage the athlete to participate in other events. For example, the sprinter who trains extremely hard but seldom wins in competition should be encouraged to run in longer events, such as the mile, in which he or she may be more successful. (For further discussion, see pp. 108–109, 239–241.)

Question: What causes local muscular fatigue?

Answer: This is not an easy question to answer. However, it would appear that the site of local muscular fatigue is confined to the contractile mechanism, as opposed, for example, to the neuromuscular junction. The most probable cause of local muscular fatigue is the accumulation of lactic acid in the muscles and blood. Remember, this kind of fatigue would follow short-term, high-intensity types of exercise. Fatigue following endurance exercise is **not** caused by lactic acid accumulation; it is probably caused by several factors, such as depletion of the muscle glycogen stores, low blood glucose, liver glycogen depletion, loss of body water (dehydration), loss of body electrolytes (e.g., salt, potassium), high body temperature, and boredom. (For further discussion, see pp. 111–114.)

Question: Do weight-training programs help improve sports performance? Don't weight lifters become "muscle-bound" and suffer a loss of flexibility?

Answer: At present, there is substantial evidence that properly designed weight-training programs may help improve performance of many sports skills (some research results, it should be noted, conflict with this finding.) One thing is certain: weight lifting does not make trainees "muscle-bound" or cause them to lose flexibility. In fact, flexibility has consistently been shown to increase following weight-training programs. The term "muscle-bound" is a misnomer and has no scientific basis. Certainly muscles increase in size (undergo hypertrophy) as a consequence of weight training, but not to the point of limiting the range of motion about a joint. (For further discussion, see pp. 156–157.)

Question: What makes a muscle stronger?

Answer: The single most important change in a muscle in relation to its strength is an increase in size (diameter) of existing fibers. This is due to a greater number of myofibrils per fiber, more total protein, and an increase in the size and strength of connective, tendinous, and ligamentous tissues. This kind of increase in the size of muscle fibers is called hypertrophy. In some animal studies, an increase in the number of muscle fibers has been found following strength-training programs. Such an effect is called longitudinal fiber splitting and would, of course, also increase the size of the muscle, but no such fiber splitting has yet been found to occur in humans. (See pp. 124–125, 153–156.)

Question: Should athletes weight-train during their seasons?

Answer: This depends on their level of strength. If they are losing strength or need to gain strength during the season, weight-training sessions should be held at least twice per week. However, if the desired strength level has already been attained through the off-season and preseason programs, then maintenance of strength should require only one workout per week. (For further discussion, see pp. 151–153.)

Question: Is there one kind of weight-training program that is best for athletes? If so, what makes the program the best?

Answer: There are advantages and disadvantages to each of the four basic kinds of programs: isotonic, isometric, isokinetic, and eccentric. However, it would appear that isokinetic training programs are somewhat better than the other programs in promoting both muscular strength and muscular endurance. But it should be pointed out that the availability of isokinetic equipment is rather limited in comparison to the other methods. In addition, nearly all world-class, competitive lifters still use free weights (isotonics) as the method of choice for strength development. It is very possible that there may not be a single method that is best for all athletes. (For further discussion, see pp. 145–148.)

Question: Does it matter whether slow or fast isokinetic training is used?

Answer: Yes. Training at slow speeds of movement (24–36° of movement per sec) produces gains in force (strength) only at slow movement speeds, whereas training at fast speeds (greater than 100° of movement per sec) produces strength gains at all speeds of movement at and below the training speed. Therefore, training with fast speeds will ensure that: (1) greater force may be applied no matter at what speed it is being applied; and (2) greater speeds of movement will be possible no matter what degree of force is applied. (For further discussion, see pp. 141–144.)

Question: Can both muscular endurance and strength be gained from a single weight-resistance program?

Answer: Yes. It has been found that both strength and muscular endurance can be gained from a single program consisting of high-resistance and low-repetition loads. Generally, endurance can also be gained from low-resistance and high-repetition loads whereas strength cannot. (For further discussion, see pp. 153–157.)

Question: What is circuit training? Is it effective in preparing athletes for competition?

Answer: Circuit training consists of exercises carried out at a number of "stations," at each of which the athlete performs a given activity, usually within a specified time period. The activities consist mainly of weight-resistance exercises; however, running, swimming, cycling, calisthenics, and stretching exercises may also be included. Therefore, circuit training may be designed to increase muscular strength, muscular endurance, flexibility, and cardiorespiratory endurance—provided that running, swimming, cycling, or similar endurance activities are involved.

Circuit training may be recommended as an effective training technique, particularly for off-season programs, for athletes whose sports require high levels of muscular strength, power, and endurance, but lower levels of cardiorespiratory endurance. (For further discussion, see pp. 148–150.)

Question: Does the use of anabolic-androgenic steroids increase strength and muscle mass?

Answer: The practice of taking steroids does not always lead to increased muscular mass and strength. Such a practice may in fact constitute a serious health hazard for the user. Taking steroids for the sole purpose of improving athletic performance should **never** be sanctioned by any individual or athletic organization. (For further discussion, see pp. 157–159.)

Question: Do weight-training programs affect male and female athletes differently?

Answer: In general, no. However, it does appear that muscular hypertrophy in women is somewhat less pronounced than in men, even when their gains in relative strength are similar. The reason for this is not known, although testosterone, a male sex hormone, may be involved. Normally, the levels of testosterone are lower in women than in men. Incidentally, the so-called masculinizing effect of weight-training on women simply does not exist. (For further discussion, see pp. 150–151 and 155.)

Question: Do athletes have to weight-train every day in order to gain their desired level of strength?

Answer: No. Actually, weight training every day in conjunction with the other training demands of a given sport is not recommended. Chronic fatigue, which may develop under these conditions, will, in most cases, cause a noticeable decrease in performance. The recommended frequency of weight training is three days per week. (For further discussion, see pp. 131, 138 and 144.)

Question: Is is true that muscular strength may be significantly increased when isometric tension is held for 6 sec at two thirds of maximum strength once a day for five days per week?

Answer: Yes. However, it should be mentioned that several studies have shown that greater strength gains may be obtained by training five days per week using five to ten maximal contractions held for 5 sec each. (For further discussion, see pp. 135–140.)

Question: How long does it take for weight-training programs to produce noticeable gains in strength?

Answer: With just about any type of weight-resistance program, strength gains may be noticeable within four weeks of training when the training frequency is three times per week. Further strength gains will be observed as training goes on (e.g., at the end of eight weeks). (For further discussion, see pp. 131, 138, 144, and 147.)

Questions Related to the Oxygen Transport System

Question: Does pulmonary ventilation limit performance?

Answer: Not normally, at least not in healthy individuals. (For further discussion, see p. 165.)

Question: It is common to see pure oxygen being administered to professional athletes during time-outs and during rest breaks. Does this practice aid in recovery or performance?

Answer: The answer depends on whether the athletes are competing at sea level or at altitudes well above sea level. At sea level, the partial pressure of oxygen in the air is high enough to very nearly fully saturate hemoglobin with oxygen. Therefore, at sea level, it is not possible to combine significantly more oxygen with hemoglobin by raising the partial pressure through breathing pure oxygen. The small amount of additional oxygen that will actually be physically dissolved in plasma (less than 2 ml per 100 ml of blood) is helpful, but dissolved oxygen still only represents less than 10% of the total amount of oxygen carried by the blood. Research has shown that breathing 100% oxygen at sea level during time-outs and rest periods does not enhance recovery or performance.

On the other hand, at altitudes above sea level, where the partial pressure of oxygen in the air is reduced, breathing 100% oxygen will significantly increase the oxygen-carrying capacity of the blood. Under high-altitude conditions, supplemental oxygen during time-outs should aid the recovery and thus the performance of the athlete. (For further discussion, see pp. 173–174 and 194–196.)

Question: How does cigarette smoking affect performance?

Answer: Cigarette smoking limits performance, both by increasing the smoker's airway resistance and by decreasing the amount of oxygen that can be carried in the blood. Increased airway resistance is specifically the result of long-term smoking; if severe enough it can lead to decrements in endurance performance. (It is interesting to note that some of the added resistance caused by smoking can be noticeably reduced by abstinence from smoking for 24 hr prior to performance. Thus, endurance athletes who will not or cannot "kick the habit" may aid their performances by not smoking on the day of competition.)

As for reductions in the amount of oxygen that can be carried in the blood, this effect is produced by a by-product of cigarette smoke: carbon monoxide (CO). Carbon monoxide has a greater capacity for combining with hemoglobin than does oxygen. Therefore, when both CO and O_2 are present, as when a smoker inhales, carbon monoxide is quicker to combine with hemoglobin. Oxygen and carbon monoxide cannot be carried simultaneously by hemoglobin; as a result, the oxygen-carrying capacity of blood is reduced. (For further discussion, see pp. 167–168 and 174.)

Question: What is second wind? What are its causes?

Answer: Second wind usually involves a sudden transition from a feeling of distress or fatigue during the early portions of prolonged exercise to a more comfortable feeling later in the exercise. As the term itself suggests, respiratory adjustments are probably responsible for the transition to a feeling of comfort; additional causes of second wind might include the removal of lactic acid, adequate warm-up, relief from muscular fatigue, and psychological factors. (For further discussion, see p. 168.)

Question: What is a stitch in the side? What are its causes?

Answer: A stitch in the side is a sharp pain in the side or rib cage. It usually occurs early in exercise and generally subsides as exercise continues. In some individuals, the pain is so great that they must slow down or stop exercising altogether. The pain is thought to be related to a lack of oxygen in the diaphragm and intercostal muscles due to insufficient blood flow. How to prevent a stitch in the side from occurring remains as problematic as how to get rid of it once it appears. (For further discussion, see p. 169.)

Question: What exactly is blood doping?

Answer: Blood doping is the removal and subsequent reinfusion of blood, undertaken for the purpose of temporarily increasing blood volume and, most importantly, the number of red blood cells. Overloading the blood with red blood cells (which contain hemoglobin) should increase the oxygen-carrying capacity of the blood and, theoretically at least, lead to improved endurance performance. Although blood doping has been shown to improve endurance performance, no coach should recommend it. Blood doping is illegal in Olympic competition. (For further discussion, see pp. 174-176.)

Question: What is meant by the anaerobic threshold?

Answer: The anaerobic threshold is defined as that intensity of workload or oxygen consumption in which anaerobic metabolism (accumulation of lactic acid in the blood) is accelerated. It is much higher in endurance athletes than in other athletes or untrained individuals. The anaerobic threshold is an important physiological capacity for success in endurance performance. (For further discussion, see pp. 190-191.)

Question: How important is the maximal aerobic power ($\dot{V}O_2$max) to success in endurance performance?

Answer: The $\dot{V}O_2$max is actually one of three functional capabilities of the oxygen transport system that are important with respect to endurance performance (the other two are the anaerobic threshold and the efficiency of the oxygen transport system). There is generally a positive relationship between $\dot{V}O_2$max and endurance performance. However, among internationally prominent endurance athletes, such a relationship is not necessarily of a very high degree. In these individuals, a high anaerobic threshold might be more important. This idea is supported by the fact that Derek Clayton, one of the world's fastest marathoners, has only an average $\dot{V}O_2$max for a marathoner, but he can utilize 86% of the $\dot{V}O_2$max without accumulating much lactic acid. In marathon runners, efficiency—that is, the amount of oxygen required to run a given distance at a given speed—is about 5 to 10% better (less oxygen is required) than in other runners. (For further discussion, see pp. 187-194.)

Question: What are amphetamines? Do they improve performance?

Answer: Amphetamines are stimulant drugs that produce effects rather like those induced by actions of the sympathetic nervous system. Such effects include increases in alertness, heart rate, cardiac output, blood pressure, and metabolism. While scientific investigations of the effects of amphetamines on endurance performance are not complete, most current studies show little, if any, positive effects. It should be emphasized that regardless of the effects, taking any drug for the sole purpose of improving athletic performance should not be encouraged. (For further discussion, see p. 194.)

Question: When athletes are to compete at high altitudes, what should they be told about the effects of altitude on performance?

Answer: If the altitude is above 4000 to 5000 ft, the athletes should be told that their endurance performance may not be as good as at sea level or lower altitudes. They should also be told that they might feel more tired (i.e., their ventilation and heart rates will be higher) after completing a workout (or after exerting themselves for any reason). Nonendurance events (e.g., those lasting less than 2 min) should not be affected, and athletes should be told. (For further discussion, see pp. 194-197 and 249-250.)

Question: Will endurance performance at an altitude above sea level improve or get worse as one spends more time at this altitude?

Answer: Performance will generally improve as one's stay at a moderate altitude continues. This improvement is attributable to a process called acclimatization. During acclimatization, several physiological changes occur that allow more oxygen to be carried in the blood. One of the more rapid changes involves an increase in the number of red blood cells and thus in the amount of hemoglobin available. Significant improvements in performance due to acclimatization may be seen following a stay of several weeks at a moderate altitude; however, endurance performance will never be quite as good as at sea level, no matter how well acclimatized the athlete. At very high altitudes—over 10,000 ft—performance does not always improve with acclimatization. (For further discussion, see pp. 196-197 and 249-250.)

Questions Related to Aerobic and Anaerobic Training

Question: What is meant by the specificity of training?

Answer: This simply means that most changes produced as a result of training will be specific to the type of training program used. For example, a training program consisting of repeated sprints will develop those specific physiological capabilities required for sprinting. Training programs involving swimming will develop those capabilities required for swimming but not those required for running or cycling. Isometric strength may best be developed through isometric rather than isotonic training programs. (Another type of specificity is clearly demonstrated in athletes who participate in back-to-back seasonal sports. The football player who is in excellent condition for playing football, for instance, can hardly run the length of the court on the first day of basketball practice.) (For further discussion, see pp. 202-205.)

Question: What guidelines should be followed when selecting training programs for athletes?

Answer: One of the first considerations in selecting training programs for athletes is metabolic specificity. That is, the training program selected should be one that will lead to an increase in the physiological capacity of the energy system most used in the sport for which the program is being designed. This means that coaches should have an idea of which energy systems are used predominantly in the sport or sports that they coach. This kind of information is available from Table 9-2, p. 207.)

When it is known on which energy systems the training emphasis is to be placed, the next step is to select the training method most likely to produce the desired change. The choice of training method can be made on the basis of the information provided in Tables 9-3 and 9-4 on pages 208 and 210-211. A final consideration involves incorporating into the training program a core of exercises that closely resemble actions used in the sport for which the athlete is being trained. (For further discussion, see pp. 206-219.)

Question: What is interval training? What are its advantages?

Answer: Interval training programs consist of repeated bouts of exercise alternated with periods of relief (the relief periods usually consist of light or mild exercise). This system of training was developed mostly by track-and-field and swimming coaches. The biggest advantage of the interval training system is that it develops all three energy systems. (See pp. 209, 211, 212, and 213.)

Question: What is the value of a warm-up?

Answer: A warm-up serves to:

1. Increase body and muscle temperatures, a change which facilitates enzyme function, increases blood flow, and makes more oxygen available to the muscles.

2. Lessen the danger of the athlete's actual event (strenuous exercise performed abruptly—that is, without warm-up—may be associated with inadequate blood flow to the heart).

3. Reduce the likelihood of injuries to muscles and joints.

4. "Adjust" the athlete to performing psychologically (athletes may have a difficult time without prior warm-up). (For further discussion, see pp. 220–223 and 224.)

Question: What kinds of exercises should an adequate warm-up program contain?

Answer: Stretching activities, calisthenics, and formal activity, in that order. The most important activity is stretching. Good stretching routines may take 20 to 30 min to complete. (For further discussion, see pp. 220–223, 224, and App. E.)

Question: What kinds of exercises should an adequate warm-down program contain?

Answer: It is recommended that warm-down be similar to warm-up, but with the exercises arranged in reverse order. In this case, the formal activity and stretching activities should be considered the most important phases. (See pp. 222–223 and 224.)

Question: What should athletes do about training during the off-season?

Answer: Generally, during the off-season, athletes should engage in training programs that require only that they keep moderately active and, perhaps of most concern, keep their body weights at or reasonably near "playing weight." An off-season training program might consist of:

1. A weight-training program designed to increase strength and endurance in those muscle groups most involved in the athlete's particular sport.

2. A six- to ten-week conditioning regimen of low intensity and moderate frequency (sessions scheduled no more than twice a week).

3. Participation in sports activities and recreational games, including the athlete's specific sport. (For further discussion, see pp. 223–224.)

Question: What is "athlete's heart?"

Answer: "Athlete's heart" is an old term once used to refer to the cardiac hypertrophy (increased size of the heart) seen in most athletes. Its original connotation was pejorative—that is, it was thought that cardiac hypertrophy resulting from athletic training was pathological and thus dangerous. Of course, it is known today that cardiac hypertrophy resulting from chronic exercise training greatly improves the performance of the heart. (For further discussion, see pp. 231–233.)

Question: Are training frequencies of two and even three times per day more effective than a frequency of one session per day?

Answer: Research on this subject is slight. However, present evidence indicates that training more than once a day is not necessarily more productive than training in single daily sessions. However, two sessions per day are often necessary for endurance runners and swimmers, to allow for their rather large volume of training. Remember, too many training sessions—in whatever combination—will increase the risk of chronic fatigue. (For further discussion, see pp. 213–214.)

Question: What factor has the greatest influence on the magnitude of the effects of training?

Answer: Although several factors (e.g., frequency and duration of training) are influential, the most important factor in training is probably intensity. Training intensity has particularly substantial influence on the effects of interval training programs. (For further discussion, see pp. 215–217.)

Question: Since training intensity is so important, how may the proper intensity level be determined?

Answer: The easiest way for coaches and athletes to ascertain the proper intensity level is to gauge the heart-rate response during exercise. Specifically, for endurance athletes, the intensity should be such that the heart rate during exercise is 85 to 90% of the maximal level. (The maximal heart rate may be estimated by subtracting the athlete's age from 220). For those athletes using sprint-training programs, the heart rate during exercise should be 180 beats per min or greater. (For further discussion, see pp. 218–219.)

Question: Do men and women respond differently to training programs?

Answer: There are no major differences between the training responses of women and men exposed to the same relative training stress. (For further discussion, see pp. 241–248.)

Question: Does the menstrual cycle affect athletic performance?

Answer: No. For the majority of young female athletes, performance is not affected by the menstrual cycle. By the same token, mild exercise does not appear to have a significant effect on menstrual disorders. In fact, dysmenorrhea (painful menstruation) is less common in physically active women than in those who are sedentary. However, heavy, intensive training has been found to induce amenorrhea (abnormal cessation of menstruation) in some athletes, particularly long-distance runners, joggers, and gymnasts. The amenorrhea is temporary and uncomplicated and disappears upon cessation of heavy training. (For further discussion, see pp. 243–247.)

Question: Are there any supplemental training methods that will increase running speed?

Answer: Among the popular methods used for increasing running speed are towing (by an automobile), downhill running (ramp running), uphill running, and treadmill sprinting. Some coaches and athletes have had success in increasing sprinting speed using these methods. Not a lot of research has been done on this topic. It should be mentioned here that supplemental treadmill running (not sprinting), from which a sense of running pace and rhythm may be gained, might help improve the performance of distance runners. (For further discussion, see pp. 248–249.)

Question: Can a combination of training at sea level and at higher altitudes enhance the effects that training has on endurance performance at sea level?

Answer: Theoretically, this should be true. However, research results appear to be about evenly split. The important thing to remember here is that the altitude must not be too high—not above about 7500 ft (2400 m). Other factors to consider are the length of time spent continuously above sea level (not more than four weeks) and the need to maintain a regular training schedule at sea level. (For further discussion, see pp. 249–251.)

Question: Should there be any difference in the training frequencies of endurance athletes and nonendurance athletes?

Answer: Yes. It is recommended that endurance athletes train four to five days per week. For runners and swimmers, this frequency may be increased to six or even seven days per week for short periods. For nonendurance athletes, training three days per week should be sufficient. (For further discussion, see p. 219.)

Questions Related to Nutrition and Sports Performance

Question: Is it true that athletes who are engaged in vigorous training programs need large quantities of supplemental protein?

Answer: No. The protein requirement of athletes, even during heavy training, is the same as that of nonathletes (1 g protein per kg of body weight). The consumption of excessive quantities of protein, particularly in the forms of pills and powders, during athletic training is neither required nor recommended. (For further discussion, see pp. 258–259.)

Question: Many coaches, and even some physicians, advise athletes to supplement their diets with large amounts of vitamins and minerals. Is such supplementation necessary?

Answer: No, not according to scientific evidence. Contrary to what many athletes and coaches believe, taking vitamins and minerals in quantities above the minimum required daily does not improve physical performance. In fact, excessive accumulation of the fat-soluble vitamins (A, D, E, and K), which are stored in the body, can cause toxic effects. The recommended minimum daily allowances are easily met through a varied normal diet. (One exception may be the iron requirement of female athletes, particularly those who have heavy menstrual blood losses. Following heavy physical training, women have been found to have significantly decreased levels of iron in the blood. However, since overdoses of iron can be toxic, iron supplements should be taken only at the advice of a physician.) (For further discussion, see pp. 261–264.)

Question: What about the nutritional needs of the athlete? Are they different from those of the nonathlete?

Answer: Yes and no. From a nutritional standpoint, athletes are not different from anybody else. However, their caloric needs are generally much greater (5000 to 7000 kcal per day during heavy training). It should be mentioned here that in order to consume 5000 to 7000 kcal per day, athletes may need to eat five or six meals per day. (For further discussion, see pp. 264–265, 270.)

Question: What exactly is glycogen loading, or supercompensation? Does it affect performance?

Answer: Glycogen loading is a technique of dietary manipulation, usually combined with exercise, that increases stores of muscle glycogen (with exercise, levels are raised to two to three times normal). The technique can take three different forms: (1) a high-carbohydrate diet is followed for three or four days; (2) muscles are depleted of glycogen by exhaustive exercise, after which the individual follows a high-carbohydrate diet for three days; or (3) exercise is used to deplete muscles of glycogen, whereupon a diet high in fat and protein is followed for three days, after which a high-carbohydrate diet is consumed, also for three days. Although a positive relationship between muscle glycogen stores and endurance performance has been firmly established, glycogen loading does not always prove effective for all athletes who try it. For example, a feeling of stiffness and heaviness is often associated with glycogen loading, since water is stored with the extra glycogen. Moreover, persistent glycogen loading may cause chest pains and myoglobinuria. (For further discussion, see pp. 274–277.)

Question: Of what should the pregame meal consist?

Answer: First, it should be emphasized that no known foods, when taken several hours prior to competition, will lead to "super" performances. Carbohydrates should be the major constituents of the so-called pregame meal and may be consumed up to 2½ hr before competition. However, it should be cautioned that consumption of large amounts of sugar, particularly in liquid or pill form, less than an hour prior to exercise is not recommended (see next question and answer). Fats should be consumed well before competition (at least three to four hours prior to the event) because they are digested slowly. Finally, the athlete's diet on the day of competition should not be drastically different from his or her normal diet. (For further discussion, see pp. 279–280.)

Question: Some people argue that taking dextrose pills, honey, and other large doses of sugar, 30 to 45 min prior to endurance competition, will improve performance. Is this true?

Answer: No. In a recent study, it was found that insulin production was stimulated by the ingestion of 75 g (2.6 oz) of sugar 45 min before the start of a 30-min bout of exercise. The result was that the availability of blood-borne glucose during exercise was actually decreased. Greater dependence was placed on muscle glycogen for energy, thus depleting muscle glycogen sooner and, in turn, hastening fatigue. (For further discussion, see p. 279.)

Question: Are liquid pregame meals a good idea?

Answer: For most athletes, yes. There are several liquid formulas available today that can serve as excellent pregame meals (Ensure,

Ensure Plus, Nutriment, Sustagen, and SustaCal). Palatable and easily digested, liquid pregame meals provide nutritional balance and contribute to energy intake, hydration, and relief of hunger, with little risk of causing gastrointestinal disorders. In using the liquid meal, it should be remembered that a period of adjustment will be needed, since, for most athletes, a liquid meal will be a new experience. The coach should thus introduce the liquid meal early in the season. (For further discussion, see p. 279.)

Question: Should sugar be ingested during prolonged endurance performances?

Answer: Yes. It is generally agreed that ingestion of some liquid glucose during prolonged exercise will help spare muscle glycogen and delay or prevent hypoglycemia, two effects that should help reduce fatigue. The recommended concentration of sugar is 2.5 g per 100 ml of water; too much sugar retards gastric emptying. (For further discussion, see pp. 280–282.)

Question: It has been rumored that drinking a cup or two of coffee before an endurance event may improve performance. Is this true?

Answer: Yes. Recent evidence has indicted that caffeine is "ergogenic," or "work-producing"; specifically, caffeine is an effective aid to endurance performance. It has been estimated that the performance time of an athlete who has had a cup of coffee before an endurance event such as the 26-mile marathon may be improved (i.e., reduced) by as much as 10 min. (For further discussion, see p. 282.)

Question: What effect does alcohol ingestion have on sports performance?

Answer: Acute ingestion of small amounts of alcohol has a deleterious effect upon reaction time, coordination, accuracy, balance, strength, power, local muscular endurance, speed, and cardiovascular endurance. (For further discussion, see pp. 282–283.)

Questions Related to Body Composition and Weight Control

Question: What are the major components of the body? How do they relate to athletic performance?

Answer: The body's two major components are fat and fat-free weight (also called lean body mass). The amount of stored body fat is determined by both the number and size of the fat-storing cells. Once adulthood is reached, the number of fat cells is fixed and cannot be changed. Fat-free weight, or lean body mass, reflects mainly the skeletal muscle mass, with the weight of other tissues and organs, such as bone and skin, included as well. Athletes are generally lower in body fat and higher in fat-free weight than are nonathletes. Fat-free weight is positively related to athletic performance. Since women generally have a greater relative body fat and a lesser absolute fat-free weight component, they are at a disadvantage in most sports activities. (For further discussion, see pp. 286–288.)

Question: Is there any simple way for coaches to assess the body composition of their athletes?

Answer: Yes. Body composition may be reasonably estimated from measurements of subcutaneous fat as reflected by skinfold thicknesses. Although some practice is required, this method has been successfully used by many physicians, trainers, coaches, and physical educators. The most accurate way to assess body composition is by underwater weighing. Unfortunately, this method requires special equipment and skilled technicians. (For further discussion, see pp. 289–295.)

Question: How might knowing the body composition of athletes help the coach in preparing them for competition?

Answer: There are many ways that coaches may help their athletes prepare for competition by knowing their body composition. For example, the effectiveness of a training program may be assessed by watching changes in body fat and fat-free weight. (In this regard, training can be made appropriate not to total body weight but to body composition.) Wrestling coaches in particular have found that information relative to the amount of fat is most important in making decisions as to the weight class in which their wrestlers should belong. (For further discussion, see pp. 294–295.)

Question: What are the most important considerations when an athlete needs to gain weight?

Answer: First of all, an athlete should gain fat-free weight rather than fat. Secondly, in order to gain weight, caloric intake must be greater than caloric expenditure. In order to gain 1 lb of fat-free weight (mainly muscle), an excess intake of about 2500 kcal is required. It is recommended that not more than 2 or 3 lb per week be gained. To ensure that the excess calories will be laid down primarily as muscle, a vigorous training program, particularly of weight training, should be undertaken during the high-caloric diet period. (For further discussion, see pp. 302–303.)

Question: What should athletes be told about losing body fat?

Answer: First, any athlete who has a measured or estimated body fat of less than 7% should not be encouraged to lose body fat except under medical advisement. Second, to lose one pound of fat requires an excess expenditure of 3500 kcal. Third, an ideal rate of loss is 2 to 3 lb per week. Fourth, the caloric deficit should be made up from an increased expenditure and a reduced dietary intake of calories. (For further discussion, see pp. 297–302.)

Question: Is there a safe way for wrestlers to lose weight?

Answer: Yes. Estimates of minimal weights can be predicted from anthropometric measures. In addition, the American College of Sports Medicine has issued a position statement concerning weight loss in wrestlers. Every wrestling coach is urged to read this statement carefully and adhere to its recommendations. (For further discussion, see pp. 303–311.)

Questions Related to Water Needs and Heat Illness

Question: What are the physiological effects of dehydration?

Answer: The effects of dehydration or excessive loss of body water are: (1) a reduction in muscular strength; (2) a decrease in work performance times (the athlete cannot work as long); (3) lower plasma and blood volumes; (4) a reduction in cardiac functioning during submaximal work conditions; (5) a lower oxygen consumption; (6) an impairment of thermoregulatory processes; (7) a decrease in renal blood flow and in the volume of fluid filtered by the kidney; (8) a depletion of liver glycogen stores; and (9) an increase in the amount of electrolytes lost from the body. (For further discussion, see p. 315.)

Question: Is wearing a rubber sweatsuit during practice sessions an effective way for athletes to lose weight?

Answer: Absolutely not! All that will be lost is water (sweat), not real weight. In particular, body fat will not melt nor will it be lost in any other way if one wears a rubber sweatsuit. Deliberately causing excessive water loss through sweating for purposes of losing weight is a very hazardous practice. It does nothing but provoke serious heat illness and other related health problems. (For further discussion, see pp. 316–319.)

Question: Should athletes be allowed to drink water during practice sessions and competition?

Answer: Yes. The availability of water should be unrestricted during athletic practices and games. Water breaks should be scheduled every 10 to 15 min, and the athletes should be encouraged to drink small amounts (3 to 6 oz) at each break. This procedure is more physiologically sound than having a break every hour or so, during which athletes might gulp copious amounts of water. (For further discussion, see pp. 320–321.)

Question: Does the drinking of cold water during practices or competitions cause stomach cramps?

Answer: No. Stomach cramps are thought to be more a problem of the volume of water consumed than the water's temperature. It is interesting to note that cold (45 to 55°F) drinks have been shown to empty from the stomach faster than warmer drinks. (For further discussion, see p. 321.)

Question: Are salt tablets necessary for athletes during hot weather?

Answer: Generally not. More water than salt is lost through sweating. Taking salt tablets, particularly without adequate water, is far worse than taking no salt tablets at all. Salt obtained through the diet is usually sufficient for most athletes. (For further discussion, see p. 320.)

Question: What does a program of heat acclimatization involve?

Answer: Heat acclimatization improves the functioning of the circulatory and sweating mechanisms responsible for dissipating heat, thus minimizing increases in skin and body temperatures. Acclimatization can be induced by means of a four- to eight-day conditioning program in which exercises are made progressively more demanding and are performed in the heat. The first workout in such a program might consist of an abbreviated period of exercise performed in shorts; workouts on succeeding days can be lengthened by 10 to 20 min each day until full practice sessions are possible. During the acclimatization period, adequate water should be available; withholding water retards the acclimatization process. (For further discussion, see pp. 321–325.)

Question: What are the signs and symptoms of heat illness?

Answer: Early warning symptoms of heat illnesses include the following: hair on the chest and arms stands on end (piloerection); a chill is felt; there is throbbing pressure in the head; and nausea and unsteadiness are present. Every coach and athlete should be able to recognize these symptoms immediately: they represent an emergency—a particularly dangerous one if heat stroke is present. Heat stroke is the most severe heat illness because the sweating mechanism breaks down; the victim has a dry, warm skin, and the body temperature mounts rapidly (if it exceeds 105°F, irreversible changes can occur). In addition, the victim loses consciousness. (For further discussion, see p. 330.)

Question: What can the coach do when someone is stricken with heat illness?

Answer: Act quickly as follows:

1. Remove all the victim's clothing immediately.

2. Provide cooling at once by whatever means are available (e.g., garden hose, containers of ice water, or cold shower).

3. Summon an emergency vehicle and notify the hospital of a possible heat casualty.

4. While en route to the hospital, use sponges or towels to apply ice water continuously and generously to the victim.

(For further discussion, see pp. 330–331.)

APPENDIX A

Journal Abbreviations and Titles*

Abbreviation	Full Title
Acta Med. Scand.	Acta Medica Scandinavica
Acta Physiol. Scand.	Acta Physiologica Scandinavica
Acta Rheumatologica Scand.	Acta Rheumatologica Scandinavica
Advances Internal Med.	Advances in Internal Medicine
Am. J. Anat.	American Journal of Anatomy
Am. J. Clin. Nutri.	American Journal of Clinical Nutrition
Am. J. Physiol.	American Journal of Physiology
Am. J. Phys. Med.	American Journal of Physical Medicine
Ann. Intern. Med.	Annals of Internal Medicine
Ann. N.Y. Acad. Sci.	Annals of the New York Academy of Science
Ann. Rev. Physiol.	Annual Review of Physiology
Arbeitsphysiol.	Arbeitsphysiologie
Arch. Environ. Health	Archives of Environmental Health
Arch. Phys. Med. Rehabil.	Archives of Physical Medicine and Rehabilitation
Aust. J. Health Phys. Educ. Rec.	The Australian Journal of Health, Physical Education and Recreation
Aust. J. Sports Med.	Australian Journal of Sports Medicine
Can. J. Appl. Sport Sci.	Canadian Journal of Applied Sport Sciences
Europ. J. Appl. Physiol.	European Journal of Applied Physiology (formerly Arbeitsphysiol. and Int. Z. Angew Physiol.)
Fed. Proc.	Federation Proceedings
Int. Z. Angew Physiol.	Internationale Zeitschrift fur Angewandte Physiologie
Israeli J. Med. Sci.	Israeli Journal of Medical Sciences
J. Am. Coll. Health Assoc.	Journal of the American College Health Association
J.A.M.A.	Journal of the American Medical Association
J. Amer. Phys. Therapy Assoc.	Journal of the American Physical Therapy Association

*Journals for which full titles have been given in text are not included here.

J. Appl. Physiol.	Journal of Applied Physiology
J. Appl. Physiol.: Respirat. Environ. Exercise Physiol.	Journal of Applied Physiology: Respiratory, Environmental and Exercise Physiology (formerly J. Appl. Physiol.)
J. Drug Issue	Journal of Drug Issues
J. Lipid Res.	Journal of Lipid Research
J. Phys. Educ. Rec.	Journal of Physical Education and Recreation
J. Physiol.	Journal of Physiology
J. Sports Med.	Journal of Sports Medicine and Physical Fitness
Med. Sci. Sports	Medicine and Science in Sports
Med. Sci. Sports Exercise	Medicine and Science in Sports and Exercise (formerly Med. Sci. Sports)
Mod. Med.	Modern Medicine
Obstet. Gynecol.	Obstetrics and Gynecology
Ohio State Med. J.	Ohio State Medical Journal
Orthop. Clin. N. Am.	The Orthopedic Clinics of North America
Res. Quart.	Research Quarterly
Scand. J. Clin. Lab. Invest.	Scandinavian Journal of Clinical and Laboratory Investigation
Scand. Arch. Physiol.	Scandinavian Archives of Physiology
Sports Med. Bull.	Sports Medicine Bulletin

APPENDIX B

Symbols and Abbreviations

ADP adenosine diphosphate

ATP adenosine triphosphate

a-$\bar{v}O_2$diff arterial-mixed venous oxygen difference

bg black-globe temperature (radiant energy)

°C degrees Celsius (centigrade)

CA carbonic anhydrase

Ca^{++} calcium ion

cm^3 or cc Cubic centimeter

cm centimeter

CO_2 carbon dioxide

d distance

db dry bulb

F force

f frequency of breathing per minute

°F degrees Farenheit

FFA free fatty acids

FFW fat-free weight

FT (or FG) fast-twitch muscle fibers or motor units (or fast, gly-colytic fibers)

F_x fractional concentration of gas

g gram or grams

H^+ hydrogen ion

Hb hemoglobin

HbO_2 oxyhemoglobin

HCO_3^- bicarbonate ion

Hg mercury

HR heart rate

H_2CO_3 carbonic acid

H_2O water

kcal kilocalorie

kcal/min kilocalories per minute

kg kilogram

LA lactic acid

ml milliliter

m meter

max$\dot{V}O_2$ or $\dot{V}O_2$max maximal volume of oxygen consumed per minute during exercise

ml milliliter

mm millimeter

Na^+ sodium ion

O_2 oxygen

P power

P_B barometric pressure

PC phosphocreatine

P_{CO_2} partial pressure of carbon dioxide

Pi inorganic phosphate

P_{N_2} partial pressure of nitrogen

P_{O_2} partial pressure of oxygen

P_x partial pressure of gas

$\dot{Q}$ cardiac output

RM repetition maximum

sec second

ST (or SO) slow-twitch muscle fibers or motor units (or slow, oxidative fibers)

SV stroke volume

t time

TV tidal volume

V volume

$\dot{V}_E$ minute ventilation, or amount of air expired in one minute

$\dot{V}O_2$ volume of oxygen consumed per minute

$\dot{V}O_2$max or max$\dot{V}O_2$ maximal volume of oxygen consumed per minute during exercise

wb wet bulb

WBGT wet-bulb globe temperature

WBT wet-bulb temperature

Description of Weight-Lifting Exercises

The weight-resistance exercises mentioned in Chapter 7 are performed as described below. The principle muscles involved in each of the exercises are presented in Table C-1. The exercises are listed in alphabetical order for both their descriptions and the muscles involved. The major muscles of the human body are shown in Figure C-1.

Arm Curl (Fig. C-2)

This exercise is performed with a barbell.
From a standing position, hold the barbell in front of the thighs with arms fully extended and the hands in a supinated grip ("underhand" grip). Raise the barbell to the chest by flexing the elbows. While lifting, stand erect and keep the elbows in toward the sides. Repeat.

Back Hyperextension (Fig. C-3)

This exercise is performed with a free weight.
Lie face down with the upper body extending over the edge of a table and with a partner holding the legs. Hold the weight behind the neck and lower the head toward the floor. On returning, raise the head and arch the back as much as possible. Repeat.

Bench Press (Fig. C-4)

This exercise is performed with a barbell.
Lie on the back on a bench, holding the barbell over the chest with the arms extended, shoulder-width apart, and the hands in a pronated (overhand) grip. Lower the barbell to the chest and return. Repeat.

Bent-Arm Pullover (Fig. C-5)

This exercise is performed with a barbell.
Lie on the back on a bench, holding the barbell over the head with elbows

Table C-1: Principle Muscles Involved in Various Weight-Resistance Exercises

Exercise	Primary Muscles
Arm curl	Biceps, brachialis, brachioradialis
Back hyperextension	Erector spinae, gluteus maximus, hamstrings
Bench press	Anterior deltoid, pectoralis major, triceps
Bent-arm pullover	Deltoid, pectoralis major, teres major, latissimus dorsi, triceps
Bent-knee sit-up	Rectus abdominis, obliques, psoas major
Bent-over rowing	Latissimus dorsi, teres major, brachialis, trapezius, posterior deltoids
Dumbbell swing	Triceps, sacrospinalis
Good morning exercise	Quadriceps, gluteus maximus, hamstrings, erector spinae
Heel (toe) raise	Gastrocnemius, soleus
Incline press	Upper pectoralis major, anterior deltoid, triceps
Knee (leg) extension	Quadriceps
Lateral arm raise	Deltoid, supraspinalis
Leg curl (knee flexion)	Hamstrings
Leg raise	Abdominals
Neck extension	Deep posterior muscles, cervical region
Neck flexion	Sternocleidomastoid
Parallel bar dip	Triceps, deltoids
Power clean	Quadriceps, gluteus maximus, hamstrings, deltoids
Power snatch	Quadriceps, gluteus maximus, hamstrings, deltoids
Press behind neck	Deltoids, triceps
Pulldown lat machine	Latissimus dorsi
Reverse curl	Biceps, brachialis, brachioradialis, extensor carpi muscles
Reverse wrist curl	Extensor carpi muscles
Shoulder shrug	Upper trapezius, levator scapulae, rhomboids
Squat	Gluteus maximus, quadriceps, erector spinae
Standing (overhead) press	Deltoid, supraspinatus, triceps
Stiff-legged dead lift	Erector spinae, gluteus maximus, hamstrings
Straight arm pullover	Deltoid, pectoralis major, teres major, latissimus dorsi, triceps
Triceps extension	Triceps
Upright rowing	Deltoid, supraspinalis, biceps
Wrist curl	Flexor carpi muscles
Wrist roller	Extensor carpi muscles, flexor carpi muscles

at 90° angles and the hands in a pronated grip about shoulder-width apart. Lower the barbell over and behind the head as far as possible. Return to the starting position.

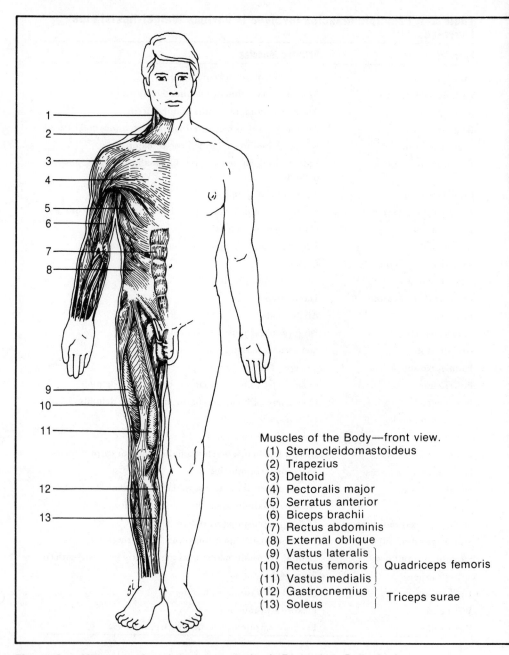

Muscles of the Body—front view.
(1) Sternocleidomastoideus
(2) Trapezius
(3) Deltoid
(4) Pectoralis major
(5) Serratus anterior
(6) Biceps brachii
(7) Rectus abdominis
(8) External oblique
(9) Vastus lateralis ⎫
(10) Rectus femoris ⎬ Quadriceps femoris
(11) Vastus medialis ⎭
(12) Gastrocnemius ⎫ Triceps surae
(13) Soleus   ⎭

Figure C-1 Major muscles of the human body: A, Front view; B, back view.
(Adapted from Falls, H.B., A.M. Baylor, and R.K. Dishman: *Essentials of Fitness*.
Philadelphia, Saunders College Publishing, 1980, pp. 64–65).

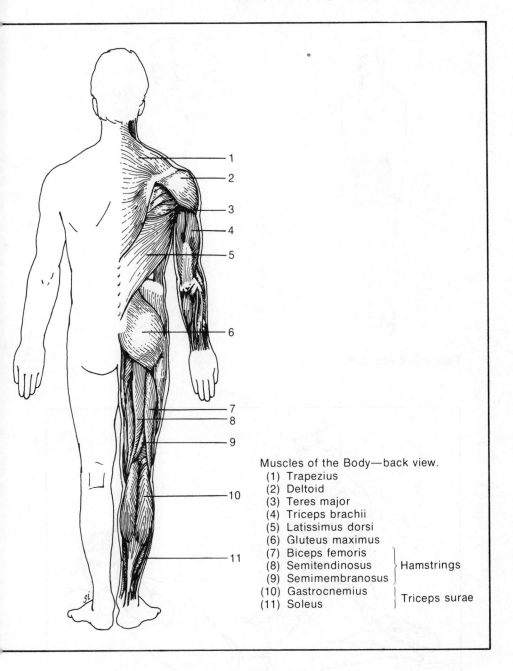

Muscles of the Body—back view.
(1) Trapezius
(2) Deltoid
(3) Teres major
(4) Triceps brachii
(5) Latissimus dorsi
(6) Gluteus maximus
(7) Biceps femoris
(8) Semitendinosus   } Hamstrings
(9) Semimembranosus
(10) Gastrocnemius   } Triceps surae
(11) Soleus

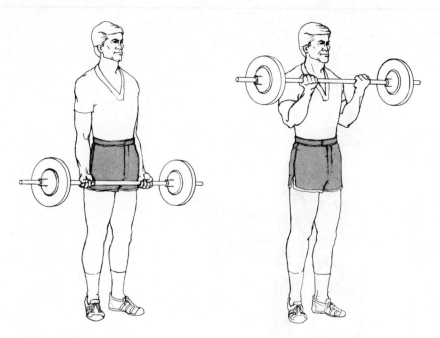

Figure C-2 Arm curl.

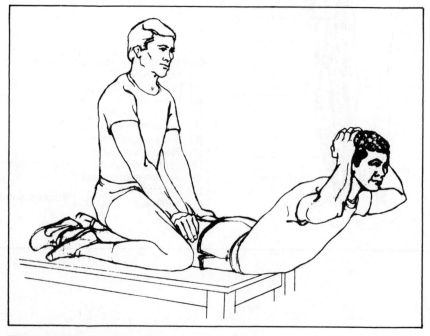

Figure C-3 Back hyperextension.

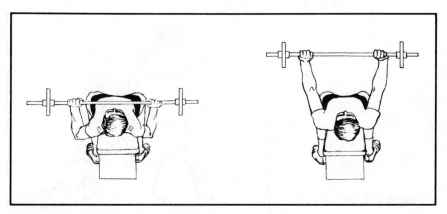

Figure C-4 Bench press.

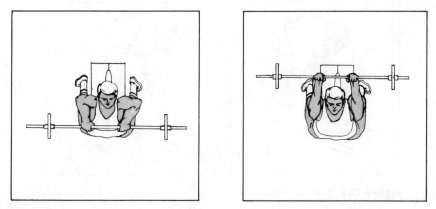

Figure C-5 Bent-arm pullover. The grip shown here is called a pronated grip.

Bent-knee Sit-ups (Fig. C-6)

Perform a regular sit-up but with the knees bent at approximately 90°.

Bent-over Rowing (Fig. C-7)

This exercise is performed with a barbell.

Flex the knees at a 45° angle and bend over from the hips until the back is parallel to the floor. With arms extended, grab the barbell with the hands pronated and lift to the chest and return.

Dumbbell Swing

This exercise is performed with a dumbbell loaded with weights in the middle.

While standing, grasp the dumbbell with both hands, using a pronated

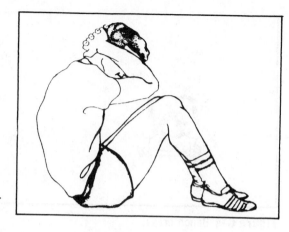

Figure C-6 Bent-knee sit-up.

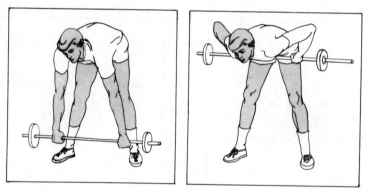

Figure C-7 Bent-over rowing.

grip. Swing the dumbbell overhead and lower it to behind the neck so the elbows are pointing straight up. Keep the head erect and the feet more than shoulder-width apart. Now extend the arms, swinging the dumbbell forcefully overhead in a large arc; continue the arc downward until the dumbbell goes between the legs. With the same momentum, return it in the same arc to the position behind the neck. Repeat.

Good Morning Exercise

This exercise is performed with a barbell.

Grasp the barbell in a pronated grip and rest it across the shoulders and behind the neck while standing erect. Bend forward from the hips with legs straight until the trunk is parallel to the floor and return to starting position. Repeat.

Heel (Toe) Raise (Fig. C-8)

This exercise is performed with a barbell.

With the barbell held across the shoulders and behind the neck, place the balls of the feet on a board about two inches high so that the heels are off the board. Rise up on the toes as far as possible; then lower the heels to the floor. Repeat.

Incline Press

This exercise is a bench press (see earlier description) performed on an inclined bench (head raised above the feet).

Knee (Leg) Extension

This exercise is performed with a leg machine.

Sit on the edge of the leg machine with the knees flexed at about 90°. Extend the knees fully, then return. (If a leg machine is not available, the exercise may be performed by placing appropriate weights on the foot or ankle and sitting on the edge of a table.)

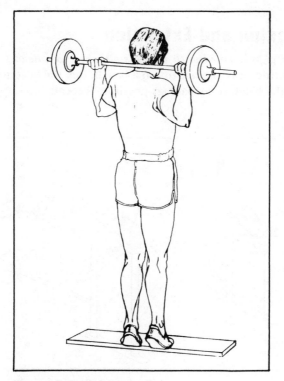

Figure C-8 Heel (tow) raise.

Lateral Arm Raise

This exercise is performed with dumbbells.

Stand erect with arms at the sides and dumbbells in each hand. Raise the dumbbells laterally with arms straight to about shoulder level. Return to starting position and repeat.

Leg Curl (Knee Flexion) (Fig. C-9)

This exercise is performed with a leg machine.

Lie face down on the edge of a table or leg machine. Flex the knees as far as possible and return. Repeat.

Leg Raise

Lie on the floor on the back with legs straight and hands behind the neck. Raise the legs until they are approximately perpendicular to the floor. Lower, then repeat.

Neck Flexion and Extension

This exercise is performed with weights attached to a head harness.

While sitting or lying face up on a bench, flex the head to the chest and then extend the head as far back as possible. Repeat.

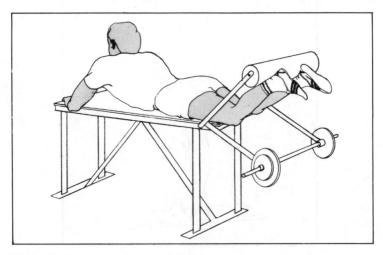

Figure C-9 Leg curl (knee extension).

Parallel Bar Dip

This exercise is performed with parallel bars.

Grab the parallel bars with your hands and jump up, supporting your body weight with both arms extended and locked. Lower the body (dip) until the elbows are flexed at about 90° and return. Repeat.

Power Clean (Fig. C-10)

This exercise is performed with a barbell.

With the barbell resting on the floor in front of the feet, bend forward at the hips with the knees straight. Grasp the barbell in a pronated grip and pull it up to the chest, keeping it close to the body. Now throw the elbows under the bar and stand straight up. Repeat.

Power Snatch

This exercise is performed with a barbell.

With the barbell resting on the floor in front of the feet, bend forward at the hips with knees slightly flexed. Grasp the barbell in a pronated grip and

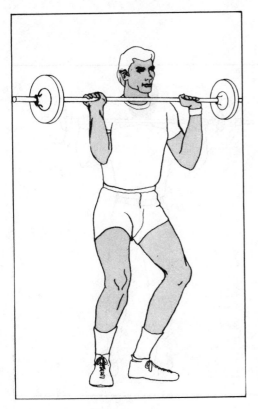

Figure C-10 Power clean.

raise it to the knees by raising head, shoulders, and hips simultaneously. As the bar passes the knees, swing the hips forward and upward toward the bar and assume a squat or split position while continuing to lift the bar toward the head. Complete the lift by locking the arms at full length overhead and stand erect. Repeat.

Press Behind Neck (Fig. C-11)

This exercise is a standing (overhead) press, in which the barbell is lowered behind the neck rather than in front of the chest.

Pulldown Lat Machine (Fig. C-12)

This exercise is performed with a lat machine.

Sit on the end of a bench or kneel on the floor. Grasp the bar of the lat machine in a pronated grip, with the hands more than shoulder-width apart. Pull the bar down behind the head until it touches the base of the neck and shoulders. Return to starting position and repeat.

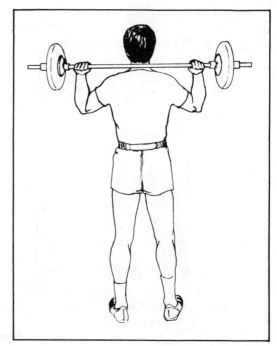

Figure C-11 Press behind neck.

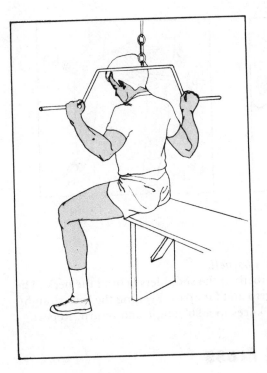

Figure C-12 Pulldown lat machine.

Reverse Curl

This exercise is performed with a barbell.

From a standing position, hold the barbell in front of the thighs with arms fully extended and the hands in a pronated grip. Raise the barbell to the chest by flexing the elbows. While lifting, stand erect and keep the elbows in toward the sides. Repeat. This exercise is the same as the arm curl except for the grip.

Reverse Wrist Curl (Fig. C-13)

This exercise is performed with a barbell.

Grasp the barbell in a pronated grip and sit with the forearms on the thighs so that the wrists and hands extend over the knees. Flex and extend the wrists as far as possible without raising the forearms from the thighs. Repeat.

Shoulder Shrug

This exercise is performed with a barbell.

From a standing position, grasp the barbell in a pronated grip, with arms extended so that the barbell is resting in front of the thighs. Now, shrug the shoulders up and back as far as possible. Repeat.

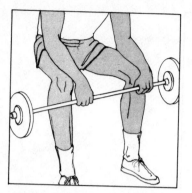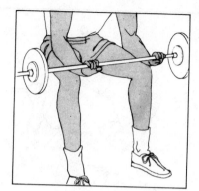

Figure C-13 Reverse wrist curl.

Squat (Fig. C-14)

This exercise is performed with a barbell.

Standing erect, place the barbell on the shoulders behind the neck. The hands should be in a pronated grip and far apart. Keeping the back straight, lower the weight by flexing the knees to a 90° angle and return. Repeat.

Standing (Overhead) Press

This exercise is performed with a barbell.

Stand erect and hold the barbell in front of the chest in a pronated grip, with the hands about shoulder-width apart. Raise the weight overhead by fully extending the arms, then return. Keep the back straight and do not bend the knees (see Fig. C-11). Repeat.

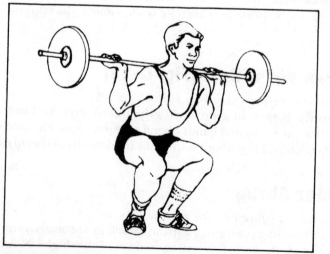

Figure C-14 Squat.

Stiff-Legged Dead Lift
(Fig. C-15)

This exercise is performed with a barbell.

Start from a standing position holding the barbell in a pronated grip, with the arms extended and shoulder-width apart so that the barbell is resting in front of the thighs. With the knees locked, bend forward at the hips, lowering the barbell until it just touches the floor. Raise the weight by straightening the body. Repeat.

Straight Arm Pullover

This exercise is performed with a barbell.

Lie on the back on a bench. Hold the barbell above the chest in a pronated grip. With arms fully extended, first lower the barbell to a position behind the head, then raise the barbell back over the chest and lower it slowly to the thighs. Raise the barbell off the thighs and repeat.

Triceps Extension (Fig. C-16)

This exercise is performed with a lat machine.

While standing, grasp the bar of the lat machine in a pronated grip, keeping the hands closely together. The bar should be at about face level. Pull the bar downward as far as possible without bending the hips or knees. Return to the starting position and repeat.

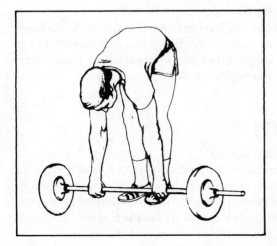

Figure C-15 Stiff-legged dead lift.

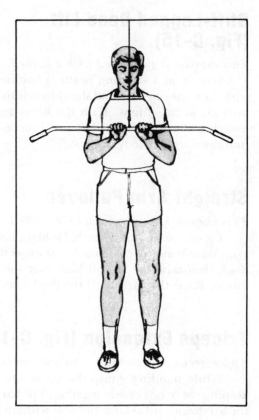

Figure C-16 Triceps extension.

Upright Rowing

This exercise is performed with a barbell.

Stand with the barbell held at hip level in front of and close to the body, keeping the hands close together (almost touching) and in a pronated grip. Lift the barbell to chin height, keeping the elbows out so that the barbell stays close to the body; then lower it to hip level. Repeat.

Wrist Curl (Fig. C-17)

This exercise is performed with a barbell.

Grasp the barbell in a supinated grip and sit with the forearms on the thighs so that the wrists and hands extend over the knees. Flex and extend the wrists as far as possible without raising the forearms from the thighs. Repeat. To include the fingers, hold the barbell on the tips of the fingers with hands open but cupped. Make a fist and then flex and extend the wrist.

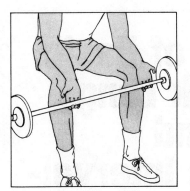
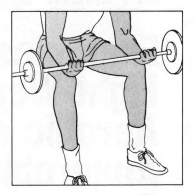

Figure C-17 Wrist curl.

Wrist Roller (Fig. C-18)

This exercise is performed with a bar that has weights hanging on a rope from its center.

   While standing, grasp the bar in a pronated grip and first raise the weights by rolling the rope up with the wrist and then lower the weights by unrolling the rope. Repeat.

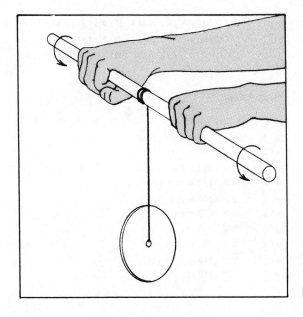

Figure C-18 Wrist roller.

Examples of Basic Eight-Week Long Aerobic and Anaerobic Interval-Training Programs

The following sample programs should be suitable for use in the preseason for men and women athletes. Running times have been included for completeness, but more than likely will have to be adjusted to fit the individual needs of the athletes involved. Suggested methods for determining the proper running speeds were given in Chapter 9, p. 218. The daily programs are given in prescription form as defined in Table 9-6 (p. 213). Each training session should be preceded by an adequate warm-up period and followed by an adequate warm-down period.

Aerobic Program

The training frequency is given as five days per week. If only four days are desired, day 5 may be dropped. Also, the first two weeks of the program are relatively easy, in order to provide time for gradual adjustments to full intensity levels.

Day		Prescription First Week
1	Set 1 Set 2	4 × 220 at easy (1:3)* 8 × 110 at easy (1:3)
2	Set 1 Set 2	2 × 440 at easy (1:3) 8 × 110 at easy (1:3)
3	Set 1 Set 2	2 × 440 at easy (1:3) 6 × 220 at easy (1:3)
4	Set 1 Set 2	1 × 880 at easy 6 × 220 at easy (1:3)
5	Set 1 Set 2	2 × 440 at easy (1:3) 8 × 110 at easy (1:3)

*Work-relief ratio.

Day	**Prescription**	
	Second Week	
1	Set 1	2 × 880 at easy (1:3)
	Set 2	2 × 440 at easy (1:3)
2	Set 1	6 × 440 at easy (1:3)
3	Set 1	3 × 880 at easy (1:3)
4	Set 1	1 × 2640 at easy
5	Set 1	6 × 440 at easy (1:3)

Third Week

1	Set 1	2 × 660 at 2:15*(4:30)
	Set 2	2 × 440 at 1:20 (2:40)
2	Set 1	4 × 220 at 0:38 (1:54)
	Set 2	4 × 220 at 0:38 (1:54)
	Set 3	4 × 220 at 0:38 (1:54)
3	Set 1	1 × 880 at 3:00 (3:00)
	Set 2	2 × 440 at 1:20 (2:40)
4	Same as day 1	
5	Same as day 3	

Fourth Week

1	Set 1	3 × 660 at 2:10 (4:20)
	Set 2	3 × 440 at 1:20 (2:40)
2	Set 1	4 × 220 at 0:38 (1:54)
	Set 2	4 × 220 at 0:38 (1:54)
	Set 3	4 × 220 at 0:38 (1:54)
	Set 4	4 × 220 at 0:38 (1:54)
3	Set 1	2 × 880 at 2:55 (2:55)
	Set 2	2 × 440 at 1:20 (2:40)
4	Same as day 1	
5	Same as day 3	

Fifth Week

1	Set 1	4 × 660 at 2:05 (4:10)
	Set 2	2 × 440 at 1:20 (2:40)
2	Set 1	4 × 220 at 0:37 (1:51)
	Set 2	4 × 220 at 0:37 (1:51)
	Set 3	4 × 220 at 0:37 (1:51)
	Set 4	4 × 220 at 0:37 (1:51)
3	Set 1	2 × 880 at 2:55 (2:55)
	Set 2	2 × 440 at 1:20 (2:40)
4	Same as day 1	
5	Same as day 3	

Sixth Week

1	Set 1	4 × 660 at 2:00 (4:00)
	Set 2	2 × 440 at 1:18 (2:36)

*Minutes:seconds.

Prescription

Day			
	Sixth Week *(continued)*		
2	Set 1	4 × 220 at 0:36	(1:48)
	Set 2	4 × 220 at 0:36	(1:48)
	Set 3	4 × 220 at 0:36	(1:48)
	Set 4	4 × 220 at 0:36	(1:48)
3	Set 1	2 × 880 at 2:50	(2:50)
	Set 2	2 × 440 at 1:18	(2:36)
4	Same as day 1		
5	Same as day 3		

Seventh Week

Day			
1	Set 1	2 × 880 at 2:45	(2:45)
	Set 2	2 × 440 at 1:16	(2:32)
2	Set 1	4 × 220 at 0:35	(1:45)
	Set 2	4 × 220 at 0:35	(1:45)
	Set 3	4 × 220 at 0:35	(1:45)
	Set 4	4 × 220 at 0:35	(1:45)
3	Set 1	1 × 1320 at 4:30	(2:15)
	Set 2	2 × 1100 at 3:40	(1:50)
4	Same as day 1		
5	Same as day 3		

Eighth Week

Day			
1	Set 1	2 × 880 at 2:40	(2:40)
	Set 2	2 × 440 at 1:16	(2:32)
2	Set 1	4 × 220 at 0:34	(1:42)
	Set 2	4 × 220 at 0:34	(1:42)
	Set 3	4 × 220 at 0:34	(1:42)
	Set 4	4 × 220 at 0:34	(1:42)
3	Set 1	1 × 1320 at 4:24	(2:12)
	Set 2	2 × 1100 at 3:34	(1:47)
4	Same as day 1		
5	Same as day 3		

Anaerobic Program

As mentioned in Chapter 9, the frequency of anaerobic training need be only three days per week. However, notice that the first two weeks of workouts are relatively easy and are conducted five days per week. With sprint training, it is extremely important to gradually progress toward full intensity. If this is not done, then extreme muscular soreness and even injury will often result.

Prescription

Day			
	First Week		
1	Set 1	4 × 220 at easy	(1:3)*
	Set 2	8 × 110 at easy	(1:3)

*Work-relief ratio.

	Prescription	
Day	**First Week** *(continued)*	
2	Set 1	2 × 440 at easy (1:3)
	Set 2	8 × 110 at easy (1:3)
3	Set 1	2 × 440 at easy (1:3)
	Set 2	6 × 220 at easy (1:3)
4	Set 1	1 × 880 at easy
	Set 2	6 × 220 at easy (1:3)
5	Set 1	2 × 440 at easy (1:3)
	Set 2	6 × 220 at easy (1:3)

Second Week

1	Set 1	2 × 880 at easy (1:3)
	Set 2	2 × 440 at easy (1:3)
2	Set 1	6 × 440 at easy (1:3)
3	Set 1	3 × 880 at easy (1:3)
4	Set 1	1 × 2640 at easy
5	Set 1	6 × 440 at easy (1:3)

Third Week

1	Set 1	8 × 110 at 0:20*(1:00)
2	Set 1	6 × 110 at 0:20 (1:00)
	Set 2	6 × 110 at 0:20 (1:00)
3	Set 1	8 × 110 at 0:20 (1:00)
	Set 2	8 × 110 at 0:20 (1:00)

Fourth Week

1	Set 1	4 × 220 at 0:40 (2:00)
	Set 2	8 × 110 at 0:20 (1:00)
	Set 3	8 × 110 at 0:20 (1:00)
2	Set 1	4 × 220 at 0:40 (2:00)
	Set 2	8 × 110 at 0:20 (1:00)
	Set 3	8 × 110 at 0:20 (1:00)
3	Set 1	4 × 220 at 0:40 (2:00)
	Set 2	8 × 110 at 0:20 (1:00)
	Set 3	8 × 110 at 0:20 (1:00)

Fifth Week

1	Set 1	4 × 220 at 0:40 (2:00)
	Set 2	4 × 220 at 0:40 (2:00)
	Set 3	8 × 110 at 0:20 (1:00)
2	Set 1	4 × 220 at 0:40 (2:00)
	Set 2	4 × 220 at 0:40 (2:00)
	Set 3	8 × 110 at 0:20 (1:00)
3	Set 1	4 × 220 at 0:40 (2:00)
	Set 2	4 × 220 at 0:40 (2:00)
	Set 3	8 × 110 at 0:20 (1:00)

*Minutes:seconds.

Prescription

Day		Sixth Week		
1	Set 1	4 ×	220 at 0:38	(1:54)
	Set 2	4 ×	220 at 0:38	(1:54)
	Set 3	8 ×	110 at 0:18	(0:54)
2	Set 1	4 ×	220 at 0:38	(1:54)
	Set 2	4 ×	220 at 0:38	(1:54)
	Set 3	8 ×	110 at 0:18	(0:54)
3	Set 1	4 ×	220 at 0:38	(1:54)
	Set 2	4 ×	220 at 0:38	(1:54)
	Set 3	8 ×	110 at 0:18	(0:54)

Seventh Week

Day				
1	Set 1	4 ×	220 at 0:35	(1:45)
	Set 2	8 ×	110 at 0:15	(0:45)
	Set 3	10 ×	55 at 0:08	(0:24)
	Set 4	6 ×	55 at 0:08	(0:24)
2	Set 1	4 ×	220 at 0:35	(1:45)
	Set 2	8 ×	110 at 0:15	(0:45)
	Set 3	10 ×	55 at 0:08	(0:24)
	Set 4	6 ×	55 at 0:08	(0:24)
3	Set 1	4 ×	220 at 0:35	(1:45)
	Set 2	8 ×	110 at 0:15	(0:45)
	Set 3	10 ×	55 at 0:08	(0:24)
	Set 4	6 ×	55 at 0:08	(0:24)

Eighth Week

Day				
1	Set 1	4 ×	220 at 0:35	(1:45)
	Set 2	8 ×	110 at 0:15	(0:45)
	Set 3	10 ×	55 at 0:08	(0:24)
	Set 4	6 ×	55 at 0:08	(0:24)
2	Set 1	4 ×	220 at 0:35	(1:45)
	Set 2	8 ×	110 at 0:15	(0:45)
	Set 3	10 ×	55 at 0:08	(0:24)
	Set 4	6 ×	55 at 0:08	(0:24)
3	Set 1	4 ×	220 at 0:35	(1:45)
	Set 2	8 ×	110 at 0:15	(0:45)
	Set 3	10 ×	55 at 0:08	(0:24)
	Set 4	6 ×	55 at 0:08	(0:24)

Some Suggested Stretching Exercises

As mentioned in Chapter 9, stretching exercises for most sports should involve the major muscle groups and joints of the body, including the neck, back, hamstrings, gastrocnemius, Achilles tendon, chest, hips, groin, spine, quadriceps, shoulders, arms, ankles, abdominals, knees, and toes. Each stretching exercise should be performed **without** bobbing or jerking, and with the final stretched position held for 20 to 30 sec. Each exercise may be repeated five or six times. Stretching should be performed before as well as after training and competition (warm-up and warm-down). Adequate stretching routines may require a total of 20 to 30 min to complete.

The following stretching exercises are only suggestions. Many other exercises may be used with the same general results.

Achilles Tendon, Gastrocnemius (Fig. E-1)

Stand several feet in front of a wall with the feet several inches apart. Place outstretched hands on the wall, keeping the feet flatly on the floor. Gradually move away from the wall by backing up but keep the feet flatly on the floor. Hold the final stretched position. Each day try to increase the distance you move from the wall.

Neck

For stretching the neck, rotate the head, first in one direction, then in the other. Rotate slowly and repeat several times.

Back (Fig. E-2)

Lying on the back with the arms extended to the sides, bring the knees toward the chin as far as possible without raising the arms off the floor. Hold position, then repeat.

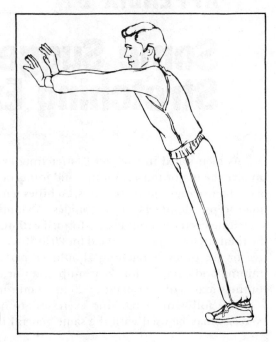

Figure E-1 Achilles tendon and gastrocnemius stretch.

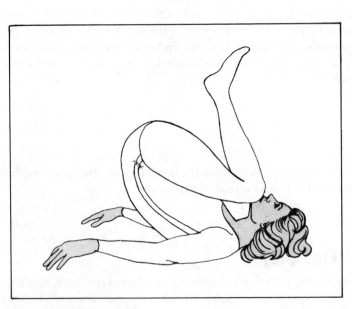

Figure E-2 Back stretch.

Hamstrings (Fig. E-3)

Sitting on the floor with the legs spread, first reach for one foot, hold, then reach for the other and hold. Each time you reach, attempt to touch and hold the head and chest as closely as possible to the thigh of the leg you are trying to hold at the foot. Repeat—that is, continue reaching first for one foot and then the other.

Groin (Fig. E-4)

Sit on the floor with the soles of the feet touching in front of you. Gradually push down on the knees as far as possible. Hold the final stretched position. Each day try to push the knees closer to the floor.

Spine, Waistline (Fig. E-5)

Sit on the floor with the right leg straight and cross it with the left leg, placing the left foot flatly on the floor. With the right hand, reach around the left leg toward your left hip. Put the left arm directly behind you and slowly turn the head. Sit up straight, looking over the left shoulder. Hold, then stretch the other side by crossing the right leg over the left.

Quadriceps (Fig. E-6)

Lying on your left side, flex the knee of your right leg and grab the ankle with the right hand. Gradually move the hips forward until a good stretch is felt on the thigh. Hold. Repeat for the left leg by lying on your right side.

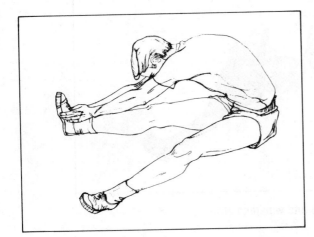

Figure E-3 Hamstring stretch.

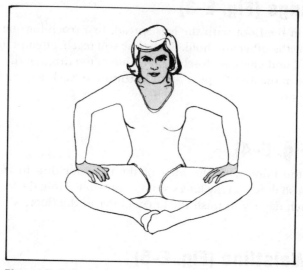

Figure E-4 Groin stretch.

Shoulder, Chest (Fig. E-7)

Stand with the feet several inches apart, with hands in front and the elbows raised to the side. Keep the head up and pull the elbows back as far as possible and hold. Repeat several times.

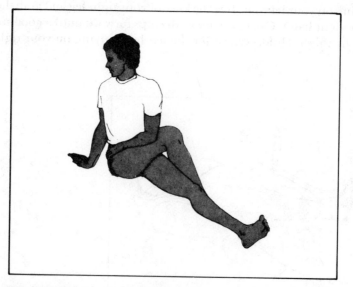

Figure E-5 Spine and waistline stretch.

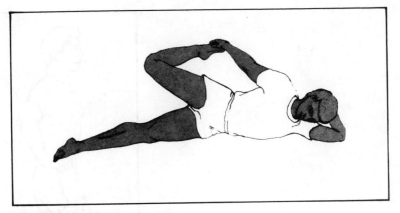

Figure E-6 Quadriceps stretch.

Ankle (Fig. E-8)

Standing with the weight on the right foot, place the ball of the left foot on the floor, transferring the weight to it gradually. Alternate by placing the ball of the right foot on the floor and transferring the weight to it from the left foot. Gradually increase the tempo to a jog.

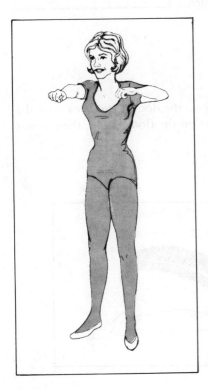

Figure E-7 Shoulder and chest stretch.

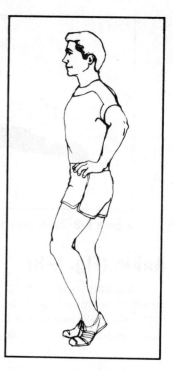

Figure E-8 Ankle stretch.

Abdominals (Fig. E-9)

Kneel by placing the hands and knees on the floor. Lean back onto the heels, extend the arms, and place the chest on the floor. Hold, then repeat several times.

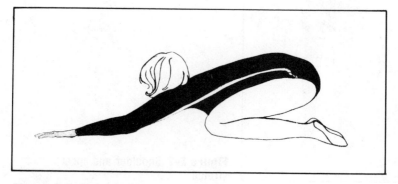

Figure E-9 Abdominal stretch.

Hips (Fig. E-10)

Lie on the back and raise the feet straight into the air, supporting the hips with the hands. Point the toes and touch first one foot to the floor above the head, hold, then do the same with the other foot. Repeat.

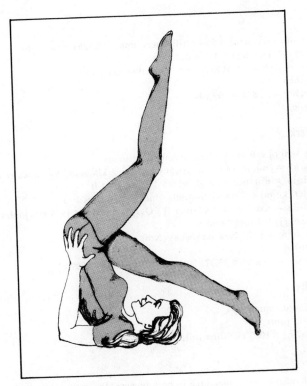

Figure E-10 Hip stretch.

APPENDIX F

Units of Measure

Distances

1 inch = 2.54 centimeters (cm) = 25.4 millimeters (mm) = 0.0254 meters (m)
1 foot = 30.48 cm = 304.8 mm = 0.304 m
1 mile = 5280 ft = 1760 yds = 1609.35 m = 1.61 kilometers (km)
1 cm = 0.3937 inch
1 m = 39.37 inches = 3.28 ft =1.09 yds
1 km = 0.62 mile

Energy and Work

Work = energy = application of a force through a distance
1 kilocalorie (kcal) = amount of energy required to heat 1 kilogram (kg) of water 1° centigrade
1 foot-pound (ft-lb) = distance through which 1 lb moves 1 ft
1 kilogram-meter (kg-m) = distance through which 1 kg moves 1 m
1 kcal = 3086 ft-lbs = 426.4 kg-m = 0.2 liter (L) O_2 consumed = 4.1855 kiloJoules (kJ)
1 kJ = 1000 joules (J) = 0.23892 kcal
1 ft-lb = 0.1383 kg-m = 1.356 Newton-meters (Nm)
1 kg-m = 7.23 ft-lbs
1 L O_2 consumed = 5.05 kcal = 15.575 ft-lbs = 2153 kg-m = 21.237 kJ

Volume (Capacity)

1 pint = 0.473 L = 0.5 quart (qt)
1 qt = 0.946 L = 2 pints
1 liter (L) = 1.057 qt = 1000 milliliter (ml)

Power

Power = work divided by time; measured in horsepower (HP), watts, etc.
1 HP = 33,000 ft-lbs/min = 4.564 kg-m/min = 746 watts
1 watt = 44.22 ft-lbs/min = 6.118 kg-m/min = 0.0013 HP.
1 ft-lb per min (ft-lb/min) = 0.1383 kg-m/min = 0.00003 HP = 0.0226 watt
1 kg-m/min = 7.23 ft-lbs/min = 0.00022 HP = 0.1635 watt
1 L O_2 consumed/min = 5.05 kcal/min = 15.575 ft-lbs/min = 2153 kg-m/min

Velocity

1 foot per second (ft/sec) = 0.3048 m/sec = 18.3 m/min = 1.1 km per hour (km/hr) = 0.68 mile/hr (mph)
1 mph = 88 ft/min = 1.47 ft/sec = 0.45 m/sec = 26.8 m/min = 1.61 km/hr
1 km/hr = 16.7 m/min = 0.28 m/sec = 0.91 ft/sec = 0.62 mph

Weights

1 ounce (oz) = 0.0625 lb = 28.35 grams (g) = 0.028 kg
1 pound (lb) = 16 oz = 454 g = 0.454 kg
1 g = 0.035 oz = 0.0022 lb = 0.001 kg
1 kg = 35.27 oz = 2.2 lb = 1000 g

Temperature

$0°C = 32°F$
$100°C = 212°F$
$273°K = 0°C = 32°F$
$°C = (°F - 32) \times 5/9$
$°F = (9/5 \times °C) + 32$

Glossary

A-band That area located in the center of the sarcomere containing both actin and myosin.

Acceleration sprints Bouts of running in which the running speed is gradually increased from jogging to striding and finally to full sprinting.

Acclimatization Physiological adjustments brought about through continued exposure to a different climate or altitude.

Acetylcholine A chemical substance involved in several important physiological functions, including transmission of an impulse from one nerve fiber to another across a synapse. The latter function qualifies acetylcholine as a **transmitter substance**.

Adenosine diphosphate (ADP) A complex chemical compound which when combined with inorganic phosphate forms ATP.

Adenosine triphosphate (ATP) A complex chemical compound that is formed with the energy released from food and that is stored in all cells, particularly muscle cells. Only with the energy released from the breakdown of this compound can the cell perform work.

Actin A protein contained in the myofibril and involved in muscular contraction.

Action potential The electrical activity that develops in a muscle or nerve as a result of reversal of polarity or depolarization.

Adipocyte A fat cell; a cell that stores fat.

Adipose tissue Fat tissue.

Aerobic In the presence of oxygen.

Aerobic glycolysis The incomplete breakdown of glycogen or glucose to pyruvic acid. Part of the aerobic or oxygen system.

Alactacid oxygen debt That portion of oxygen used to resynthesize and restore ATP and PC in muscle following exercise (i.e., during recovery).

Altitude sickness Illness resulting from exposure to diminished oxygen pressure at high altitudes. Symptoms include nausea, vomiting, headache, rapid heart rate, and loss of appetite.

Alveolar-capillary membrane The thin layer of tissue dividing the alveoli and the pulmonary capillaries; the site at which gas exchange between air and blood occurs.

Alveolar ventilation Movement of air into and out of the alveoli.

Alveoli Tiny terminal air sacs in the lungs. Between the alveoli (singular: alveolus) and the pulmonary-capillaries is the alveolar-capillary membrane (see preceding definition).

Amenorrhea An abnormal cessation of menstruation.

Amino acids Nitrogen-containing compounds that form the building blocks of proteins.

Amphetamines Synthetic drugs closely related to epinephrine; they produce stimulation of the central nervous system.

Anabolic "Tissue-building"—that is, conducive to the constructive process of metabolism (other processes of metabolism are called "catabolic," meaning "breaking down").

Anaerobic In the absence of oxygen.

Anaerobic glycolysis The incomplete chemical breakdown of carbohydrate. The anaerobic reactions in this breakdown release energy for the manufacture of ATP as they produce lactic acid (anaerobic glycolysis is also known as the lactic acid system).

Anaerobic threshold That intensity of workload or oxygen consumption in which anaerobic metabolism (accumulation of lactic acid in the blood) is accelerated.

Androgenic Of or characterized by the development of the male secondary sex characteristics.

Aorta The major artery supplying the body tissues with arterial blood. It arises from the left ventricle of the heart.

Arterial-mixed venous oxygen difference (a-$\bar{v}O_2$diff) The difference in the oxygen content of arterial and mixed venous blood.

Association fibers Neural fibers connecting the motor and premotor areas.

ATP-PC System An anaerobic energy system in which ATP is manufactured when phosphocreatine (PC) is broken down. This system represents the most rapidly available source of ATP for use by muscle. Activities performed at maximum intensity in a period of 10 sec or less derive energy (ATP) from this system.

Atria (atrium = singular) The two (left and right), small, upper chambers of the heart.

Atrioventricular node (A-V node) A specialized area of heart tissue which is part of the nervous conduction system of the heart.

Autonomic nervous system An involuntary system that aids in controlling movement, secretion by the visceral organs, urinary output, body temperature, heart rate, blood flow, and blood pressure. The system is termed "involuntary" because it functions without one's conscious direction (one does not have to "think" about heart rate, for instance, for the heart to beat.)

Axon A nerve fiber.

Barometric pressure The pressure exerted by the atmosphere. At sea level it is 14.7 lb per square inch, or 760 mm or mercury.

Betz cells Motor neurons located in the primary motor area of the brain (cortex).

Bicarbonate ion (HCO$_3^-$) A by-product of the dissociation (ionizing) of carbonic acid.

Biopsy The removal and examination of tissue from the living body.

Black-bulb (globe) temperature The temperature of the air as affected by heat from the sun (radiant heat), measured by the warming of a thermometer that has a black (more sunlight-absorbent) bulb.

Black-bulb (globe) thermometer See preceding definition.

Blood doping The removal and subsequent reinfusion of blood and/or blood cells, undertaken for the purpose of temporarily increasing blood volume and the number of red blood cells.

Blood glucose The level of sugar in the blood.

Blood pressure The driving force that moves blood through the circulatory system. Systolic pressure (the higher pressure) is reached when blood is ejected into the arteries; diastolic pressure (the lower pressure) is reached when the blood drains from the arteries.

Body composition The component parts of the body—mainly fat and fat-free weight.

Bradycardia A decreased or slowed heart rate.

Calorie A unit of work or energy equal to the amount of heat required to raise the temperature of 1 g of water 1° C.

Capillaries Small vessels in a fine network located between arteries and veins.

Carbamino compounds The end product obtained from the chemical combination of carbon dioxide (CO_2) with plasma proteins and/or hemoglobin (Hb).

Carbohydrate A chemical compound containing carbon, hydrogen, and oxygen. Some important carbohydrates are the starches, celluloses, and sugars. Carbohydrates are one of the basic food-stuffs.

Carbonic acid (H_2CO_3) A chemical formed from the reaction of CO_2 and water.

Carbonic anhydrase (CA) An enzyme found in the red blood cells that speeds up the reaction of CO_2 and water (H_2O).

Cardiac hypertrophy An increase in the size of the heart.

Cardiac output ($\dot{Q}$) The amount of blood pumped in 1 min by either the left or right ventricle of the heart; the product of the heart rate and stroke volume.

Cardiorespiratory Pertaining to the circulatory and respiratory systems.

Cell A small protoplasmic mass; the basic unit of tissue.

Central nervous system The portion of the nervous system consisting of the brain and spinal cord.

Cerebellum That division or part of the brain responsible for the synchronous and orderly activity of groups of muscles.

Cerebral cortex That portion of the brain responsible for mental functions, movement, visceral functions, perception, and behavioral reactions, and for the association and integration of these functions.

Circuit training A conditioning program consisting of a number of exercises performed at "stations." Usually, a given exercise is performed at a station within a specified time; then the athlete moves to the next station, with its own particular exercise and specified time, then to the next station, and so on.

Connective tissue The tissue which binds together and is the support for the various structures of the body.

Cori cycle A series of chemical reactions in which the lactic acid produced from the breakdown of muscle glycogen is converted to blood glucose in the liver.

Coupled reactions Two series of chemical reactions, one of which releases energy (heat) for use by the other.

Cross-bridges Tiny projections extending from the myosin filaments and toward the actin filaments.

Dead space Any area of the respiratory passages in which no exchange between blood and air takes place.

Dehydration The condition resulting from excessive loss of body water.

Dendrite A nerve fiber.

Diffusion The random movement of molecules due to their kinetic energy.

Doping The use of physiological substances in abnormal amounts and with abnormal methods with the exclusive aim of improving competitive performance.

Dry-bulb temperature The temperature of the air, measured with an ordinary thermometer (called a "dry-bulb" thermometer).

Dry-bulb thermometer See preceding definition.

Eccentric contraction Muscular contraction in which the muscle lengthens while developing tension.

Electrocardiogram A recording of the electrical activity of the heart.

Electrolyte A substance that ionizes in solution, such as salt (NaCl), and is capable of conducting an electrical current.

Electron A negatively charged particle.

Electron transport system A series of chemical reactions occurring in mitochondria, in which electrons and hydrogen ions combine with oxygen to form water, and ATP is resynthesized. Part of the aerobic or oxygen system.

Endocrine gland An organ or structure that produces an internal secretion (hormone).

Endomysium The connective tissue that surrounds a muscle fiber.

Endurance (aerobic) training A form of conditioning designed to increase aerobic capacity and endurance performance.

Energy The capacity or ability to perform work.

Energy (chemical) Energy associated with chemical transformations.

Energy (kinetic) Energy associated with motion.

Energy (potential) Energy by virtue of position.

Energy balance The balance that results when caloric expenditure equals caloric intake.

Energy system One of three metabolic systems involving a series of chemical reactions resulting in the formation of waste products and the manufacture of ATP.

Enzyme A protein compound that speeds up chemical reactions.

Enzyme activity A measure of the functional capabilities of an enzyme.

Epimysium A connective tissue that surrounds the entire muscle.

Ergogenic Improving work or exercise performance.

Ergometer An apparatus or device, such as a treadmill or stationary bicycle, used for measuring the physiological effects of exercise.

Evaporation The changing of a liquid to a vapor.

Extrafusal fiber A typical or normal muscle cell or fiber.

Extrapyramidal tract The area in which the axons from the neurons located in the premotor area descend to the lower motor neurons in the spinal cord.

Fartlek training See *Speed play.*

Fasciculus (muscle-bundle) The largest subunit of skeletal muscle. Muscle fibers in a fasciculus (plural: fasciculi) may number from one to over one hundred.

Fast-twitch fiber A muscle fiber characterized by fast contraction time, high anaerobic capacity, and low aerobic capacity, all making the fiber suited for high power output activities.

Fat (1) A foodstuff containing glycerol and fatty acids. (2) In the body, the soft tissue other than that making up the skeletal muscle mass and the viscera.

Fat-free weight (FFW) That portion of the body weight remaining when the weight of body fat is subtracted from the total body weight; mainly the weight of the skeletal muscle mass.

Fatigue A state of weariness, discomfort, and decreased efficiency resulting from prolonged or excessive exertion.

Fiber splitting A division of a muscle fiber or cell into two or more fibers or cells.

Flexibility The range of motion about a joint (static flexibility); opposition or resistance of a joint to motion (dynamic flexibility).

Foodstuff A substance suitable for food. Protein, carbohydrate, and fat are foodstuffs.

Foot-pound The amount of work done by a 1-lb force acting through a distance of 1 ft.

Force A push or pull exerted upon some object; an action exerted by one body on another that tends to change the state of motion of the body acted upon.

Force-velocity curve The graph of the relationship between muscular force and speed of movement.

Free fatty acid (FFA) The usable form of triglycerides.

Functional (power rack) isometrics Isometric contractions performed with weights and with the use of a device from which weights are lifted and against which weights are held (a power rack).

Gamma loop (gamma system) The neural involvement of the muscle spindles during voluntary movement.

Glucose Sugar.

Glycerol The breakdown product of triglycerides.

Glycogen A polymer of glucose stored in the body.

Glycogen loading (supercompensation) An exercise-diet procedure that elevates muscle glycogen stores to concentrations two to three times normal.

Glycogen sparing The diminished utilization of glycogen that results when other fuels are available (and are used) for activity. If, for instance, fat is used to a greater extent than usual, glycogen is "spared"; glycogen will thus be available longer before ultimately being depleted.

Golgi tendon organ A proprioceptor located within the muscle tendon.

Heat cramp A heat illness characterized by painful muscular contractions and caused by prolonged exposure to environmental heat.

Heat exhaustion A heat illness caused by fatigue resulting from prolonged exposure to environmental heat.

Heat illness Incapacitation from excessive environmental heat.

Heat stress The "load" imposed by environmental heat, evaluated in terms of the degree to which various activities become difficult or impossible to perform (without risk to health) at certain temperatures. See also *WBGT Index* and *WBT Index*.

Heat stroke An often fatal illness caused by excessive exposure to environmental heat and characterized by high body temperature, hot, dry skin, and (sometimes) delirium or unconsciousness.

Heart rate (HR) The number of times the heart beats per minute.

Hemoglobin (Hb) A complex compound found in red blood cells that contains iron (heme) and protein (globin) and is capable of combining with oxygen.

Hollow sprints Bouts of running performed two sprints at a time with a period of jogging or walking between the two sprints (a "hollow" period).

Hydrogen ion The hydrogen atom without its electron.

Hypertension High blood pressure.

Hypertrophy An increase in the size of a cell or organ.

Hyperthermia Excessively high body temperature.

Hyperventilation Excessive movement of air into and out of the lungs, caused by increased depth and frequency of breathing and usually resulting in elimination of carbon dioxide.

Hypoglycemia Low blood sugar level.

Hypotonic Having a low osmotic pressure.

Hypoxia Lack of adequate oxygen due to a reduced oxygen partial pressure.

Hypoxic Pertaining to hypoxia.

H zone The area in the center of the A band where the cross-bridges are absent.

I band That area of a myofibril containing actin and bisected by a Z line.

Innervate To supply a nerve to a bodily part.

Intercalated discs Cell membranes that connect heart muscle fibers end-to-end.

Intermittent work Exercises performed with alternate periods of relief.

Interval training An exercise program in which the body is subjected to short but regularly repeated periods of work stress interspersed with adequate periods of relief.

Intrafusal fiber A muscle cell or fiber that houses the muscle spindle.

Ion An electrically charged particle.

Isokinetic contraction Muscular contraction executed at a constant speed and in such a fashion that the tension developed by the muscle while shortening is maximal over the full range of joint motion.

Isometric contraction Muscular contraction in which tension is developed but with no change in the length of the muscle. Also referred to as a static contraction.

Isotonic contraction Muscular contraction in which the muscle shortens with varying tension while lifting a constant load. Also referred to as dynamic contraction and concentric contraction.

Kilocalorie A unit of work or energy equal to the amount of heat required to raise the temperature of 1 kg of water 1° C.

Kilogram A metric unit of weight equal to 2.2 lb.

Kinesthetic sense (kinesthesis) Awareness of body position.

Kinetic energy Energy associated with motion.

Krebs cycle A series of chemical reactions occurring in mitochondria, in which carbon dioxide is produced and hydrogen ions and electrons are removed from carbon atoms (oxidation). Also referred to as the tricarboxylic acid cycle (TCA), or citric acid cycle.

Lactacid oxygen debt That portion or component of oxygen used to remove accumulated lactic acid from the blood and muscle following exercise (i.e., during recovery).

Lactic acid (LA) A fatiguing metabolite of the lactic acid system resulting from the incomplete breakdown of carbohydrate.

Lactic acid system (LA system) An anaerobic energy system in which ATP is manufactured when carbohydrate is broken down to lactic acid. High-intensity efforts requiring 1 to 3 min to perform draw energy (ATP) primarily from this system.

Lean body mass (fat-free weight) That portion of the body weight remaining when the weight of body fat is subtracted from the total body weight; mainly the weight of the skeletal muscle mass.

Lipid Fat.

Liter A metric unit of capacity very nearly equivalent to a quart (1.0 L = 1.056 quarts). One liter equals one-thousand milliliters (ml).

Lower motor neurons Motor neurons located in the spinal cord.

Maximal oxygen consumption ($\dot{V}O_2$max) The maximal rate at which oxygen can be consumed per minute; the power or capacity of the aerobic (oxygen) system.

Medullated nerve fiber A nerve fiber containing a myelin sheath.

Metabolic fuel A chemical or food used for energy production.

Metabolism The sum total of the chemical changes or reactions occurring in the body.

Metabolite Any substance produced by a metabolic reaction.

Milliliter One thousandth of a liter (see *Liter*).

Minerals Inorganic compounds, some of which are nutrients (i.e., vital to proper bodily function). Examples of important nutrient minerals are calcium, phosphorus, potassium, sodium, iron, and iodine.

Mitochondrion (plural: mitochondria) A subcellular structure that is found in all aerobic cells and in which the reactions of the Krebs cycle and electron transport system take place.

Mitral valve A flap of tissue that prevents backflow of blood into the left atrium from the left ventricle.

Mixed diet See *Normal (mixed) diet.*

Mole The gram-molecular weight or gram-formula weight of a substance. For example, 1 mole of glucose, $C_6H_{12}O_6$, weighs $(6 \times 12) + (12 \times 1) + (6 \times 16) = 72 + 12 + 96 = 180$ g. (Calculated from atomic weights: carbon = 12, hydrogen = 1, oxygen = 16.)

Motoneuron (motor neuron, motor nerve) A nerve cell that, when stimulated, effects muscular contraction.

Motor cortex An area of the brain in which are contained specialized neurons that cause motor movement when stimulated.

Motor nerve (motoneuron, motor neuron) A nerve cell which when stimulated effects muscular contraction.

Motor unit An individual motor nerve and all the muscle fibers it innervates.

Muscle-bound A colloquial term meaning "lacking in flexibility." The term is a misnomer when applied to persons in weight-training programs, for such persons are definitely not lacking in flexibility.

Muscle bundle See *Fasciculus*.

Muscle cell (muscle fiber) The basic contractile unit at work in all activities involving flexing, extending, bending, and so on. Muscle fibers may be fast to contract or slow to contract. See *Fast-twitch fiber* and *Slow-twitch fiber*.

Muscle spindle A proprioceptor located within an intrafusal muscle fiber.

Muscular endurance The ability of a muscle or muscle group to perform repeated contractions against a light load for an extended period of time.

Myelin sheath A structure composed mainly of lipid (fat) and protein that surrounds some nerve fibers (axons).

Myocardium The heart muscle.

Myofibril That part of a muscle fiber containing two protein filaments, myosin and actin.

Myoglobin An oxygen-binding pigment similar to hemoglobin that gives the muscle fiber its red color. It acts as an oxygen store and aids in the diffusion of oxygen.

Myoglobinuria Myoglobin in the urine.

Myosin A protein contained in the myofibril and involved in muscular contraction.

Negative energy balance Less energy is consumed than expended and body weight decreases.

Nerve A cordlike structure that conveys impulses from one part of the body to another.

Nerve cell See *Neuron*.

Nerve impulse An electrical disturbance at the point of stimulation of a nerve that is self-propagated along the entire length of the axon.

Nerve fiber An axon or dendrite, each of which is capable of conducting nervous impulses.

Nervous system The system of nerves and nerve centers, including the central nervous system and the autonomic nervous system.

Neuromuscular Pertaining to the nervous and muscular systems.

Neuromuscular junction The joining of a muscle and its nerve. Also referred to as the motor end-plate and the myoneural junction.

Neuron (nerve cell) A conducting cell of the nervous system, the cell consisting of a cell body (with its nucleus and cytoplasm), dendrites, and an axon.

Newton-meter (Nm) A unit of work equal to 0.7375 foot-pounds. One foot-pound equals 1.356 Newton-meters.

Nodes of Ranvier Those areas on a medullated nerve that are devoid of a myelin sheath.

Nonmedullated nerve fiber A nerve fiber entirely devoid of a myelin sheath.

Normal (mixed) diet A diet that contributes its calories in this proportion: approximately 10 to 15% of the calories come from protein, 25 to 30% from fat, and 55 to 60% from carbohydrate.

Nutrition The process of assimilating food.

Overload To exercise a muscle or muscle group against resistance greater than that which is normally encountered. The resistance (load) can be maximal or near-maximal.

Oxidation The breakdown of a compound by the removal of electrons. In the body, this is usually done in the presence of oxygen.

Oxidize To break down a compound by the removal of electrons. In the body, this is done in the presence of oxygen.

Oxygen consumption The intake and utilization of oxygen by the body.

Oxygen debt The amount of oxygen consumed during recovery from exercise above that ordinarily consumed at rest in the same time period. There is a rapid component (alactacid) and a slow component (lactacid).

Oxygen transport system ($\dot{V}O_2$) The cardiorespiratory system, composed of the stroke volume (SV), the heart rate (HR), and the arterial-mixed venous oxygen difference (a-$\bar{v}O_2$diff). Mathematically, it is defined as $VO_2 = SV \times HR \times$ a-$\bar{v}O_2$diff.

Oxyhemoglobin (HbO_2) The chemical combination between oxygen and hemoglobin.

Oxyhemoglobin curve The graph of the relationship between the amount of oxygen combined with hemoglobin and the partial pressure of oxygen.

Partial pressure The pressure exerted by a gas in relation to its fractional concentration in a gas volume.

Perimysium The connective tissue that surrounds a muscle bundle (fasciculus).

Phosphagens Compounds that yield inorganic phosphate and release energy when broken down. ATP and PC are phosphagens.

Phosphocreatine (PC) A chemical compound that is stored in muscle and that when broken down aids in manufacturing ATP.

Plasma The liquid portion of the blood.

Polarity The property of having one end (or side) that is electrically positive and another that is electrically negative.

Polymer A complex compound formed by the combination of simpler molecules; for example, glycogen is a polymer of glucose.

Positive energy balance More energy is consumed than expended and body weight increases.

Potential energy Energy by virtue of position.

Power Work per unit of time. For example, if 1 kg is raised 1 m in 1 sec, power is expressed as 1 kg-m per sec.

Power rack isometrics See *Functional (power rack) isometrics.*

Premotor area An area that lies in front of the primary motor area and that contains motor neurons other than Betz cells.

Primary motor area That area of the brain (cortex) containing groups of motor neurons known as Betz cells.

Progressive resistance Overloading a muscle or muscle group consistently throughout the duration of a weight-resistance program.

Proprioceptors Sense organs that are found in muscle joints and tendons and that give information concerning movements and positions of the body (kinesthesis). Muscle spindles and Golgi tendon organs are examples of proprioceptors.

Pulse rate Heart rate.

Protein A basic foodstuff containing amino acids.

Psychrometer An instrument used for measuring the relative humidity of the air. It contains a dry-bulb thermometer and a wet-bulb thermometer.

Pyramidal tract The area in which the axons of the motor neurons located in the motor cortex descend to lower motor neurons that lie in the spinal cord.

Pyruvic acid The chemical precursor of lactic acid.

Radiant heat Heat radiated from the sun.

Receptor A sense organ that receives stimuli.

Red blood cells The cells in the blood that contain hemoglobin and are responsible for carrying oxygen.

Reflex An automatic response induced by stimulation of a receptor.

Relative humidity The ratio of water vapor in the air to the amount of water vapor required to saturate the air at the same temperature.

Relief interval In an interval training program, the time between work intervals as well as between sets.

Repetition maximum (RM) The maximum load that a muscle or muscle group can lift in a given number of repetitions before fatiguing. For example, an eight-RM load is the maximum load that can be lifted eight times.

Respiration Ventilation.

Residual volume Volume of air remaining in the lungs at the end of a maximal expiration.

Resting membrane potential The potential (electrical) difference existing between the inside and outside of the resting nerve fiber.

Saltatory conduction The propagation of a nerve impulse from one node of Ranvier to another along a medullated fiber.

Sarcolemma The cell membrane of a muscle fiber.

Sarcomere The smallest functional unit of muscle; the distance between two Z lines.

Sarcoplasm The protoplasm of muscle cells.

Second wind A sensation characterized by a sudden transition from an ill-defined feeling of distress or fatigue during the early portion of prolonged exercise to a more comfortable, less stressful feeling later in the exercise.

Sensory nerve A nerve that conveys impulses from a receptor to the central nervous system. Examples of sensory nerves are those excited by sound, pain, light, and taste.

Set In an interval training program, a group of work and relief intervals. In weight lifting, the number of repetitions performed consecutively without resting.

Sinoatrial node (S-A node) A specialized area of heart tissue in the posterior wall of the right atrium where the normal heartbeat is initiated. Part of the conduction system of the heart.

Skinfold A pinch of skin and subcutaneous fat from which total body fat may be estimated.

Skinfold caliper An instrument used to measure the thickness of a fold of skin (see preceding definition).

Sliding filament theory The idea that in isotonic muscular contraction the actin filaments slide over the myosin filaments toward the center of the sarcomere.

Slow-twitch fiber A muscle fiber characterized by slow contraction time, low anaerobic capacity, and high aerobic capacity, all making the fiber suited for low-power-output activities.

Specificity In terms of conditioning, the property of having effects that are directly linked to the particulars of training. An effect such as a gain in anaerobic power is linked directly to those exercises in one's training program that involve short, intense bouts of work (e.g., sprints); if the program consists only of distance runs, an anaerobic gain cannot be expected.

Speed play (fartlek) An exercise program involving alternating fast and slow running over natural terrains. It is the forerunner of the interval training system.

Sprint (anaerobic) training Conditioning designed to increase the capacity of the anaerobic system—the system needed for short, high-power activities (e.g., sprints).

Steroid A derivative of the male sex hormone testosterone, which has masculinizing properties.

Stimulus (plural: stimuli) A change in the environment that modifies the activity of cells.

Stitch-in-the-side A sharp pain in the side or rib cage.

Strength The maximal pulling force of a muscle or muscle group.

Stroke volume (SV) The amount of blood pumped by the left or right ventricle of the heart per beat.

Subcutaneous fat Fat deposits and storage beneath the skin.

Submaximal exercise Exercise demanding less than the maximal oxygen consumption of a performer.

Sympathetic nervous system The part of the autonomic nervous system that controls alertness, heart rate, blood flow, blood pressure, and metabolism.

Syncytium A merging of cells such as the muscle fibers of the heart.

Tidal volume (TV) The amount of air inspired or expired per breath.

Tissue-capillary membrane The thin layer of tissue dividing the capillaries and an organ (such as skeletal muscle); the site at which gas exchanges take place between blood and tissue.

Torque A rotary force.

Total lung volume Volume of air in the lungs at the end of a maximal expiration.

Training A program of exercise designed to improve the skills and increase the energy capacities of an athlete for a particular event.

Transmitter substance A chemical that relays electrical information either from nerve to nerve (synapse) or from nerve to muscle (neuromuscular junction). An example of a transmitter substance is acetylcholine.

Tricuspid valve A flap of tissue that prevents backflow of blood into the right atrium from the right ventricle.

Triglycerides The storage form of free fatty acids.

Underload To work a muscle or muscle group at a load that is normally encountered.

Upper motor neurons Motor neurons located in the higher centers (brain).

Vasoconstriction A decrease in the diameter of a blood vessel (usually an arteriole) resulting in a reduction of blood flow to the area supplied by the vessel.

Vasodilation An increase in the diameter of a blood vessel (usually an arteriole) resulting in an increased blood flow to the area supplied by the vessel.

Vena cava The great veins of the body that return blood from the tissues to the heart.

Ventilation The movement of air into and out of the lungs. Sometimes referred to as pulmonary ventilation and minute ventilation.

Vital capacity Maximal volume of air forcefully expired after a maximal inspiration.

Vitamins Organic nutrients in the presence of which important metabolic reactions occur.

Warm-down An exercise procedure performed immediately after training sessions or competitions for purposes of quickly removing any accumulated lactic acid from the muscles and blood.

WBGT Index A guide to the degree of comfort or stress associated with a range of temperatures taking into account the effects of radiant heat and humidity (wet-bulb-globe temperatures).

WBT Index A guide to the degree of comfort or stress associated with a range of temperatures taking into account the effects of humidity (wet-bulb temperatures). High temperatures on the Index are presented as sufficiently stressful to require limits on most (or all) activity.

Wet-bulb-globe temperature A temperature calculated from dry-bulb, wet-bulb, and black-bulb (globe) temperatures, indicative of the environmental heat load.

Wet-bulb temperature The temperature of the air in relation to the amount of water vapor that is present, measured by the cooling of a thermometer as water evaporates from a wet wick wrapped around the thermometer's bulb.

Wet-bulb thermometer See above.

Work Application of a force through a distance. For example, moving 1 kg (force) through 1 m equals 1 kg-m of work.

Work interval That portion of an interval training program consisting of the work effort.

Work-relief ratio In an interval training program, the ratio of the duration of the work interval to the duration of the relief interval.

Z line A protein band that defines the distance of one sarcomere in the myofibril.

Author Index

Numbers in *italics* refer to illustrations; numbers followed by a (t) refer to tables.

Subject Index

A

A band, *90*, 91, *92*, *93*
Abbreviation(s), used in text, 359, 361
Acceleration sprint(s), definition of, 208(t)
  prescription for, 212(t)
  sports training and, 210-211(t)
Acclimatization, *195*, 196, 321-323, 322(t), 323(t)
  altitude and, *195*, 196
  changes produced by, 322(t)
  environmental heat and, 321-323, 322(t), 323(t)
Acetylcholine, 89
Actin, 91-92, *92*, *93*, 93(t)
Action potential, 88, 89
Actomyosin, 92, 93(t)
Adenosine diphosphate (ADP), *12*, 13
Adenosine triphosphate (ATP), aerobic synthesis
    of, 16-22, *17*, *18*, *20*, *21*
  breakdown of, 12-15, *12*, *14*
  coupled reactions and, *12*, 13
  definition of, 11
  effects of training on, 227-230, 231(t)
  muscular contraction and, 91-92, 93(t)
  phosphate bond and, 12, 13
  recovery from exercise and, 59-64
  resynthesis of, 14-22
  weight-training effects and 156, 158(t)
Adipocyte(s), 287
Adipose tissue, 287
  triglyceride stores and, 52
ADP, *12*, 13
Aerobic glycolysis, definition of, 18
Aerobic metabolism, 13-14
  summary equations for, 21
Aerobic (oxygen) system, 16-22, *17*, *18*, *20*, *21*, 22(t)
  effects of training on, 214, 226-230, *230*, 231(t),
    233-240, 236(t), *238*, *239*, *240*, 249-250
Aerobic training (endurance training), 202-256. *See
    also* Training.
Afferent nerve, 86
Age, training effects and, 241, 248
Alactacid oxygen debt, 59-60, *60*, 63-64, *65*, 68
  of athletes, *65*
Alcohol, effects of, on sports performance, 282-283
Altitude, 194-197, *195*
  acclimatization to, *195*, 196
  oxygen transport and, 194-197, *195*
  performance at, 194-197, *195*
  training and, 196-197, 249-250, *251*, 251(t)
Alveolar ventilation, 167
Alveoli, 167
American College of Sports Medicine, guidelines
    for weight-loss programs, 300-302
  position statements,
    on running in the heat, 329-330
    on steroid consumption, 157-159
    on weight loss in wrestlers, 310-311

Amphetamine(s), effects of, on endurance
    performance, 194
Anaerobic glycolysis, 15
Anaerobic metabolism, 13-14
Anaerobic threshold, 190-191, *190*
Anaerobic training (sprint training), 202-256. *See
    also* Training.
Aortic valve, of heart, 179
Archery, potential energy and, 10
Arm curl, circuit training and, 149(t)
    description of, 362, *366*
    muscles involved in, 363(t)
    sports training and, 136(t)
Arm exercise, 204-205, *205*
Ascorbic acid (vitamin C), functions and source of,
    261(t)
Athlete(s), body composition of, 286-295, 294(t)
  body fat of, 287, 288, *288*, 290-291(t), 294(t)
  diet and, 269-283
  diffusion capacity of, 171-172, *172*
  fat-free weight (lean body mass) of, 287-289, *292*
  female. *See* Female athlete(s).
  fluid replacement for, 320-321, 321(t)
  lactic acid system and, 36-37, *38*
  maximal oxygen consumption of, 36-37, *38*, *39*
  muscle fibers in, types of, *107*, 108, *110-111*
  nutrition and, 258-269
  phosphagen (ATP + PC) system and, 36-37, *38*
  protein requirement for, 258-259
Athletic performance, body composition and,
    243-245, 287-292, *288*, 290-291(t), *292*
  environmental heat problems and, 316-332
  weight-training effects and, 157, 158(t)
ATP. *See* Adenosine triphosphate (ATP).
ATP + PC, concentrations of, in muscle, 14-15, *14*
ATP = PC system, 14-15, *14*, 36-37, *38*
Atrioventricular bundle, 180
Atrioventricular node (A-V node), 179
Atrium (atria), of heart, 177, *178*
Axon, 86, *87*

B

Back hyperextension, circuit training and, 149(t)
    description of, 362, *366*
    muscles involved in, 363(t)
    sports training and, 136(t)
Backstroke, weight exercises for, 136-137(t)
Baseball, energy continuum and, *31*, 35(t)
    energy systems for, 207(t)
    kinetic energy and, 10
    training methods for, 210(t)
    weight exercises for, 136-137(t)
Baseball player(s), body composition values for,
    290-291(t)
    body fat of, *288*
    fat free weight (lean body mass) of, *292*

406